THE LEGAL ASPECTS OF MIDWIFERY

SECOND EDITION

Bridgit Dimond

MA LLB DSA AHSM Barrister-at-law
Emeritus Professor of the University of Glamorgan

Foreword by
Robyn Phillips

Professional Officer for Midwifery, Welsh National Board

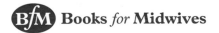
Books *for* Midwives

BOOKS FOR MIDWIVES
An imprint of Elsevier Science Limited

First edition 1994
Second edition 2002

ISBN 0 7506 5277 2

British Library Cataloguing in Publication Data
A catalogue record for this book is available from the British Library

Library of Congress Cataloging in Publication Data
A catalog record for this book is available from the Library of Congress

Note
Medical knowledge is constantly changing. As new information becomes available, changes in treatment, procedures, equipment and the use of drugs become necessary. The authors and the publishers have taken care to ensure that the information given in this text is accurate and up to date. However, readers are strongly advised to confirm that the information, especially with regard to drug usage, complies with the latest legislation and standards of practice.

 ELSEVIER SCIENCE your source for books, journals and multimedia in the health sciences

www.elsevierhealth.com

The publisher's policy is to use paper manufactured from sustainable forests

Printed in China by RDC Group Limited

for Bette

Contents

FOREWORD

I am deeply honoured to be invited to write the foreword for the second edition of The Legal Aspects of Midwifery. It gives me great pleasure to do so.

Professor Dimond is a renowned expert in the law relating to healthcare. She has published extensively on the law as it applies to a number of healthcare professions and also to specific aspects of care, for example, consent and confidentiality. Those who have had the privilege of attending Professor Dimond's lectures, study days or workshops, will appreciate the depth and vastness of her legal knowledge. She invites interaction and the law comes alive through her unique ability and commensurate skill in using participants' questions and applying her answers to practical clinical examples relevant to a specific audience. Professor Dimond has considerable experience in writing and lecturing on the law as it relates to midwifery and in discussing the issues formally and informally with midwives.

Similarly with this book. Professor Dimond engages the reader and makes the law interesting and relevant through her comprehensive and practical coverage of the subject and sound use of case study examples. The arrangement of the book into six discrete areas, each with a clear introduction and outline of what follows, enables even the novice to approach the subject with confidence. As Professor Dimond herself states, the aim is not to frighten but to inform and protect midwives and their clients. As with the first edition, the 'questions and exercises' at the end of each chapter are thought-provoking and helpful for the reader when considering their own practice. Valuable additions to this second edition include the legislative changes governing the new Nursing and Midwifery Council and professional regulation, and a separate chapter on use of complementary therapies in midwifery practice.

This book makes an important contribution to midwifery education and practice and maternity care generally. It enables midwives to understand the legal framework of their practice and to consider some of the legal and ethical issues inherent within it. The book is particularly relevant to student midwives, midwife lecturers, midwife practitioners and mothers alike.

Robyn Phillips PhD
Professional Adviser (Midwifery)
Welsh National Board for Nursing, Midwifery and Health Visiting

PREFACE TO THE SECOND EDITION

It is now eight years since the first edition of this book was published and there have been significant changes in the law, the structure and institutions of the NHS and the practice of midwifery. Unfortunately (but predictably), litigation, especially in obstetrics and midwifery, has become increasingly common, and the need for easy access to the law for every practising midwife is even more important than it was in 1994. There is clear justification for a new edition to include major changes in legislation including the Human Rights Act, the Data Protection Act 1998, and to explain the major changes which have taken place in the NHS following the Health Act 1999, including the establishment of the Nursing and Midwifery Council. Significant decisions have been made by the Court of Appeal in relation to compulsory Caesarean section and the House of Lords in relation to human rights. Gradually, the recommendations of the National Institute for Clinical Excellence are covering areas of obstetric and midwifery practice and will inevitably develop the research base for effective clinical practice. The Clinical Negligence Scheme for Trusts also is playing its part in raising standards of practice across those trusts which are members of the CNST pool. A new chapter is included on complementary therapies.

ARRANGEMENT OF THE BOOK

The law, and consequently this book, is divided into six discrete areas:

- Professional Issues: registration, education and the role of the statutory bodies, supervision, professional conduct proceedings and the Rules, Codes and the Scope of Professional Practice

- Client Rights: looking at issues from the client's perspective

- Litigation and accountability: the personal and professional accountability of the midwife in the civil and criminal courts, and issues relating to health and safety laws

- Management Issues: the organisation of the NHS, employment law, the position of the independent midwife and the regulations relating to private maternity hospitals

- Statutory Provisions: relating to births, deaths, human fertilisation and embryology, abortion and other statutes

- Specific Situations: different aspects of the midwife's role including the midwife as teacher, researcher, and in relation to children and the mentally disordered.

My aim, as always, is not to frighten the reader, but to provide information which a midwife can use with confidence, knowing that the law is there to protect her and her clients.

ACKNOWLEDGEMENTS

I would like to thank all those hundreds of midwives who, by raising their concerns with me, have provided the situations and problems which this book aims to resolve. My special thanks go to Dorothy Walters, for using her contacts with colleagues and fellow Supervisors to direct me toward some of the issues they wanted to see covered in this book, and for being such a generous source of information and help and also to Ruth Gammon for her helpful comments and Helene Shaw of the Department of Health. I would like to thank officers at the Royal College of Midwives and Royal College of Nursing, particularly Angela Perrett. I would also like to acknowledge the support and assistance of Robyn Phillips (who has provided a Foreword), and that of her predecessor as Professional Officer for Midwives at the Welsh National Board, the late Ruth Davies, who was much loved and respected. I also wish to thank my family for their constant encouragement and Bette for her great support. It is to her that this book is dedicated.

The copyright of the Stationery Office for Statute and Statutory Instruments and of the various publishers for law reports and of the Clinical Negligence Scheme for Trusts and National Health Service Litigation Authority for their reports are acknowledged. The author wishes to thank them all for being able to quote from their works.

PREFACE TO THE FIRST EDITION

I was taken to task by the former President of the Royal College of Midwives for having the temerity to write a book on legal aspects of nursing which included a chapter on midwives. I was conscious at the time of writing that book that there were so many special areas of relevance to midwives, that a book on legal aspects of midwifery was more than justified. I was therefore delighted when Henry Hochland gave me the opportunity to meet that need.

I am grateful to so many midwives and others for suggestion and comments in the preparation of this book, that it seems invidious to pick out a few names, but the following must be mentioned in particular:

Jane Winship, Ruth Davies, Dot Walters and Tessa Shellens who read the text and offered many constructive suggestions and gave much encouragement. The responsibility however for the accuracy and contents of the book remains mine.

I am also grateful to the editors and publishers of Modern Midwife, in particular Julia Magill-Cuerden and Alison Turnbull, who through my monthly articles on legal issues have given me the opportunity to research and develop some of the topics which appear in this book. I must also thank those many midwives across the country who have raised with me legal issues which are of a constant concern in their practice which form the substance of this book.

Finally I thank as always my family and friends who made the sacrifices for this to be produced.

I am grateful to you all.

ABBREVIATIONS

ACPC	Area Child Protection Committee
ACAS	Advisory, Conciliation and Arbitration Service
AID	Artificial Insemination by Donor
AIDS	Acquired Immune Deficiency Syndrome
AIH	Artificial Insemination by Husband
ARC	AIDS Related Condition
CHC	Community Health Council
CHI	Commission for Health Improvement
CPS	Crown Prosecution Service
DGH	District General Hospital
DHA	District Health Authority
DHSS	Department of Health and Social Security (Divided in 1989 into DH and DSS)
DH	Department of Health
DHA	District Health Authority
DNA	Deoxyribonucleic Acid
DSS	Department of Social Security
EC	European Community
ECR	Extra-Contractual Referral
EEC	European Economic Area
EWC	Expected Week of Confinement
FHSA	Family Health Service Authority
GP	General Practitioner
HFEA	Human Fertilisation and Embryology Authority
IV	Intravenous(ly) or Intravenous infusion
IVF	In Vitro Fertilisation
JP	Justice of the Peace
LREC	Local Research Ethics Committee
LSA	Local Supervising Authority
MHAC	Mental Health Act Commission
MHRT	Mental Health Review Tribunal
MPP	Maternity Pay Period
NHS	National Health Service

NICE	National Institute of Clinical Excellence
NMC	Nursing and Midwifery Council
NSF	National Service Framework
PCC	Professional Conduct Committee
PPC	Preliminary Proceedings Committee
PREP	Post-Registration Education and Practice
RCOG	Royal College of Obstetricians and Gynaecologists
RCM	Royal College of Midwives
RHA	Regional Health Authority
SI	Statutory Instrument
SOAD	Second Opinion Appointed Doctor
UKCC	United Kingdom Central Council for Nursing, Midwifery and Health Visiting
WHO	World Health Organisation

TABLE OF STATUTES

TABLE OF CASES

would have had an abortion if the defect had been found on a scan.

414
Royal College of Nursing of the UK v. Department of Health and Social Security
The RCN challenged the lawfulness of nurses using prostaglandins to terminate pregnancy, since nurses are not registered medical practitioners.

416
Janaway v. Salford
An NHS secretary appealed after being dismissed for refusing to type abortion referral letters.

419
R v. Price
A doctor fitted a pregnant woman with an IUD. He claimed to be unaware of the pregnancy and argued that he was preventing an implantation, not procuring a miscarriage.

420
Paton v. Trustees of the British Pregnancy Advisory Service
Mr Paton tried to prevent his wife from having an abortion. He took the case to the European Commission of Human Rights (see below).

420
Paton v. United Kingdom
Mr Paton challenged his wife's right to an abortion citing the European Convention of Human Rights, Article 8, on respect for family life.

420
Kelly v. Kelly
A father separated from his wife brought an action to stop her having an abortion in the name of the unborn child.

421
Morrow and others v. Director of Public Prosecutions
Protestors outside an abortion clinic were convicted under the Public Order Act.

432
R v. Human Fertilisation and Embryology Authority, ex parte Blood
Diane Blood claimed the right to use sperm taken from her husband shortly before his death in order to conceive his child.

434
R v. Ethical Committee of St

Mary's Hospital (Manchester)
A woman previously convicted of prostitution was denied access to fertility services.

434
R v. Sheffield Health Authority, ex parte Seale
A 37-year-old woman was refused IVF treatment by the Health Authority as their cut-off point for treatment was the age of 35.

435
R v. Secretary of State ex parte Mellor
A prisoner sought IVF facilities to inseminate his wife while he was in prison.

435
Re A (an adoption)(surrogacy)
The court ruled that a payment to a surrogate mother did not contravene the Adoption Act if it did not include an element of profit or reward.

454
Best v. Wellcome Foundation
The Irish Supreme Court held that the manufacturers were liable for the negligent release of a batch of triple vaccine which caused brain damage.

478
Hedley Byrne v. Heller & Partners Ltd.
If a reference is written negligently, the writer may be liable.

479
Spring v. Guardian Assurance plc and others
If a reference is written negligently, the writer may be liable.

479
Cox v. Sun Alliance Life Ltd.
Cox sued for damages after being given an inaccurate and defamatory reference.

501
D v. NSPCC
Following a suspected case of child abuse which is found to be unfounded, those accused do not have the right to know the names of their accusers.

505
Re C (a minor)(medical treatment - refusal of parental consent)
Parents refused to allow a liver transplant to be given to their child.

505
Re E (a minor)(wardship: medical treatment)
A child of Jehovah's Witnesses was given a blood transfusion.

521
Watling v. Gloucester County Council Employment Tribunal
An occupational therapist was dismissed for seeing private patients for alternative therapies during working hours.

522
Shakoor (adminastratrix of the estate of Shakoor (deceased)) v. Situ (T/A Eternal Health Co)
A man died of acute liver failure after using Chinese herbal medicine.

INTRODUCTION

In this Section, we explore how laws are formed and the structure of the legal system in the UK.

Chapter 1
THE LEGAL SYSTEM

WHAT IS THE LAW?

'It is against the law' is a powerful statement, and anyone making it should be able to declare the source of the law to which reference is being made. If the statement is accurate then either an Act of Parliament/Statutory Instrument (known as a statute or 'legislation') or a decided case would be cited. (See the Glossary for further explanations of legal terms.)

LEGISLATION

Legislation consists both of Acts of Parliament (with approval by the Houses of Commons and Lords, and the Queen's signature), and directives and regulations emanating from the European Community, which we as a member state are required to implement and obey.

Legislation can be primary or secondary. Primary legislation consists of Acts of Parliament, known as statutes, which come into force at a date set either in the initial Act of Parliament or subsequently fixed by order of a Minister (i.e. by Statutory Instrument). The date of enforcement is often later than the date the Act is passed by the two Houses of Parliament and signed by the Crown.

The statute sometimes gives power to a Minister to enact more detailed laws, and this is known as secondary legislation. Some regulations have to be laid before the Houses of Parliament and in certain circumstances have to receive express approval. Statutory Instruments which are quoted in the text are an example of this secondary legislation.

Section 60 of the Health Act 1999 gives power to Her Majesty to make by Order in Council provisions for the regulation of various health professions. The Order relating to the establishment of the Nursing and Midwifery Council in turn gives power to the NMC to make rules regulating the practice of midwifery (article 40(1)). Under Article 45, the approval of the Privy Council shall be required for any exercise by the Council of a power to make rules under this Order.

DECIDED CASES

The other main source of law is the decisions of the courts. This source is known as case law, or judge-made law, or the common law. The courts form a hierarchy and the highest court in this country is the House of Lords (different in composition from the House of Lords in Parliament, since only the law lords hear cases, not the bishops, hereditary peers and life peers who all sit in Parliament). If the House of Lords sets out a specific rule, then this is binding on all courts in the country, except itself – i.e. the House of Lords does not have to follow its own principles. A principle set out by a senior court is known as a precedent. Judges decide cases which may involve interpretation of Acts of Parliament, or situations where there does not appear to have been any enacted law or relevant case. Recent decisions of the House of Lords have included the Pinochet case,[1] where it was held that a ruler of another state was subject to law and could be lawfully arrested whilst a request for extradition to another state was considered. Another recent decision[2] was the ruling that an adult who lacked mental competence to give consent to admission, could be admitted to a psychiatric hospital without being placed under the Mental Health Act 1983.

Following the Hillsborough football disaster, the House of Lords had to rule on whether it was lawful to withdraw artificial feeding from a patient in a persistent vegetative state.[3] It held that artificial feeding for Tony Bland could cease, on the basis that that was in his best interests. (This case is considered in Chapter 9.)

Each decision of the courts is reported, so that lawyers and judges can refer to the case and the principles it established (known as the ratio decidendi) can be applied to any matters in dispute. If there is a dispute between a case and a statute, the latter would take priority: judges have to follow an Act of Parliament. Parliament can enact legislation which would overrule a principle established in the courts.

Appeals can be made to the European Court of Justice in Luxembourg which gives interpretations of European laws. Their decisions are binding on the courts of member states.

THE HUMAN RIGHTS ACT 1998

This country was a signatory of the European Convention in 1951 and accepted the articles on human rights. However, the Convention was not incorporated into our law at that time. If a person considered his or her rights had been infringed then he or she had to take the case to Strasbourg, to the European Court of Human Rights, to argue the case there. Parliament has now passed the Human Rights Act 1998. This came into force on 2nd October 2000 for England and Wales (in Scotland the Act came into force earlier, on devolution). It is discussed in detail in Chapter 6, and the Articles of the European Convention on Human Rights, set out in Schedule 1 to the Human Rights Act 1998, can be found in Appendix 1 to this book.

The Act:

– requires all public authorities to implement the articles of the European Convention on Human Rights

– gives a right to anyone who alleges that a public authority has failed to respect those rights to bring an action in the courts of this country, and

– enables judges who consider that legislation is incompatible with the Articles of the Convention to refer that legislation back to Parliament.

CHANGES TO THE LAW

Law is dynamic. As conflicts and disputes arise and are brought before the courts, the judges have to decide in the light of existing statutes and decided cases which are binding upon them, the principles which apply. In that sense there is always a law, the judges simply declare it. New legislation is enacted which may overrule existing case law, change existing statutes and statutory instruments or fill gaps created by technological developments. (See for example Chapter 27 and laws relating to embryology and genetic developments.)

EFFECT OF THE EUROPEAN COMMUNITY

Since the United Kingdom signed the Treaty of Rome in 1972, the UK has become one of the member states of the European Community. The effect of this is that the UK is now subject to the laws made by the Council of Ministers and the European Commission. In addition, secondary legislation of the European Community in the form of regulations is binding on the member states. Directives of the Community must be incorporated by Act of Parliament into the law of each member state. (See for example the European Directive 80/155/EEC Article 4, which sets out the definition of the activities of a midwife.)

CRIMINAL LAWS AND CIVIL LAWS

A major distinction in the law of the United Kingdom is that between criminal laws and civil laws.

CRIMINAL LAWS

These laws, mostly derived from statutes, create offences which can be followed by criminal proceedings in the form of a prosecution. An example of a statutory provision giving rise to criminal proceedings is Article 43 of the Nurses, Midwives and Health Visitors Order[4] which makes it a criminal offence for a person other than a registered midwife or doctor, or student of either, to attend a woman in childbirth, except in an emergency (see Chapter 25).

An example of case law which gives rise to criminal proceedings is the definition of murder which was set out in a case in the 17th century. Most of our criminal laws are enforced by prosecutions brought by the Crown Prosecution Service, which was created in 1985. Other bodies also have powers to prosecute in specific cases, eg. the Health and Safety Inspectorate, the National Society for the Prevention of Cruelty to Children, and Environmental Health Officers.

There are other criminal laws such as those created by Local Authority powers known as by-laws, which create local offences. There is also a right of an individual to bring a private prosecution, but this can be costly and of uncertain benefit.

CIVIL LAWS

These are laws (both statutory and case law) which enable citizens to claim remedies against other citizens or organisations as a result of a civil wrong. A large group of civil wrongs are known as torts, of which negligence is the main one, but the group also includes action for breach of statutory duty, nuisance and defamation. Actions for breach of contract are not included in the definition of tort.

An example of a statute which can give rise to civil action is the Congenital Disabilities Act 1976, which gives a child who is born alive the right to sue in respect of negligence which led to him or her suffering from a congenital defect. (This is considered in Chapter 17.)

An example of a case which applies to civil proceedings is that of Whitehouse v. Jordan[5] in which an obstetrician was sued for negligence on the grounds that he had allegedly pulled too long and too hard in a trial of forceps. The House of Lords held that an error of clinical judgement may or may not be evidence of negligence, and that it had not been established that Dr Jordan failed to follow the reasonable standard of care required in the circumstances, based on the approved standard of practice at the time. (The case is considered in detail in Chapter 14.)

Some acts may be actionable as both a criminal offence and a civil wrong. For example, in Chapter 7, the action for trespass to the person is discussed. This action can be brought where treatment is given without the consent of the individual and in the absence of other factors which would be a defence to the action (eg. acting out of necessity). A trespass may however also be a criminal act of assault, and there could be a prosecution in the criminal courts. It can be seen from this that there is not necessarily a moral difference between a crime and a civil wrong.

WHAT ABOUT ETHICS?

Some civil and criminal wrongs may also be ethically wrong. Some may not be considered as ethical issues. For example, failure to register the birth of a baby may not give rise to ethical issues if it has occurred simply from absent-mindedness. It would however be a criminal offence. In this book we are concerned with the law and therefore there can be little discussion of ethical issues. However, the reader is referred to the Reading List for sources on ethics in midwifery. Codes of Practice and conduct are not in themselves 'laws'. They do however provide guidance for professional practice, and could be used in evidence in civil or professional conduct proceedings to demonstrate that reasonable practice has not been followed. This is further discussed in Chapter 5.

LEGAL PERSONNEL

Lawyers in this country are trained as solicitors or barristers. The former, in the past, have had direct dealings with clients and arranged with barristers (known as Counsel) for the paperwork to be drafted and for representation of the client in court. Now, increasingly, solicitors are being trained for advocacy and have rights of presenting a case in court. Eventually this may lead to a single legal profession.

Solicitors and barristers share a common foundation training: either a law degree or success in the Common Professional Examination. Then would-be solicitors undertake practical training with a firm of solicitors, and take the Law Society's Part 2 examination, called the Legal Practice Course, whilst would-be barristers study for the Bar with the Council for Legal Education and are then 'called' to the bar after having dined on a specified number of occasions at one of the Inns of Court to which they must belong. A barrister who wishes to practice must then undertake pupillage where they are attached to a practising barrister. Senior barristers are eligible to 'take silk', i.e. they become Queen's Counsel (QC) appointed by the Lord Chancellor.

LEGAL AID AND CONDITIONAL FEES

Major changes have been made to the legal aid system under the Access to Justice Act 1999.

Part I of the Act provides for two new schemes, replacing the existing legal aid scheme, to secure the provision of publicly-funded legal services for people who need them. It establishes a Legal Services Commission to run the two schemes, and enables the Lord Chancellor to give the Commission orders, directions and guidance about how it should exercise its functions. It requires the Commission to establish, maintain and develop a Community Legal Service. The Community Legal Service fund will replace the legal aid fund in civil and family cases. The Commission will also be responsible for a Criminal Defence Service, which will replace the current legal aid scheme in criminal cases. The new scheme is intended to ensure that people suspected or accused of a crime are properly represented, while securing better value for money than is possible under the legal aid scheme. The Legal Services Commission will be empowered to secure these services through contracts with lawyers in private practice, or by providing them through salaried defenders (employed directly by the Commission or by non-profitmaking organisations established for the purpose).

Part II of the Access to Justice Act 1999 makes changes to facilitate the private funding of litigation. A scheme known as 'no win, no fee' or conditional fee system has been introduced. By this system, potential litigants can agree with lawyers terms on which they will be represented. Insurance cover is taken out to meet the expenses of witnesses and other costs arising, in case the action is lost. The 1999 Act amends the law on conditional fee agreements between lawyers and their clients; in particular it allows the additional fees payable to a solicitor in a successful case in a 'no win, no fee' agreement to be recovered from the other side. In a recent court decision, the Court of Appeal has agreed that the cost of taking out insurance at a reasonable premium could be recovered from the losing party.[6]

It is impossible in a work of this size to deal adequately with the complexities of the legal system and the procedures which are followed. The interested reader is therefore referred to the works in the list of Further Reading.

QUESTIONS AND EXERCISES

1. Look at the Glossary and identify the words and terms with which you are not familiar.

2. Try and arrange a visit to a court of law, and make notes of the procedure which is followed, the language used, the level of formality followed (eg. in clothes which are worn) and the purpose of the proceedings. What preparations would you need to make if you were required to give evidence?

3. Obtain a copy of Schedule 1 to the Human Rights Act 1999 and consider those articles which would appear to be relevant to the practice of midwifery and the rights of the woman.

References

1 R v. Evans and others ex parte Pinochet Ugarte. Times Law Report 26 November 1998 HL

2 R v. Bournewood Community and Mental Health NHS Trust ex parte L [1998] 1 All ER 634 HL

3 Airedale NHS Trust v. Bland [1993] 1 All ER 821

4 The Nursing and Midwifery Order 2001. SI 2002 No 253

5 Whitehouse v. Jordan [1981] 1 All ER 267

6 Callery v. Gray; Russell v. Pal Pak Corrugated Ltd. Times Law Report 18 July 2001

PROFESSIONAL ISSUES

In this Section, professional issues relating to midwifery practice are considered. The first chapter looks at the role of the NMC in the registration and education of midwives. The next chapter considers those aspects which relate to the Supervisor of Midwives and the Local Supervising Authority. The last two chapters consider the regulations which relate to professional conduct proceedings and the nature of the Midwives Rules, the Midwife's Code of Practice, the Scope of Professional Practice and other NMC (formerly UKCC) guidance.

Chapter 2
MIDWIFERY:
PROFESSIONAL REGULATION

This chapter considers the following topics:

– What is a midwife?

– Role constitution and function of the statutory bodies

– The Midwifery Committee of the NMC

– Registration and false claims to registration

– Pre-registration education and training

– Post-registration education and practice (PREP)

WHAT IS A MIDWIFE?

The origin of the term in Middle and Old English means 'with a woman' (Middle and Old English mid = with; Middle English wif = a woman). Churchill's medical directory gives a present day meaning as 'a healthcare worker who may or may not be formally trained and is not a physician, that delivers babies and provides associated maternal care'.

The same directory defines midwifery as 'the practice of obstetrics by a midwife', a definition which may not be universally accepted in view of the present debate concerning the separate role of obstetricians and midwives in childbirth.

The definition adopted by the World Health Organisation from the International Conference of Midwives (1972) and the International Federation of Gynaecologists and Obstetricians (1973) as adapted in 1991 and 1992 is set out in the beginning of the Midwife's Code of Practice.[1]

The definition includes the following:

She must be able to give the necessary supervision, care and advice to women during pregnancy, labour and the postpartum period; to conduct deliveries on her own responsibility and to care for the newborn and the infant.

Care includes:

- preventative measures
- the detection of abnormal conditions in mother and child
- the procurement of medical assistance
- the execution of emergency measures in the absence of medical help
- health counselling and education, not only for the women, but also within the family and community
- Antenatal education and preparation for parenthood, certain areas of gynaecology, family planning and child care.

Article 4 of the European Community Midwives Directive 80/155/EEC, which defines the activities of a midwife, is also set out at the beginning of the Midwife's Code of Practice and is shown in Box 2.1.

Box 2.1 Activities of a midwife laid down by the EC

Member states shall ensure that midwives are at least entitled to take up and pursue the following activities:

- to provide sound family planning information and advice

- to diagnose pregnancies and monitor normal pregnancies; to carry out examinations necessary for the monitoring of the development of normal pregnancies

- to prescribe or advise on the examinations necessary for the earliest possible diagnosis of pregnancies at risk

- to provide a programme of parenthood preparation and a complete preparation for childbirth including advice on hygiene and nutrition

- to care for and assist the mother during labour and to monitor the condition of the fetus in utero by the appropriate clinical and technical means

- to conduct spontaneous deliveries including where required an episiotomy and in urgent cases a breech delivery

- to recognise the warning signs of abnormality in the mother or infant which necessitate referral to a doctor and to assist the latter where appropriate; to

▶ take the necessary emergency measures in the doctor's absence, in particular the manual removal of the placenta, possibly followed by manual examination of the uterus

– to examine and care for the newborn infant; to take all initiatives which are necessary in case of need and to carry out where necessary immediate resuscitation

– to care for and monitor the progress of the mother in the postnatal period and to give all the necessary advice to the mother on infant care to enable her to ensure the optimum progress of the newborn infant

– to carry out the treatment prescribed by a doctor

– to maintain all necessary records.

The UKCC has updated[2] its requirements for pre-registration midwifery programmes, following the report of its Commission for Education, Fitness for Practice.

There is no doubt that in relation to normal births, the duties set out above are extremely comprehensive. Although midwives in this country have not enjoyed a smooth path historically, as *The Art and Science of Midwifery* by Louise Silverton[3] shows, they do at present enjoy a higher status and protection in law than their colleagues in America.[4] Their present situation in law contrasts greatly with the limited recognition of the scope of midwifery in certain American states quoted by Louise Silverton.[5] She cites the situation in California where the state law which governs the practice of nurse-midwives, prohibits them from using any instrument to assist the birth of the child (with the exception of used those to clamp and cut the umbilical cord) or from prescribing or administering, either before or during birth, drugs or medications other than laxatives or disinfectants. Reference could also be made to the gripping thriller by Chris Bohjalian, *Midwives*,[6] a novel about a midwife in Vermont and her prosecution following a home delivery as a contrast between the legal position of midwives in that state of the United States and in the UK.

MIDWIVES IN THE UNITED KINGDOM

In the period 1st April 2000 – 31st March 2001[7] there were 90,378 midwives on the effective register (164 male and 90,214 female) and 33,291 were registered as practising midwives (93 male and 33,198 female). The UKCC notes that the number of practising midwives forms only 36.84% of the total number of midwives holding effective registration, and that their number has fallen by 1.79% compared with the previous year. Of the practising midwives:

- 27,772 were shown as working in the NHS hospital and/or community (2,233 trust only, 2 community only)

- 2,099 were employed by the midwifery bank

- 622 were midwife teachers

- 504 were employed by an agency

- 121 were employed by a family practitioner

- 121 were employed in a private institution

- 63 were self-employed in private practice.

The totals are more than those registered to practise, since some midwives undertake more than one kind of practice.

The total number of midwives who work part-time has been increasing over the years so that in 2000-2001 they constitute more than half of the practising midwives. 49% were described as full-time and 51% as part-time, compared with 66.4% full-time and 33.6% part-time in 1988.

NHS MATERNITY STATISTICS

The statistics published by the Department of Health[8] show that between 1989/90 and 1997/8 the Caesarean rate increased from 11.3% to 18.2%, and provisional figures for 1999/2000 suggest a further rise to over 20%. The proportion of women staying in hospital for 4 days or more after delivery fell from 38% to 21%. The figures thus show an increased level of surgical intervention in delivery, and a faster turnover of women in hospital. Both figures suggest an increase of pressure on the midwives working in delivery units. Issues relating to Caesarean section are considered in Chapter 6.

ROLE CONSTITUTION AND FUNCTION OF THE STATUTORY BODIES

In April 2002 the Nursing and Midwifery Council began its work, taking over from the UKCC as the registration body for nurses, midwives and health visitors. It had existed in shadow form since May 2001 when the Department of Health announced the appointment of the President, members and alternates. Existing guidance from the UKCC will remain effective until such time as the NMC replaces it.

The events leading up the establishment of the NMC were as follows:

The Government commissioned an independent review of the Nurses, Midwives and

Health Visitors Act 1997 from JM Consulting Ltd. Its report was published in February 1999. The Government accepted its main recommendations, that the UKCC and the four National Boards should be replaced by a smaller, more strategic Nursing and Midwifery Council with stronger lay input and ultimate ownership of the setting and monitoring of standards of training and conduct. Following publication of the Department of Health's Modernising Regulation[9] consultation document, draft orders were published in April 2001 and, after a further consultation period, came into force in April 2002 (The Nursing and Midwifery Order 2001 Statutory Instrument 2002 No 253).

The constitution of the NMC is shown in Box 2.2.

Box 2.2 Constitution of the NMC (Schedule 1 Part 1 to the Orders in Council)

The Council shall consist of:

- 12 members who are appointed by the Council on being elected under the electoral scheme ('Registered members')

- 11 members who are appointed by the Privy Council. ('lay members')

Alternate members

In addition the Council shall appoint 12 members of the Council (referred to as 'alternate members') who have been elected under the election scheme, who may not attend or vote at a Council meeting unless their corresponding registrant member is unable to do so.

THE ELECTION SCHEME

The details for this are set out in Paragraph 2 of Schedule 1. The Council has the power to provide rules for the scheme but the scheme must provide for:

(a) A person seeking election as a registrant member or alternate member:

  i. is registered in the part of the register for which he seeks election but no person may be elected for more than one part of the register at a time

  ii. in respect of a national constituency, lives or works wholly or mainly in that national constituency

  iii. is not the subject of any allegation, investigation or proceedings concerning his fitness to practise; and

iv. is wholly or mainly engaged in the practice, teaching or management of the profession in respect of which he is registered and seeks election or in research in those fields;

(b) At least one registrant member and one alternate member shall be appointed from each part of the register and the number of members from each part shall be equal

(c) at least one member shall be elected from each of the national constituencies for each part of the register

(d) a person may only vote:

i. in respect of one part of the register

ii. for candidates who represent a part of the register in which he is registered at the time of the election and

iii. for a candidate seeking election for the constituency in which he wholly or mainly lives or works or, if he does not wholly or mainly live or work in any constituency, the constituency he has selected or to which he has been assigned in accordance with prescribed criteria

(e) a person may vote even if he is residing or works outside the UK

(f) where someone ceases to be a member or alternate member a replacement may be appointed by the Council.

LAY MEMBERS

The Privy Council, after consulting such persons as it considers appropriate, shall appoint lay members from among persons who are not and never have been on the Register, and who have such qualifications, interests and experience as, in the opinion of the Privy Council, will be of value to the Council in the performance of its functions. At least one of the PC appointed members shall be appointed from each country of the UK and that member shall live or work (wholly or mainly) in the country concerned.

TENURE OF MEMBERS

Each member's term of office will be for a period of four years.

PRESIDENT

The first president was appointed after open competition. In future, members of the Council shall elect the president from amongst themselves for a term of four years.

STANDING ORDERS

The Council may make standing orders in respect of the Council, its committees and sub-committees, but not in respect of any of the Practice Committees.

The functions of the NMC which under Schedule 3 Paragraph 8(2) of the Health Act 1999 cannot be delegated to any other body are shown in Box 2.3.

Box 2.3 Functions of the NMC

- Keeping the register of members admitted to practice

- Determining the standards of education and training for admission to practice

- Giving advice about standards of conduct and performance

- Administering procedures (including making rules) relating to misconduct, unfitness to practice and similar matters.

PERFORMANCE OF FUNCTIONS

Under Article 3(4) and (5) of the Order the Council is required to follow several stipulations in performing its functions. These are shown in Box 2.4.

Box 2.4 NMC performance of functions

The main objective of the Council in exercising its functions shall be to safeguard the health and wellbeing of persons using or needing the services of registrants.

(b) In exercising its functions, the Council shall:(a) Have proper regard to the interests of all registrants and prospective registrants and persons referred to in paragraph (4) in each of the countries of the UK and to any differing considerations applying to the professions to which this Order applies and to groups within them and co-operate wherever reasonably practicable with:

▶
i.   employers and prospective employers of registrants

ii.   persons who provide, assess or fund education or training for registrants or prospective registrants, or who propose to do so

iii.   persons who are responsible for regulating or co-ordinating the regulation of other health and social care professionals, or of those who carry out activities in connection with services provided by those professions or the professions regulated under this Order.

The NMC is also required to inform and educate registrants and the public about its work (Article 3(13) of the Order).

Before establishing any standards or giving guidance the Council shall consult representatives of any group of persons it considers appropriate, including, as it sees fit representatives of:

– registrants or classes of registrants

– employers of registrants

– users of the services of registrants, and

– persons providing, assessing or funding education or training for registrants and prospective registrants.

The Council shall publish any standards it establishes and any guidance it gives (Article 3(15)).

POWERS OF THE COUNCIL

The powers of the Council are set out in Paragraph 15 of Schedule 1 Part 1 of the NMC Order 2001 (SI 2002 No 253). They include power to borrow, to appoint such staff as it may determine necessary, to pay salaries, pensions, fees and allowances for members and to set up or abolish any of its committees except statutory committees. Where it appears to the Council that any statutory committee is failing to perform its functions adequately, the Council may give a direction as to the proper performance of those functions. Where it has given directions but is satisfied that the committee has failed to comply with the direction, the Council may exercise any power of that committee or do any act or other thing authorised to be done by that committee.

STATUTORY COMMITTEES

These are the following:

– Investigating Committee

– Conduct and Competence Committee

– Health Committee

– Midwifery Committee.

The Investigating Committee, the Conduct and Competence Committee and the Health Committee are also referred to as the 'Practice Committees'. Their constitution and functions are explained below.

THE MIDWIFERY COMMITTEE OF THE NMC

Part VIII of the Order for the NMC sets out the statutory provisions relating to midwifery. Article 41 states that the role of the Midwifery Committee shall be to advise the Council, at the Council's request or otherwise, on any matter affecting midwifery. The Council is required to 'consult the Midwifery Committee on the exercise of its functions in so far as it affects midwifery including any proposal to make rules under Article 42'.

Article 42 is shown in Box 2.5.

Box 2.5 Article 40

1. In addition to its functions under other provisions in this Order, the Council shall by rules regulate the practice of midwifery and the rules may in particular:

   (a) Determine the circumstances in which and the procedure by means of which a midwife may be suspended from practice

   (b) require midwives to give notice of their intention to practise to the Local Supervising Authority (LSA) for the area in which they intend to practise

   (c) require midwives to attend courses of instruction in accordance with the rules.

2. If rules are made requiring midwives to give the notice referred to in 1(b) above, the LSA shall inform the Council of any notices given to it under those rules.

The role of the Local Supervising Authority under Article 43 is discussed in the next chapter.

The NMC has the power to make provision by standing orders for the composition, members, quorum, procedure, standards for the attendance and performance of members and the performance of the functions of the Midwifery Committee. The Chairman is required to be a member of Council and the majority of members must be practising midwives. The Council must have regard to the guidance issued by the Commissioner for Public appointments when selecting non-Council members for the Committee. No person who is a member of the Council or the Midwifery Committee by virtue of his membership of any profession may take part in any proceedings of the Committee in any period during which he is the subject of any investigations, proceedings or a determination against him concerning his fitness to practise his profession. The powers of the Midwifery Committee may be exercised even though there is a vacancy among its members. No proceedings of the Midwifery Committee shall be invalidated by any defect in the appointment of a member.

REGISTRATION

Under Article 4 the NMC is required to appoint a Registrar to hold office for such period and on such terms as the Council may determine and who shall have such functions as the Council may direct. Article 5 requires the Council to establish and maintain a register of qualified nurses and midwives. The Council shall from time to time establish the standards of proficiency necessary to be admitted to the different parts of the Register, being standards it considers necessary for safe and effective practice under that part of the Register.

The Register shall show, in relation to each registrant, such address and other details as the Council may prescribe.

The Register may be divided into such parts as the Privy Council may by order determine, on a proposal by the Council or otherwise (Article 6(1)). Each part shall have a designated title indicative of different qualifications and different kinds of education or training, and a registered professional is entitled to use the title corresponding to the part of the Register in which he is registered. Rules can be made under Article 7 for the keeping of the Register.

ACCESS TO THE REGISTER

The Council shall make the Register available for inspection by members of the public at all reasonable times and shall publish the Register in such manner and at such times as it considers appropriate (Article 8).

REGISTRATION

Under Article 9, a person seeking admission to a part of the Register shall be entitled to be registered in that part if the application is made in the prescribed form and manner and the applicant:

(a) satisfies the Registrar that he holds an approved qualification awarded:

  i. within such period not exceeding five years, ending with the date of the application, as may be prescribed; or

  ii. before the prescribed period mentioned above and he has met such requirements as to additional education, training, and experience as the Council may specify under article 19(3)

(b) satisfies the Registrar in accordance with the Council's requirements mentioned in Article 5 that he is capable of safe and effective practice as nurse or midwife and

(c) has paid the prescribed fee.

RENEWAL OF REGISTRATION

Under Article 10, provisions for renewal of registration and readmission require the applicant to satisfy the Registrar, in addition to other requirements, that he has met any prescribed requirements for continuing professional development within the prescribed time.

Under Article 11, visiting EEA (European Economic Area) nurses and midwives are deemed to be registered.

PRE-REGISTRATION EDUCATION AND TRAINING

Article 13 defines what is meant by an approved qualification. The definition is shown in Box 2.6.

Box 2.6 Approved qualification (Article 13)

1. For the purpose of this Order a person is to be regarded as having an approved qualification if:

(a) he has a qualification awarded in the UK which has been approved by the Council as attesting to the standard of proficiency it requires for admission to the part of the Register in respect of which he is applying

(b) he is an EEA national and has a qualification of the kind mentioned in Article 14; or

(c) he has, elsewhere than in the UK, undergone training in nursing or midwifery and either:

    i.   holds a qualification which the Council is satisfied attests to a standard of proficiency comparable to that attested by a qualification referred to in sub-paragraph (a); or

    ii. the Council is not so satisfied, but the applicant has undergone in the UK or elsewhere such additional training and experience as satisfies the Council, following any test of competence as it may require him to take, that he has the requisite standard of proficiency for admission to the part of the register in respect of which he is applying; and in either case

    iii. he is not an EEA national or exempt person and he satisfies prescribed requirements as to knowledge of English.

The NMC shall determine procedures to assess whether qualifications granted by institutions outside the UK and experience of practice outside the UK are of a comparable standard to those approved in the UK and shall, where it sees fit, keep a list of comparable qualifications which it shall keep under review.

EDUCATION AND TRAINING

Article 15 gives the responsibility to the Council from time to time to establish:

(a) the standards of education and training necessary to achieve the standards of proficiency it has established under Article 5(2)

(b) the requirements to be satisfied for admission to, and continued participation in, such education and training which may include requirements as to good health and good character.

These standards shall be set out in rules made by the Council and shall include such matters as the outcomes to be achieved by that education and training. The Council is required to ensure that universities and other bodies concerned with such education and training are notified of the NMC's standards and requirements and take appropriate steps to ensure that these standards and requirements are met. The information which the Council must give to any institution providing the education, training or test of competence is set out in Article 17.

Article 18 covers the refusal or withdrawal of approval of courses, qualifications and institutions.

Under Article 19, the Council may make rules requiring registered nurses and midwives to undertake such continuing professional development as it shall specify in standards. The rules may, in particular, make provision with respect to registrants who fail to comply with any requirements of the rules including provision for their registration to cease to have effect.

Under Article 20, the National Assembly for Wales may create or designate a body with which the Council may enter into any such arrangements as are referred to in Article 15(6) of the Order in order to perform its functions under Article 15(5)(b) in respect of the standards established under article 15(1) or 19(4) or (6).

VISITORS

The Council may appoint persons (Visitors) to visit any place at which any relevant education and training, examinations or test of competence is given or to be given (Article 16).

REQUIREMENTS FOR PRE-REGISTRATION MIDWIFERY PROGRAMMES

These have been set out by the UKCC under cover of Registrar's Letter 25/2000.

Guiding principles are set for the basis of midwifery competencies. These are:

– demonstrate a woman-centred approach to care based on partnership, which respects the individuality of the woman and her family

– promote ethical and non-discriminatory practices

– reflect the quality dimension of care through the setting and maintenance of appropriate standards

– develop the concept of lifelong learning in students, encompassing key skills including communications and teamwork

– take account of the changing nature and context of midwifery practice

– base practice on the best available evidence.

Competencies are defined as the skills and ability to practise safely and effectively without the need for direct supervision. The UKCC required the pre-registration midwifery programmes to be designed to enable the student to achieve the competencies under the direction of a practising midwife and to assume on registration the responsibilities and accountability for her practice as a midwife. The guidance refers to the definition of a midwife and her activities as set out in the European Union Midwives Directive and shown above in Box 2.1.

POST-REGISTRATION EDUCATION AND PRACTICE (PREP)

The United Kingdom Central Council had published in March 1994 the standards it had set in relation to post-registration education and practice for registered practitioners.[10] A summary is shown in Box 2.7.

Box 2.7 Summary of PREP scheme

1. Nurses, midwives, and health visitors will be required to complete to remain on the register:

   (a) a minimum of 5 study days every three years

   (b) a Notification of Practice form

   (c) a Return to Practice programme if they have been out of practice for five years or more, and

   (d) a Personal Professional Profile.

2. New standards for specialist post-registration education have been set.

IMPLICATIONS OF PREP FOR MIDWIVES

Until recently, midwives were the only group of practitioners registered by the UKCC who had statutorily to comply with minimum standards of post-registration training and education. PREP now sets standards for all the practitioners registered by the UKCC. A PREP handbook was published by the UKCC in January 2001[11] which was designed to consolidate everything the practitioner needed to know about PREP standards and guidance. It also advised that practitioners can contact the UKCC's professional advice service in confidence.

There are two separate PREP standards:

– The PREP (practice) standard. This requires midwives to have practised for a minimum of 100 days (750 hours) in the five years prior to the renewal of registration and to submit the notification of intention to practise form annually in accordance with Rule 36 of the Midwives Rules.

– The PREP (continuing professional development) standard (CPD). This must be undertaken and recorded over the three years prior to the renewal of registration. Registrants are required to declare on their notification of practice (NOP) form that they have met this requirement when they renew their registration. The standard requires the practitioner:

  - to undertake at least five days of learning activity relevant to her practice during the three years prior to the renewal of registration

  - to maintain a personal professional profile (PPP) of her learning activity

  - to comply with any request from the UKCC to audit how these requirements have been met.

The Handbook states that although there is no set format for the PPP, a template is suggested on pages 8-11. The template provides a way of recording each of the activities which have been completed, where the practitioner was practising when these activities took place, of what the learning activity consisted and how the learning related to practice.

The requirement of a personal professional profile underlines the emphasis on the practitioner being responsible for her own development and competence. It is part of the philosophy set out in The Scope of Professional Practice (see Chapter 5) which requires the practitioner to be accountable and responsible for the development of her own professional practice. Many different schemes for the structure of the personal professional profile have been marketed. The NMC may make further changes in the content of the personal professional profile.

ADVANCED MIDWIFERY AND NURSING PRACTICE

The Council recognises that many practitioners will undertake additional studies in pursuit of advanced midwifery and nursing practice and such studies are likely to be at Masters level. The Council does not, however, at this stage, propose a formal preparation and qualification with explicit links with the Council's register for advanced midwifery practice.

In April 2001, the UKCC published a document bringing together all its guidance relating to specialist practice, preparatory to providing further clarification of the UKCC standards for specialist practice.[12] This covers the areas shown in Box 2.8.

Box 2.8 UKCC standards for specialist practice

- PREP

- Recording the qualification of specialist practice

- Transitional arrangements 1.11.95-31.10.98

- Preparation for specialist practice

Standards for specialist community nursing education and practice

- General practice nursing

- Community mental health nursing

- Community learning disabilities nursing

- Public health nursing/health visiting

- Occupational health nursing

- Community nursing in the home/district nursing

- School nursing

Annexe 1 Health visitor training rules

Annexe 2 Parts of the UKCC Register

THE FUTURE

The NMC is only just established and therefore most of the current rules and guidance derive from the thinking of the UKCC. Inevitably over time the NMC will stamp its own character on this material and within its statutory framework take further the work of regulation and protecting the public.

QUESTIONS AND EXERCISES

1. If you were to stand for election to the NMC, what duties would you expect to undertake?

2. To what extent do you consider the Midwifery Committee is able to protect the educational and practice standards of registered midwives?

3. The National Boards were abolished at the end of March 2002. Who now undertakes the functions which they formerly carried out?

4. In what respects do you consider that the NMC is better organised to carry out the statutory functions of regulating the profession of midwifery than its predecessor the UKCC?

References

1 UKCC. 1988. *Midwives Rules and Code of Practice*. London: UKCC

2 UKCC. 2000. *Requirements for pre-registration midwifery programmes*. Registrar's Letter 25/2000

3 Silverton L. 1993. *The Art and Science of Midwifery*. Hemel Hempstead: Prentice Hall

4 Bryce R. 26 July 1993. *The Guardian* page 31 described how five women in Los Angeles are facing upto six years in prison for operating an independent birthing centre. The US has no national qualification standards for lay midwives (as distinct from certified nurse-midwives) so their work is regulated by individual states.

5 Silverton L. 1994. The enhanced role of the midwife. In: *Expanding the Role of the Nurse*. Hunt G and Wainwright P (eds). Oxford: Blackwell Scientific Publications

6 Bohjalian C. 1998. *Midwives: a novel*. New York: Vintage Contemporaries

7 UKCC. *Annual Report April 2000 – 31 March 2001*. Part 4

8 Department of Health. *Statistical Bulletin. NHS Maternity Statistics England 1995/6-1997/8*

9 NHS Executive. 2000. *Modernising Regulation: The New Nursing and Midwifery Council*. London: DoH

10 UKCC. 1994. *The Future of Professional Practice: The Council's Standards for Education and Practice following Registration*. London: UKCC

11 UKCC. 2001. *The PREP Handbook*. London: UKCC

12 UKCC. 2001. *Standards for specialist education and practice*. London: UKCC

Chapter 3
MIDWIFERY SUPERVISION

Midwives are unique amongst health professionals in having a system of supervision prescribed by statute. It was initiated under the Midwives' Act 1902 which set up medical and non-medical Supervisors of Midwives. No specific qualifications were required for the latter and this defect was addressed under the Midwives' Act 1936 which required that Supervisors of Midwives had adequate experience of midwifery. The present arrangements for midwifery supervision are set up under the Health Act 1999 and the Orders in Council made under that Act which amend the Nurses, Midwives and Health Visitors Act 1997. Further modifications may take place as the new Nursing and Midwifery Council takes up its duties in April 2002. Reference should be made to *Developments in the Supervision of Midwives* edited by Mavis Kirkham for an overview of supervision.[1] The English National Board issued guidelines for midwives on the statutory supervision of midwives which clarified the role of the Supervisor.[2]

Some acknowledge supervision to be such a useful system that they advocate its extension to other health professionals. Others, particularly independent midwives, whose clients may come from a variety of districts and who therefore may find that they are reporting to more than twenty Supervisors of Midwives, wish to see radical changes in the supervisory system, if not its abolition. The aim of this chapter will be to collate the statutory and guidance provisions relating to the appointment and role of the Supervisor of Midwives, and discuss these in relation to the legal issues which arise and the present debate as to the future role of supervision. Of particular value as reference material is the English National Board pack, Preparation of Supervisors of Midwives.[3]

This chapter looks at:

– The statutory framework for supervision

– The definition and functions of the Local Supervising Authority

– The appointment and role of the Supervisor of Midwives

– The duty of the midwife in relation to the LSA and Supervisor of Midwives

– Legal aspects of the supervision of midwifery

– The future.

THE STATUTORY FRAMEWORK FOR SUPERVISION

There is a statutory requirement for the establishment of Local Supervising Authorities (LSAs) and for the appointment of Supervisors of Midwives. This is laid down in the Order in Council set up under the Health Act 1999. Provision is given in the Articles of the Order in Council for rules relating to supervision to be made which have binding force. The principal Rules were enacted in 1983 but were amended in 1998. The Rules are in turn amplified by the guidance given in the Midwife's Code of Practice (most recent edition 1998). The Code does not have statutory force, but clearly failure to follow the Code will be taken into account in any investigation and/or hearing of misconduct. Part of the Code relates to the amplification of the Rules, the rest relates to practice but not to the Rules. Discussion of the Rules and the Codes can be found in Chapter 5.

THE PRINCIPAL LEGISLATION

The following provisions are made under Part VIII of the Orders in Council.[4]

Article 42

1. The Council shall by rules regulate the practice of midwifery and the rules may in particular:

    (a) determine the circumstances in which and the procedure by means of which a midwife may be suspended from practice

    (b) require midwives to give notice of their intention to practice to the Local Supervising Authority (referred to in this part as 'the LSA') for the area in which they intend to practise

    (c) require midwives to attend courses of instruction in accordance with the rules.

2. If rules are made requiring midwives to give the notice referred to in 1(b) above, the LSA shall inform the Council of any notices given to it under those rules.

DEFINITION AND FUNCTIONS OF THE LOCAL SUPERVISING AUTHORITIES (LSAS)

The definition of the LSA is given in Schedule 4 of the Nurses, Midwives and Health Visitors Statutory Instrument[4] and is shown below:

LSA means:

– In England and Wales, Health Authorities

– In Scotland, Health Boards, and

– In Northern Ireland, Health and Social Services Boards.

Provisions relating to the local supervision of midwives are made under Part VIII of the Orders in Council,[4] made under the Health Act 1999 and shown in Box 3.1.

Box 3.1 Duties of Local Supervising Authorities

Article 43

1. Each Local Supervising Authority shall:

    (a) exercise general supervision, in accordance with rules under Article 42 over all midwives practising in its area

    (b) where it appears to it that the fitness to practise of a midwife in its area is impaired, report it to the Council, and

    (c) have power in accordance with the Council's rules to suspend a midwife from practice.

2. The Council may prescribe the qualifications of persons who may be appointed by the LSA to exercise supervision over midwives within its area, and no person shall be so appointed who is not qualified.

3. The Council may by rules from time to time establish standards for the exercise by LSAs of their functions and may give guidance to LSAs on these matters.

At the time of writing the NMC has not enacted any new rules in relation to the supervision of midwifery and the role of the LSA but these can be expected as it takes up its duties. The existing Rules and guidance in the Code of Practice as drafted in 1998 will be quoted in this book.

THE MIDWIVES RULES

The Midwives Rules give powers to the LSA and regulate

- notification of intention to practice

- suspension from practice by a LSA

- the right to require the midwife to be medically examined, and

- the inspection of premises and equipment.

Notification of intention to practice

It is the statutory duty of a midwife who intends to practice to notify her intention to do so, to the Local Supervising Authority. Rule 36 sets out the provisions in relation to this duty. The LSA has a duty to notify Council of notices received by it under this rule. There is provision in Rule 36(2) for the notice to be given, in an emergency, after the time when she commences to practise, provided that it is given within 48 hours of that time. Under Rule 45, which covers the discharge of statutory functions by a Local Supervising Authority, each Local Supervising Authority shall ensure that, in respect of practising midwives within its area, there is published in writing at least once every two years

- the date in the month of March by which notice of intention to practice under Rule 36(1)(b) must be received by it, and

- the name or office of the person to whom the said notice must be sent.

Suspension from practice

It must be clarified that there are various forms of suspension.

- There is suspension from practice by the LSA, which is the subject of this discussion. Suspension from practice must, however, be distinguished from two other forms of suspension:

- The right of an employer to suspend from the workplace an employee who is alleged to be in breach of the terms of the contract of employment, or incapable by reason of physical or mental disability to perform her functions adequately. This is considered in Chapter 22 and can apply to all employees.

- The NMC (formerly UKCC) power to suspend from the Register or make an interim suspension (see Chapter 4). The effect of suspension from the Register is that the practitioner is no longer able to work as a registered practitioner, and this will inevitably mean that she would be suspended or dismissed from her employment. This applies to all registered practitioners.

Guidance on suspension from practice of midwives and interim suspension of Registration for Nurses, Midwives and Health Visitors is given by the UKCC.[5]

Suspension from practice by the LSA, which is under consideration here, does not necessarily involve the other forms of suspension.

Rule 38 of the Midwives Rules is set out in Box 3.2.

Box 3.2 Suspension from practice by LSA (Rule 38 of Midwives Rules)

1. It shall be the duty of the LSA to suspend a midwife from practice when necessary for the purpose of preventing the spread of infection, whether or not she has contravened any of the rules laid down by the UKCC.

2. The LSA may suspend from practice until any proceedings or investigations have been determined:

    (a) a midwife against whom it has reported a case for investigation to the UKCC

    (b) a midwife who has been referred to the Professional Conduct Committee of the Council...

    (c) a midwife who has been referred to the Health Committee of the Council...

3. A LSA in discharging any duty imposed on it by Section 15 2(b) of the Act, or in exercising the power given in paragraphs 1 and 2 of this rule to suspend a midwife from practice shall:

    (a) immediately notify the midwife concerned in writing of any decision to suspend her and the reason for such suspension, and

    (b) in respect of a suspension authorised by Paragraph 2 of this rule forthwith report any such suspension and the grounds thereof to the UKCC.

Once the midwife has been reported to the NMC under Rule 38(2) the procedures set down in the Councils' Professional Conduct Rules (see Chapter 4) must continue to be pursued even if the decision to suspend the midwife from practice is subsequently revoked by the LSA.

The power of suspension set out in Box 3.4 covers both employed midwives within the NHS and independent midwives who practice in the district of the LSA.

It should be noted that the LSA MUST suspend the midwife from practice when necessary for the purpose of preventing the spread of infection. However, there is a discretionary power given in relation to suspension where investigations or professional conduct proceedings are taking place or where there has been a referral to the Health Committee (see Chapter 4). The discretionary nature of the power in these circumstances is emphasised in the Registrar's letter:

'If the LSA chooses to suspend a midwife from practice the decision must be able to be justified as being in the interest of the public or the practitioner.'

The Registrar's letter points out that the power cannot be delegated to a Supervisor of Midwives and its decision is only effective within the geographical area in which it has jurisdiction.

There are at any one time only a tiny number of midwives who are suspended from practice.

Duty to be medically examined

The LSA also has the power to request a medical examination of a practising midwife. This is set out in Paragraph 39 of the rules and is shown in Box 3.3.

Box 3.3 Duty to be medically examined (Rule 39)

A practising midwife shall, if the LSA deems it necessary for preventing the spread of infection, undergo medical examination by a registered medical practitioner.

Rule 39 is part of the concern in relation to public health of the possibility that the midwife could be a cause of infection for her clients. The wording, however, is interesting. The Rule places a clear duty upon the midwife, if the LSA deems it necessary, to undergo medical examination. The LSA is not given the power to force the medical examination, but clearly if the midwife is in breach of the Rules then this could be grounds for suspension from practice as set out in Rule 38. No other health professional is placed under a similar statutory duty, though many codes of professional conduct may give guidance on the importance of a medical examination being undertaken.

Inspection of premises and equipment

Under Rule 43, the practising midwife must permit inspection and examination of her premises and equipment etc. This rule is set out in Box 3.4.

Box 3.4 Inspection of premises and equipment (Rule 43)

1. A midwife shall give to her Supervisor of Midwives, the LSA and the UKCC every reasonable facility to inspect her methods of practise, her records, her equipment and such part of her residence as may be used for professional purposes.

2. A midwife shall use her best endeavours to permit inspection from time to time by a midwifery officer, who shall be a practising midwife, of the UKCC or of an authority designated by the UKCC, of all institutional premises in which she practises other than the private residence of the mother and baby.

There are no additional powers of enforcement given by either the Act or the Rules in relation to the inspection of premises, and it is assumed that the midwife will obey the obligations placed upon her under the rules, since she can be removed from the Register for professional misconduct (see Chapter 4). No offences are created under the Act other than those in relation to registration and to attendance at childbirth (see Chapter 25). The aim of the legislation is not to create criminal offences in relation to enforcement but to secure self-regulation of the profession through the powers given to the NMC and its committees.

Local Supervising Authority: Information

Rule 45 was added in the changes made in 1993 and requires the LSA to publish the information shown in Box 3.5.

Box 3.5 Discharge of functions by a LSA (Rule 45)

(a) The LSA must ensure that, in respect of practising midwives within its area, there is published in writing at least once every two years:

    i.   the date in the month of March by which notice of intention to practise under Rule 36 must be received by it

    ii.   the name or office of the person to whom the said notice must be sent.

(b) the means by which it will:

    i.   investigate any prima facie case of misconduct, and

    ii.   determine whether to suspend a midwife from practise pursuant to Section 15 2(c) of the Act.

(c)

    i.   a list of Supervisors of Midwives whom it has appointed, and

    ii.   details of how it will provide midwives with continuous access to a Supervisor of Midwives.

(d) Details of how the practice of midwives will be supervised.

(e) All policies which it has formulated affecting the practice of midwives.

APPOINTMENT AND ROLE OF THE SUPERVISOR OF MIDWIVES

It was the aim of the UKCC that for effective supervision to be achieved, each Supervisor of Midwives should supervise no more than 40 practising midwives and this has been recommended to LSAs (see Paragraph 33 of the Midwife's Code of Practice.) The aim is to allow both effective supervision and adequate support for midwives practising within and outside the NHS. There has been a considerable improvement in these figures, and the wide variation across the UK in the supervisor-midwife ratio has (with the exception of Northern Ireland) almost disappeared. The figures for 2000-2001[6] showed the number of midwives per supervisor as:

– 18 England

– 30 Northern Ireland

– 21 Scotland

– 19 Wales

giving an average of 19 midwives per supervisor across the UK. (In 1988 the figures were 46 England, 73 Northern Ireland, 117 Scotland and 46 Wales, a total of 51 UK.)

Regulations relating to the appointment of Supervisors are set out in Rule 44 which is shown in Box 3.6.

Box 3.6 Appointment of Supervisors (Rule 44)

1. A person to be appointed by a LSA in accordance with Section 15(3) of the Act shall

    (a) be a registered and practising midwife

    (b) either:

        i.   have three years experience as a practising midwife of which at least one shall have been in the period of two years immediately preceding the appointment, or

---

     ii.   obtain such further midwifery experience, and within such period, as may be required by Council, and

(c) have successfully completed a course described in Paragraph 2 within the three year period prior to the appointment unless, in an individual case (and, in particular, in the case of a national of an EEA state or other person entitled to be treated, for the purpose of the appointment as a Supervisor of Midwives, no less favourably than a national of such a state, having regard to any enforceable Community law right or any enactment giving effect to a Community obligation) the Council decides otherwise.

2.   Course referred to in Paragraph 1(c) shall be

   (a) provided at an institution approved by a National Board

   (b) of no fewer than 100 hours duration, and

   (c) designed to enable the midwife to achieve the following outcome:

     i.   an understanding of the way in which the supervision of midwives enhances standards of care

     ii.   an understanding of the application of the law relevant to midwifery practice and the supervision of midwives

     iii. the ability to provide professional support to practising midwives relevant to maintaining and promoting standards of care

     iv. the ability to encourage midwives to use their experience in practice to enhance their professional development, and

     v.   an understanding of accountability and professional responsibility as a Supervisor of Midwives.

3.   A Supervisor of Midwives shall complete, as part the requirements of Rule 9(2)(a)(ii)(aa), at least 15 hours' study relating to the supervision of midwives in each registration period of her appointment, unless the Council, in an individual case, decides that such a study may be reduced.

An important change was effected in 1993 by the deletion of the possibility of the person appointed undertaking a course of instruction within 12 months of appointment. Now the person appointed must have completed such a course within the three years preceding the appointment. As Paragraph 32 of the Code points out, selection of the Supervisor must be from experienced midwives 'who have been appropriately trained to undertake this role'.

The Midwife's Code of Practice (Paragraphs 30-34) expands on Rule 44.

The UKCC recommended that the LSA function should be undertaken by a practising midwife, who is professionally experienced in the supervision of midwives. This person should be deployed at LSA level as the designated responsible officer and the relationship between such a midwife and the local Director of Nursing/Midwifery is of particular importance.

National Boards (or the agency taking over their functions following the establishment of the NMC) are required to provide LSAs with advice and guidance about the exercise of their functions.

THE DUTIES OF THE SUPERVISOR OF MIDWIVES

These are shown in Box 3.7 and incorporate both the Rules and the Code. They basically cover the functions of fulfilling statutory responsibilities, duties in relation to professional standards, communications, interpersonal communication, and education and development.[9]

Box 3.7 Duties of Supervisor of Midwives

1. To provide direct access to herself from all midwives within her area of responsibility. The latter should be defined by the LSA.

2. To monitor standards of practise.

3. To monitor the practice of all midwives under her responsibility.

4. To see the midwives for whom she is responsible at least annually.

5. To check all records relating to midwifery practice of those she supervises.

6. To be familiar with all maternity services in the area.

7. To ensure with the midwife effective communication in order that any problems can be shared and resolved. A key and important aspect of the supervisory function is that it enables this process (Code Paragraph 34). (The duty under the previous edition upon the midwife to initiate such communication when she considers it appropriate has been removed, see Paragraph 3.7.6 1991 edition.) The emphasis in the current edition of the

▶

Code is on reciprocity in communication. Paragraph 34 is shown in full below.

8. To be a supportive colleague, counsellor, an advisor to the midwife and develop this in order to promote a positive working relationship which is conducive to maintaining and improving standards of practice and care (Code Paragraph 34).

9. To ensure that effective communication links exist between themselves, LSAs, those engaged in determining health service policy, and medical staff in order that relevant issues are appropriately addressed and resolved (Code Paragraph 34).

10. To ensure that she is familiar with, and where possible has been involved in the formulation of, the policies, information and guidance available from LSAs. (See Rule 45 and Paragraph 35 of the Code.)

11. To report alleged misconduct to the LSA and advise the LSA.

12. Where the Supervisor of Midwives is also a manager, she may (depending upon the disciplinary procedure of the trust/employer) suspend a midwife from work. If appropriate she would report this to the LSA which could then determine whether the midwife should also be suspended from practice in accordance with Rule 38.

13. To meet regularly with the LSA and other Supervisors of Midwives.

14. To update local policies on the administration of medicines.

16. To monitor record keeping and practices.

17. Training:

   (a) To ensure that midwives comply with the statutory duties on refresher courses

   (b) To ensure that she herself is updated (see Rule 44 above).

18. To be an authorised person in whose presence drugs can be destroyed under Regulation 26 of the Misuse of Drugs regulations. NB: the Supervisor of Midwives cannot be the person to whom unwanted controlled drugs can be surrendered (Code Paragraph 18).

The NMC has a duty to provide the LSA with advice and guidance in respect of the exercise of their functions.

Supervisors should have access to this information and to any other relevant information that LSAs may hold (Code of Practice Paragraph 32).

PERSONAL CONTACT BETWEEN SUPERVISOR AND MIDWIFE

Paragraph 34 of the Code of Practice sets out in detail the nature of the relationship between supervisor and midwife, and is shown in full in Box 3.8.

Box 3.8 Relationship between supervisor and midwife (Paragraph 34 of the Code of Practice)

You should contact your Supervisor of Midwives on all such matters as required by the Midwives Rules. You and your Supervisor of Midwives, through your respective roles, should work towards a common aim of providing the best possible care for mothers and babies. You and your Supervisor of Midwives have a mutual responsibility for effective communication between yourselves in order that any problems can be shared and resolved. Your Supervisor of Midwives should give you support as a colleague, counsellor and advisor. This should be developed in order to promote a positive working relationship which is conducive to maintaining and improving standards of practice and care. Supervisors of Midwives should ensure that effective communications exist between themselves, LSAs, those engaged in determining health services policy and medical staff in order that relevant issues are appropriately addressed and resolved.

DUTY OF MIDWIFE IN RELATION TO THE LSA AND SUPERVISOR OF MIDWIVES

To assist the reader, a compilation of the duties of the midwife (taken both from the Rules and the Code) in relation to supervision is set out in Box 3.9. Further discussion can be seen in the chapters relating to records, drugs and professional practice.

Box 3.9 Duties of midwife in relation to her Supervisor of Midwives[8]

(a) Give notice of her intention to practice to the Supervisor of Midwives in the district (i.e. the geographical jurisdiction of the Supervisor of Midwives) in

---

which she intends to work. (Rule 36, explained in Paragraphs 5 and 6 of the Midwife's Code of Practice.) Notice must be given in the prescribed form. Where the midwife works in more than one district or LSA, she must notify her intention to practise to the Supervisor of Midwives in each different district or LSA (Paragraph 5 of the Code).

(b) Notify change of name and address to the NMC and the supervisor or supervisors.

(c) If she is working outside the UK but intends to practise within the UK, keep evidence and records of her length, type and place of midwifery experience outside the UK for consideration/verification by the National Board (or the body assuming its functions) in relation to appropriate refresher course requirements (Code Paragraph 7).

(d) Maintain and develop competence acquired during initial and subsequent training (Code Paragraph 13).

(e) She should consult her Supervisor of Midwives with regard to what training and experience would be needed for the acquisition of new skills (Code Paragraph 14). (The changes brought about by PREP are considered in Chapter 2.)

(f) In an emergency or where a deviation from the norm which is outside her current sphere of practice becomes apparent in the mother or baby during the antenatal, intranatal or postnatal periods, a practising midwife shall call a registered medical practitioner or such other qualified health professional who may reasonably be expected to have the requisite skills and experience to assist her (Rule 40).

(g) Official records cannot be destroyed and the midwife must transfer to the LSA or her employing authority, if she finds it impossible or inconvenient to preserve her official records safely, her official records. The transfer must be recorded (Rule 42(3)).

(h) Immediately before ceasing practice, a midwife employed by a health authority or NHS trust shall transfer her official records to the LSA recording the details (Rule 42(4)).

(i) A self-employed midwife, immediately before ceasing to practise, must ensure that her official records are kept in a safe place and she may transfer them to the LSA. The transfer must be recorded (Rule 42(5)).

(j) When attending a mother having a home birth, the midwife should find out whether or not a registered medical practitioner is available for referral, to

▶

> attend or to be on call if required. The registered medical practitioner should normally be from the obstetric list in those parts of the UK where such a list is held. When the support of a registered medical practitioner is not available, the midwife should discuss the situation in advance whenever possible with her Supervisor of Midwives and agree and record appropriate arrangements to provide advice and support as necessary (Code Paragraph 36).

LEGAL ASPECTS OF THE SUPERVISION OF MIDWIFERY

The Supervisor of Midwives is not vicariously liable for the negligence of the midwife. The midwife must accept personal responsibility and accountability for her actions. If she is at fault she cannot lay the blame upon the Supervisor of Midwives and argue that the supervisor should have told her otherwise or warned her of certain dangers.

On the other hand, the Supervisor of Midwives may be the manager of the midwife. In this situation, there may be matters relating to resources which are properly the responsibility of the manager. The midwife would have to show that she drew any dangers relating to the health and safety of mother and child to the attention of the manager and did all that she reasonably could to ensure that the clients were safe.

NEGLIGENCE BY THE SUPERVISOR OF MIDWIVES

If the Supervisor of Midwives is negligent in carrying out her duties as set out in the rules, the Code of Practice and the LSA, then she may face professional conduct proceedings before the Conduct and Competence Committee of the NMC (see Chapter 4) as being guilty of professional misconduct. Unless harm has been caused as a reasonably foreseeable result of her negligence she is not likely to face civil proceedings for compensation for the harm arising from her negligence.

If she has misinformed the midwife, who as a result of reliance upon the supervisor's information, has caused harm to the mother or baby, then the midwife, if sued for negligence, would have to show that reliance upon the supervisor's information was reasonable and would have been the practice followed by any responsible midwife. This might be difficult to establish.

The Supervisor of Midwives is not an employee of the LSA and receives no additional pay for carrying out duties in relation to the supervision of midwives. It is unlikely, therefore, that the LSA would be responsible for the actions under the concept of vicarious liability. If, of course, the LSA had reasonable grounds for believing the supervisor to be carrying out her duties negligently or improperly, it could terminate the appointment and appoint another Supervisor of Midwives. There may, however, be vicarious liability of the NHS trust as employer of the Supervisor of Midwives, if it is a recognised part of her contract that she acts as a Supervisor of Midwives appointed by the LSA.

Is there a legal relationship between Supervisor of Midwives and midwife? The conclusion from the rules and the Code of Practice is that it is not the intention of the NMC (UKCC) to create a legal relationship between them so that either one could sue the other. The Supervisor of Midwives is not professionally accountable for the professional standards of practice of the midwife she supervises, but she is answerable in her own right for failings in her role as Supervisor of Midwives to the NMC and to the LSA. She is also answerable to her employer as a practising midwife.

EMPLOYMENT SITUATION OF SUPERVISORS OF MIDWIVES

Whilst the supervisors are appointed by the LSA, they rarely receive any payment from the LSA but are usually employed by the NHS Trust. It is helpful if their work as Supervisor of Midwives is recognised by their employer and included in their contract of employment with the trust, so that the trust would be seen to be vicariously liable both for their work as a midwife within the trust and also for their activities as a supervisor. In addition, the contract would clearly have to give them time to undertake their work of midwifery supervision.

SUPERVISORS OF MIDWIVES AND LINE MANAGEMENT SUPERVISION

Supervisors of midwives might, in addition to being the midwifery supervisor for an individual midwife, also be her line manager. Where there is this dual role it is important if possible to keep them separate, so that the midwife is aware when the other midwife is acting as her line manager rather than as her Supervisor of Midwives. The distinction between the two roles is not always clear to midwives, as research carried out by Barbara Burden and Tricia Jones shows.[9]

The UKCC has issued a position statement[10] providing advice for the Local Supervising Authorities and Supervisors of Midwives and setting out the recurring issues and themes of the reports considered by the Midwifery Committee. It identifies major issues relating to clinical practice, women's experience of care, organisational issues, and lists those issues particularly relevant to midwifery practice, Supervisors of Midwives, midwifery managers and midwifery educationalists. A similar position paper is provided for NHS employers[13] which is considered in Chapter 21.

THE FUTURE

The debate over the role of the Supervisor of Midwives is ongoing. In 1998 the ENB supported research into the evaluation of the impact of the supervision of midwives on professional practice and the quality of midwifery care, which considered a range of different models of supervision of midwives.[12] Further research of the kind carried out by Elizabeth Gaffney,[13] where midwives are asked what they want from their supervisors, is essential to ensure that supervision of midwives in the future is designed to meet the clinical needs of midwives and to support their professional practice. The ENB has also investigated the extent to which statutory supervision of midwives enables midwives to contribute to the work of primary care groups and health improvement programmes[14] (see Chapter 21).

The clinical supervision as reflective practice recommended by the UKCC for non-midwife practitioners is very different from the system of midwifery supervision, and there may be continuing debate over the preferred form of supervision. As clinical supervision is increasingly introduced for nurses and health visitors, the pressure grows to redefine the role of the Supervisor of Midwives.[15] It is likely that consideration by the NMC of the role of Supervisors of Midwives will be one of their first priorities.

QUESTIONS AND EXERCISES

1. How do you see the future of supervision?

2. You are considering becoming a Supervisor of Midwives. Prepare a protocol for the role of the Supervisor of Midwives.

3. Identify the issues which you, as a practising midwife, would wish to take to a Supervisor of Midwives.

4. Identify the advantages and disadvantages of the system of supervision and consider ways, if any, of overcoming the disadvantages.

References

1 Kirkham M. 2000. *Developments in the Supervision of Midwives*. Oxford: Books for Midwives Press

2 English National Board. 1996. *Supervision of Midwives*. London: ENB

3 English National Board. 1992. *Preparation of Supervisors of Midwives: an open learning programme*. London: ENB. The four modules cover the statutory basis to the role of the supervisor; the role in supporting good midwifery practice; the role and responsibility in dealing with alleged professional misconduct; and the role in professional development.

4 The Nursing and Midwifery Order 2001. SI 2002 No 253

5 UKCC. 1994. Registrar's letter 10/1994

6 UKCC. Annual Report April 2000 – 31 March 2001. Part 4

7 ENB. 1991. *Supervision of Midwives: ENB Advice and Guidance to LSAs.* London: ENB

8 See also the list of responsibilities set out in the ENB paper Supervision of Midwives (as above)

9 Burden B and Jones T. 1999. Midwives' perceptions of supervisors and managers. *British Journal of Midwifery,* 7(9), 547-52

10 UKCC. 2001. *Strengthening and supporting the midwifery contribution to maternity care for women and their families.* Registrar's Letter 23/2001

11 UKCC. 2001. *Strengthening and supporting the midwifery contribution to maternity care for women and their families.* Registrar's Letter 22/2001

12 Stapleton H, Duerden J and Kirkham M. 1998. *Evaluation of the impact of the supervision of midwives on professional practice and the quality of midwifery care.* London: ENB; enb.resources@easynet.co.uk

13 Gaffney E. 1998. What do midwives want from their supervision? *The Practising Midwife,* 1(10), 24-6

14 English National Board. 2000. Midwives and Public Health: an identification of the extent to which statutory supervision of midwives enables midwives to contribute to the work of primary care groups and health improvement programmes. London: ENB

15 Deery R. 1999. Improving relationships through clinical supervision: Part 1. *British Journal of Midwifery,* 7(3), 160-3; Part 2 *British Journal of Midwifery,* 7(4), 251-4

Chapter 4

PROFESSIONAL ACCOUNTABILITY AND THE NMC

The midwife, as a registered practitioner, is accountable to the NMC for her conduct. This chapter looks at the principles and procedures relating to misconduct in the light of the changes brought about by the Health Act 1999 and Statutory Instrument 2002 No 253.[1]

Accountability in relation to the civil and criminal courts is considered in Section 3 to the book and accountability in relation to the employer is considered in Section 4 Chapter 22.

The topics covered in this chapter are shown below. Other functions and powers of the NMC are considered in Chapter 2. The role of the Supervisor is considered in Chapter 3.

The topics covered in this chapter are:

– The function of the NMC in maintaining standards

– The Investigating Committee

– The Conduct and Competence Committee

– The Health Committee

– Procedural rules for the investigation of allegations

– A case of alleged misconduct.

THE FUNCTION OF THE NMC IN MAINTAINING STANDARDS

The NMC has the duty of giving advice about standards of conduct and performance and administering procedures (including making rules) relating to misconduct, unfitness to practise and similar matters. (Schedule 3 Paragraph 8 of the Health Act 1999.)

Under Article 21 of the Nursing and Midwifery Order 2001 SI 2002 No 253.

1. The Council shall

    (a) establish and keep under review the standards of conduct, performance and ethics expected of registrants and prospective registrants and give them such guidance on these matters as it sees fit; and

    (b) establish and keep under review effective arrangements to protect the public from persons whose fitness to practise is impaired.

2. The Council may also from time to time give guidance to registrants, employers and such other persons as it thinks appropriate in respect of standards for the education and training, supervision and performance of persons who provide services in connection with those provided by registrants.

3. Before establishing any standards or arrangements mentioned in paragraph (1), the Council shall consult the Conduct and Competence Committee in addition to the persons mentioned in Article 3(14).

ALLEGATIONS

The provisions of article 22 apply where any allegation is made against a registered person to the effect that:

(a) his fitness to practice is impaired by reason of:

    i.   misconduct

    ii. lack of competence

    iii. a conviction or caution in the UK for a criminal offence; or a conviction elsewhere for an offence, which if committed in England and Wales, would constitute a criminal offence

    iv. his physical or mental health, or

    v.   a determination by a body in the UK responsible under any enactment for the regulation of a health or social care profession to the effect that his fitness to practise is impaired, or a determination by a licensing body elsewhere to the same effect;

(b) an entry in the register relating to him has been fraudulently procured or incorrectly made.

Article 22 also applies even if the allegation is based on a matter alleged to have occurred outside the UK or at a time when the person against whom the allegation is made was not registered.

Under Article 22(4) rules may provide that where a Practice Committee finds that a person has failed to comply with the standards mentioned in Article 21(1), such failure shall not be taken of itself to establish that his fitness to practise is impaired, but may be taken into account in any proceedings under this Order.

PROCEDURE FOLLOWING ALLEGATION

If the allegation relates to a fraudulent entry in the Register, then it is referred to the Investigating Committee.

In other cases, the allegation is referred to:

i. persons appointed by the Council in accordance with any rules made under Article 23 or

ii. a Practice Committee.

HEARINGS ARE TO BE HELD

(a) in the UK country in which the registered address of the person concerned is situated; or

(b) if he is not registered and resides in the UK, in the country in which he resides; or

(c) in any other case, in England.

PUBLICATION OF DECISIONS

Under Article 22(9) the Council is required to publish without delay particulars of any Orders and decisions made by a Practice Committee and of its reasons for them.

The Council may also disclose to any person any information relating to a person's fitness to practise which it considers it to be in the public interest to disclose.

SCREENERS

The NMC may by rules provide for the appointment of screeners to whom allegations may be referred. A screener may be a member of Council, and of any of its committees except a Practice Committee. Employees of Council are prohibited from being screeners.

There must be a panel of at least two screeners considering an allegation; one of the panel must be a lay person and one must be a registrant from the same field as the person concerned. The number of registrants on the panel cannot exceed the number of lay persons.

THE FUNCTIONS OF THE SCREENERS

The functions of the screeners include the following:

–   considering the allegation and establishing whether, in their opinion, power is given by the Order to deal with it if it proves to be well founded

–   if the power is given, of referring the matter together with a report of the results of their consideration to such Practice Committee as they see fit

–   if the power is not given, of closing the case

    -   where there are two screeners, the lay person agrees, or

    -   where there are more than two screeners, it is the decision of the majority

–   If either of these conditions is not satisfied, the screeners may refer the matter to the Practice Committee where requested to do so by a Practice Committee, of mediating in any case with the aim of dealing with the allegation without it being necessary for the Health Committee or the Conduct and Competence Committee as the case may be to reach the stage at which it would arrange a hearing in accordance with article 32(2)(f)

–   In the event that mediation fails, of referring the matter back to the Practice Committee which referred it to the Screeners.

No person may act as a Screener or sit on a Practice Committee in respect of a particular case if he has been involved in that case in any other capacity.

THE INVESTIGATING COMMITTEE

The Investigating Committee is required to investigate any allegation appropriately referred to it (Article 26). Following the referral it shall:

- Notify without delay the person against whom the allegation is made and invite him to submit written representations within a prescribed period

- Where it sees fit, notify the person making the allegations of these representations and invite him to deal within a specified period with any points raised by the Committee in respect of those representations.

- Take such other steps as are reasonably practicable to obtain as much information as possible about the case

- Consider in the light of the information which it has been able to obtain and any representations or other observations, whether in its opinion there is a case to answer or an entry has been fraudulently procured or incorrectly made.

The NMC has the power to draw up rules to make provision for the procedure to be followed by the Investigating Committee. Article 25 gives the Council power to to require disclosure of documents by any person who is believed to be able to supply information or produce any document which appears relevant to the discharge of any functions of the Practice Committee. No person can be required to disclose information which is prohibited by or under any other enactment.

CASE TO ANSWER

Where the Investigating Committee reaches a decision that there is a case to answer, it shall notify in writing both the registered professional concerned and the person making the allegation of the decision, giving its reasons.

The Investigating Committee must then undertake mediation or refer the case to:

- screeners, for them to undertake mediation

- the Health Committee

- the Conduct and Competence Committee.

Alternatively, it may make an interim order under Article 31 (see below).

This does not apply in the case of a fraudulent entry on the Register, where if the Investigating Committee are satisfied that this has occurred, it can make an order that the Registrar remove or amend the entry. In this case the registered practitioner concerned has the right of appealing to the court under Article 38 within 28 days of the notice of the order.

NEW EVIDENCE

If new evidence becomes available the Investigating Committee can review or revoke any order it has made.

CONDUCT AND COMPETENCE COMMITTEE (CCC)

The duties of the CCC are:

– Having consulted the other Practice Committees as it thinks appropriate, advise the Council on

- the performance of the Council's functions in relation to standards of conduct, performance and ethics expected of registrants and prospective registrants

- requirements as to good character and good health to be met by registrants and prospective registrants, and

- the protection of the public from persons who are unfit to practise, and

– consider

- any allegation referred to it by the Council, Screeners, the Investigating Committee or the Health Committee, and

- any application for restoration referred to it by the Registrar.

THE HEALTH COMMITTEE

The functions of the Health Committee (Article 28) are to consider:

– any allegations referred to it by the Council, Screeners, the Investigating Committee or the Conduct and Competence Committee, and

– any application for restoration referred to it by the Registrar.

Under Article 29, the Health Committee and the Conduct and Competence Committee may:

– refer the matter to Screeners for mediation or itself undertake mediation

– decide that it is not appropriate to take further action

– issue a striking off order

– issue a suspension order (lasting upto one year)

– issue a conditions of practice order (lasting upto three years)

– issue a caution order (lasting upto five years).

If the person concerned appeals, or where new evidence becomes available then there are powers, depending upon the order and the Committee concerned, to confirm the order, extend the period for which the order has effect (subject to the maximums indicated above), reduce the period, revoke the order, vary any condition, or replace the order with another.

INTERIM ORDERS BY A PRACTICE COMMITTEE

Article 31 enables an interim suspension order to be made 'if the Committee is satisfied that it is necessary for the protection of members of the public or is otherwise in the public interest, or is in the interests of the registered professional concerned, for the registration of that person to be suspended or to be made subject to conditions'.

PROCEDURAL RULES FOR THE INVESTIGATION OF ALLEGATIONS

Article 32 requires the Council to make rules as to the procedure to be followed by the Health Committee and the Conduct and Competence Committee in considering any allegation. The required content of these rules is set out in Article 32(2).

RESTORATION TO THE REGISTER

Provision for restoration to the Register is made in Article 33. No application for restoration can be made before the end of the period of five years beginning with the date on which the striking off order was made.

LEGAL ASSESSORS

The Council is required to appoint legal assessors to advise the Screeners, the Practice Committees or the Registrar on questions of law, and to perform other functions which the Council confers on them by its rules. There are stipulations relating to who is eligible to be a legal assessor (Article 34).

MEDICAL ASSESSORS

Medical assessors are to be appointed by the Council to give advice to the same persons as the legal assessors, and there are similar provisions relating to eligibility or non-eligibility (Article 35).

REGISTRANT ASSESSORS

The Council may appoint these under Article 36. They have the general function of giving advice to the Council, the committees of the Council, Screeners or the Registrar on matters of professional practice arising in connection with any matter which the Registrar or any of the bodies is considering. They may also have other functions conferred on them by rules of Council. Conditions of eligibility for appointment as professional assessors are set.

APPEALS

Part VI of the Order lays down the rules which apply to the holding of appeals.

These cover appeals to the Council against a decision made by the Registrar and also appeals to court. The establishment of a Nursing and Midwifery Independent Tribunal which had been envisaged in the draft Order was deleted from the final Order.

A CASE OF ALLEGED MISCONDUCT

The following is an example of a case of alleged misconduct by a midwife appearing before the Professional Conduct Committee. (I am indebted to Reg Pyne, former Assistant Registrar for Standards and Ethics, UKCC, for this case.)

A 48-year-old woman appeared before the Professional Conduct Committee following an incident during the course of her professional work as a Registered Midwife some months earlier. She had come to midwifery at a mature age as a direct entrant (i.e. with no previous nursing qualification), but at the time of the incident had nine years' experience as a midwife.

She was employed as a Community Midwife in a large city, and had a student midwife attached (her first after three years without).

The charges she faced arose from allegations that she failed to urgently summon medical aid when there was evidence of likely distress, and failed to adequately supervise a student midwife (approximately two months into training).

The circumstances were as follows:

The Community Midwives used a Community/General Practitioner Unit for the deliveries for which they had a responsibility. It was located at a hospital, immediately next to and only divided by an unlocked door from the Consultant Obstetrics Unit. One night, at about 12.15am, the midwife had a call from the hospital to say that as 18-year-old woman had arrived at the Community Midwifery

Unit, and that she was one of that midwife's patients. The midwife immediately telephoned her new student (whom she had not met) and asked her to travel to the Unit. The midwife arrived at approximately 12.50am, five minutes before her student. She found that the patient was one who had made several local house moves in a short time, had never been found at home by the midwife when visiting, and had received no antenatal care. During the five minutes before the student arrived the midwife, with a little difficulty, located a fetal heart beat, which she did not record but subsequently described as 'soft but regular'. (The hospital midwife who had called her to this unexpected patient had checked when the patient arrived, and she had recorded the fetal heart as 'strong'.)

When the student arrived the midwife asked her to go through the required admission and examination procedures. One of her first actions was to take the patient's blood pressure, which she found to be significantly raised, especially the diastolic pressure. The student expressed concern at the finding which she recorded, but it was not checked, and she was told to continue with her examination. She could not find a fetal heart beat but was told that the midwife had done so, with difficulty. The student was asked if she had attached fetal scalp electrodes before, and replied that she had only watched the procedure being done. She was told to apply electrodes after completing a vaginal examination.

She tried her best to comply with the instruction, and eventually succeeded after some difficulty, the patient being in some distress and preferring to lie on her side. Some nine minutes after the scalp electrodes had been attached the student observed the recording was not being properly made, not least because the paper was 'burning' but her concern seemed not to be shared or understood. The midwife seemed content with the figures flashing on the visual recording. After a further slight delay, the student took it upon herself to go to seek aid at the Consultant Unit, whence she returned with a Midwifery Sister. The Sister immediately saw that the equipment was not properly set up, in that the paper roll was not aligned or mounted on the sprocket holes. She corrected this, and checked and corrected the attachment of the electrodes. Then, having observed the recording then showing, she said to the midwife: 'I would call for medical assistance urgently if I were you'. It was then approximately 1.25am.

The Sister departed, and the midwife told the student to continue and complete her admission procedures. These were eventually completed just before 1.45am, at which time the fetal heart recording was showing cause for real concern, and the blood pressure taken by the student indicated a further increase. Only then, with the admission/examination procedures complete in her view, did the midwife go to call the patient's General Practitioner by telephone. She found that his calls were redirected to a deputising service, to whom she then spoke. They said that the only doctor on duty with obstetric experience was engaged in another part of the city, and would not be free to leave there until about 2.10am, and would arrive at approximately 2.30am.

On her return to the ward where the patient was in the care of the student, the midwife found the situation deteriorating further. She telephoned the deputising service again, and they told her they would arrange a police escort to get the doctor there as quickly as possible.

Several minutes later (by now it was approximately 2.05am) there was a sudden prolapse of the cord. The student's immediate reaction was to apply pressure to the fetal head to prevent it constricting the cord. The midwife said that she left the student with the patient, went through the door to the Consultant Unit, and shouted 'prolapsed cord' very loudly, several times. The Sister who had visited earlier and her senior colleague rushed to the patient. They quickly assessed the situation, summoned 'hospital medical aid' (which was on call in the Unit), and moved the patient. Within minutes a Caesarean had been performed. Unfortunately the patient was delivered of a fresh male stillbirth.

The evidence to prove that the sequence of events had been as described came from the student, the Sister, a nursing officer and from the midwife herself. She denied the charges, though agreeing to the sequence of events. She insisted that they had done the right things in the right order, and that she had summoned medical aid as soon as the admission procedures were completed. The Committee found the facts proved, and considered them to constitute misconduct.

At the mitigation stage it emerged that there was considerable antipathy between the midwifery staff of the Consultant Unit and the community midwives who used the other Unit. The midwife's manager said that the midwife only rarely took the in-service training opportunities provided, and that she had required counselling on the subject of student supervision on a number of occasions, culminating in the removal of students for a significant period.

The Committee decided that the midwife should be removed from the Register.

Clearly, the Committee was not convinced that the public were safe if the midwife remained on the Register. Their concern was her total obsession with procedures and her indifference as to what was actually happening to the woman.

This case was heard before the Professional Conduct Committee, but it is also an example of a case which could result in several different hearings (it is not known whether in fact any of these other proceedings took place):

–   An action in the civil courts could be commenced by the parents. seeking to claim compensation for the death of the child.

–   The events could also lead to criminal proceedings if the Crown Prosecution Service took the view that the actions of the midwife amounted to gross negligence of criminal proportions.

- The midwife would also face disciplinary proceedings before the employer. Even if the employer were to allow her to keep her post, once she was removed from the Register she would be unable to practise as a midwife.

In the Annual Report of the UKCC for 1999/2000[2] it was reported that there was one appeal to the High Court following removal from the Register. A midwife was removed from the Register by the Professional Conduct Committee after having been found guilty on one charge of misconduct. The midwife had been employed on a night shift and the charge was that she failed to summon medical assistance when it was appropriate to do so. She challenged the decision on two grounds. The first was that there was insufficient evidence to support the charge. The High Court rejected this argument and maintained that although the Committee had heard conflicting evidence, it comprised professional people and experts in the field of midwifery who were able to assess the evidence. The second ground for appeal was that, in finding one charge not proven, the Committee had acted inconsistently in finding a second charge proven. The Court also rejected this argument, and stated that the particular charge required an intent to deceive and that the Committee was entitled to reject this charge if it considered that there was no such intent.

CONCLUSIONS

Major changes have taken place in the accountability of health professionals to their registration body. The Government's intention in the NHS Plan was to raise the standards of registered practitioners and ensure that the public were protected from those who were unworthy to be placed on, or remain on, the Register. The constitution and procedures for dealing with fitness to practice of the Health Professions Council are similar to the NMC and significant changes have taken place in the powers and procedures of the General Medical Council. There are however still considerable differences between the ways in which these registration bodies function, and there is every likelihood that as the new Councils establish themselves, they will lead to greater similarities in the state regulation of the conduct of all health professionals. This uniformity will be accelerated after the establishment of the Council for the Regulation of Health Care Professionals which is proposed in the NHS Reform and Health Care Professions Bill 2002. It will act as a central regulator for the health registration bodies.[3]

QUESTIONS AND EXERCISES

1. How would you define serious professional misconduct?

2. You are asked by a colleague who is facing professional conduct proceedings to

accompany her as a friend. Outline the stages which you would expect the hearing to follow and consider the types of evidence she would require to defend herself.

3. Evaluate the role of the Health Committee of the NMC. Do you think that there could be an overlap between the functions of the Health Committee and that of the Conduct and Competence Committee?

4. You have been fined for parking on double yellow lines whilst visiting a client in the course of your employment. To your horror, you discover that someone has reported this to the NMC. Outline the stages which will follow and the procedures which exist for each stage.

References

1 The Nursing and Midwifery Order 2001. SI 2002 No 253

2 UKCC. *Professional Conduct Annual Report 1999-2000.* London: UKCC

3 Dimond B. 2002. Law for Midwives Step by Step: Part 39 Health Professions Regulation. *British Journal of Midwifery,* 10(3)

Chapter 5

THE MIDWIVES RULES AND CODE OF PRACTICE, THE CODE OF PROFESSIONAL CONDUCT AND THE SCOPE OF PROFESSIONAL PRACTICE

The midwife is the only professional (other than the registered nurses under Part 9 (fever) of those registered by the UKCC to be subject to rules made specifically for her profession. The Midwives Rules have legal force and are binding upon the practitioner. In contrast, the Midwife's Code of Practice, The Scope of Professional Practice and the Guidelines for Professional Practice, like the other UKCC advisory papers, do not have the force of law, but failure to follow the codes could be used in evidence in proceedings for professional misconduct.

THE MIDWIVES RULES

The Rules cover education (Section A) and practice (Section B) and are referred to in relevant chapters of this book. They were revised in 1998[1] from the principal Rules approved in 1983 and revised in 1986.[2] Rule 40 sets out the responsibility of the midwife and her sphere of practice, and is shown in Box 5.1.

Box 5.1 Rule 40: A midwife's responsibility and sphere of practice

1. A practising midwife is responsible for providing midwifery care to a mother and baby during the antenatal, intranatal and postnatal periods.

2. Except in an emergency, a practising midwife shall not provide any midwifery care, or undertake any treatment which she has not, either before or after registration as a midwife, been trained to give or which is outside her current sphere of practice.

3. In an emergency, or where a deviation from the norm which is outside her

---

current sphere of practice becomes apparent in the mother or baby during the antenatal, intranatal or postnatal periods, a practising midwife shall call a registered medical practitioner or such other qualified health professional who may reasonably be expected to have the requisite skills and experience to assist her.

This will be considered in relation to The Scope of Professional Practice and the development of practice below.

THE MIDWIFE'S CODE OF PRACTICE

This sets out the Council's standards, other requirements and further information for the professional practice of each midwife. Paragraph 1 states

'As a practising midwife, you are accountable for your own practice in whatever environment you are practising. In all circumstances, the safety and welfare of the mother and her baby are of primary importance.'

The standard of practice required of the midwife is very close to that which would be applied by the civil courts in determining whether there had been negligence by a professional. (This is known as the Bolam Test and is discussed in Chapter 13.)

The Code was revised in 1998 and covers the areas shown in Box 5.2.

Box 5.2 Contents of the Midwife's Code of Practice

1. Definition and activities of a midwife

2. Matters directly related to the Midwives Rules

3. Other relevant legislation

4. Conclusion

5. Selected UKCC publications at December 1998

Reference is made in appropriate chapters to relevant paragraphs of the Code.

CODE OF PROFESSIONAL CONDUCT AND OTHER UKCC GUIDANCE AND ADVISORY PAPERS

Like all other registered practitioners, the midwife has also a duty to observe the Code of Professional Conduct and the other guidance issued by the UKCC and in due course the NMC. Whilst these do not have the force of law (i.e. breach of the Paragraphs does not automatically constitute an offence), a practitioner's failure to observe the guidance can be used in professional misconduct hearings.

THE SCOPE OF PROFESSIONAL PRACTICE

In June 1992 the UKCC published its position statement entitled The Scope of Professional Practice. This has had a profound influence on the development of professional practice. The development of professional practice is no longer to be seen as tasks delegated from doctors to practitioners. This concept of 'the extended role of the nurse' is no longer appropriate and what is required is a more dynamic situation. 'Practice must, therefore, be sensitive, relevant and responsive to the needs of individual patients and clients and have the capacity to adjust, where and when appropriate, to changing circumstances.'

Six principles are suggested to enable practice to develop safely and these are set out in Box 5.3.

Box 5.3 Principles for adjusting the scope of practice

The registered nurse, midwife or health visitor:

1. must be satisfied that each aspect of practice is directed to meeting the needs and serving the interests of the patient or client

2. must endeavour always to achieve, maintain and develop knowledge, skills and competence to respond to those needs and interests

3. must honestly acknowledge any limits of personal knowledge and skills and take steps to remedy any relevant deficits in order effectively and appropriately to meet the needs of patients and clients

4. must ensure that any enlargement or adjustment of the scope of personal professional practice must be achieved without compromising or fragmenting existing aspects of professional practice and care and that the requirements of the Council's Code of Professional Conduct are satisfied throughout the whole area of practice

▶

5. must recognise and honour the direct or indirect personal accountability borne for all aspects of professional practice, and

6. must, in serving the interests of patients and clients and the wider interests of society, avoid any inappropriate delegation to others which compromises those interests.

THE SCOPE OF PROFESSIONAL PRACTICE AND MIDWIFERY PRACTICE

The Scope of Professional Practice emphasises the paragraphs in the Midwife's Code of Practice which indicate that it is the individual midwife's responsibility to maintain and develop the competence which she has acquired during her training, recognising the sphere of practice in which she is deemed to be equipped to practise with safety and competence. It recognises that new skills may be required by some midwives because of the particular settings of their practice. Local policies which accord with the UKCC policies and standards will be important. The midwife must discuss with her supervisor the full scope of her practice where she practises outside the area of her employing authority or outside the NHS. The midwife must follow:

– the Midwife's Code of Practice

– the Code of Professional Conduct

– the principles of The Scope of Professional Practice.

The emphasis is clearly upon the personal accountability of the midwife in being responsible not only for her professional practice but also for her future development. There are obvious opportunities for the midwife in this approach. Whilst there has never been a concept of the 'expanded role of the midwife' in the sense that some of their activities are delegated from medical staff, midwifery practice has been defined by a notion of what was appropriate for an obstetrician rather than a midwife to perform. Any clear demarcation between the role of the midwife and the obstetrician is not necessarily now appropriate and the line to be drawn between the two will depend upon the experience, training skills and competence of the midwife. There may in fact be in law no specific activities which can only be performed by an obstetrician or paediatrician. The only limitations upon what the midwife can perform are where specific Acts of Parliament or regulations require certain functions to be performed by a named professional (other than the midwife). For example, the Abortion Act 1967 requires that a termination of pregnancy is carried out by a registered medical practitioner (see Chapter 26).

Provided the midwife has the training, knowledge, experience and skill to undertake new activities then she can develop in these new areas. The Scope of Professional Practice emphasises competency rather than certificates, though proof of educational training and development might still be evidenced in writing. The Government's acceptance of the Cumberlege recommendations should ensure that there is encouragement and acceptance for better use of the skills of the midwife.

The UKCC, in its publication in 1997[3] gave examples of how The Scope of Professional Practice was working. Those relating to midwifery practice included the development of a midwife-led unit in Suffolk when GPs were no longer able to provide cover. Three months' intensive preparation to develop confidence in the midwives preceded the opening of the unit. As a result, the women's choice in a rural area was maintained. In another example, a midwife in the Shetland Islands had learned the skill of ultrasound scanning.[4] She considered that women seemed to be more at ease with a midwife who was able to discuss all aspects of pregnancy. Other examples of expanded practice include midwives in Trowbridge,[5] Reading[6] and Bath[7] who have been trained in ventouse delivery through a course provided at Bournemouth University;[8] midwives who have been trained in examination of the newborn,[9] and see below for midwives acting as first assistant in theatre. The Family Planning Association has suggested that midwives could provide medical abortions.[10]

The midwife should however be aware of certain problems which she may confront in developing her practice. Those discussed here include:

– Definition of competence

– Protecting the employee who asserts her incompetence

– Resisting pressures of work

– Definition of job description.

DEFINITION OF COMPETENCE

Since the midwife is personally responsible for her own professional development she needs to have some bench mark to determine whether she has the appropriate competence to practice in a new field. Attendance of an approved course with assessment procedures may still be an important criterion for competence but it will be more difficult to assess competence in the workplace as new procedures, equipment and methods of work are introduced. The introduction of water births is one example where initially there were no clear standards or criteria for competence. The same problem confronts the employer who has the responsibility to ensure that his employees are competent, and the employer will be looking for criteria to determine the competence of new and existing employees to work in new fields of practice.

PROTECTION OF THE EMPLOYEE WHO ASSERTS HER INCOMPETENCE

If the midwife knows that she is being asked to work outside her field of competence she has a clear duty under the Rules, the Midwife's Code of Practice and The Code of Professional Conduct to make that known to her employers and to practise only within her sphere of competence. However, employees who are under pressure from other professionals or managers to work outside their sphere of competence must be protected. The midwife should make known both to her Supervisor of Midwives and also to her line manager, any unacceptable pressures upon her and potential dangers for the client. Unfortunately at present, whilst there is a legal requirement for the midwife to undertake a specific number of days of professional development to remain on the register, there is no statutory requirement for an employer to fund the cost of such professional development for a midwife, and there is inconsistency across the country over whether midwives obtain paid time off work and/or obtain the costs of any study days. Ultimately, it is the midwife's personal responsibility to ensure that she is competent and that she obtains the necessary training and supervised practice before moving into new areas.

RESISTING PRESSURES OF WORK

The employee whose scope of practice is enlarged must be protected from the dangers of lowering standards. Since the skill mix is changing and more non-registered employees are being employed in ratio to registered practitioners, new techniques and work methods will have to be devised to protect standards of practice and the patients from harm. However, the law makes illegal any delegation of the activity of attendance at childbirth to a non-midwife or non-doctor (see Chapter 25).

There are pressures on the midwife to work outside her competence, as the situation in Box 5.4 illustrates.

Box 5.4 Considerable pressure

When new laws were introduced making it illegal for the junior doctors to exceed 56 hours working per week, midwives found that they were expected to act as first assistants for an emergency Caesarean section. They asked the obstetricians if they could receive training for this role, but were told that midwives could not take on a surgical activity. What is the law?

There are clear dangers to patient safety in allowing the situation identified above to continue. Either acting as first assistant is recognised as an expanded role activity for midwives, who then receive the appropriate training, or sufficient doctors are employed to ensure that midwives would not have to take on that activity. A midwife would be entitled to refuse to act in a situation where she is not competent, unless in an emergency the risks of not acting outweighed the risks of acting. There are of course many examples of hospitals providing the training for midwives to act as first assistants in theatres. For example, the developments at the Gloucester Royal Hospital[11] enabled midwives to expand their roles to include suturing, episiotomies and perineal lacerations, assisting in theatre with Caesarean sections, and carrying out cardiotocographic interpretations, venesection and intravenous canulation.

PROTECTION OF THE EMPLOYEE

The government has recognised the need to protect staff from being victimised if they bring attention to the hazards at work. Following a consultation exercise on the Secretary of State's guidance on relations with the public and media, the NHS Management Executive issued guidance EL(93)51, published 8th June 1993. This guidance made it clear that:

'Under no circumstances are employees who express their views about health service issues in accordance with this guidance to be penalised in any way for doing so.' (Paragraph 6)

This guidance was followed by a circular bringing the Public Interest Disclosure Act 1998 to the attention of staff and requiring all NHS trusts to implement the Act.[12] All NHS employers have the responsibility for establishing a local procedure for staff to raise concerns with the management including the highest level of local management and ultimately with the Chairman of the authority or trust. Any member of staff who raises concerns is protected from victimisation. (See Chapter 22 and whistle-blowing.)

Many trusts now incorporate within their contracts of employment terms that registered practitioners should follow the professional guidance of their registration bodies as part of the contract of employment. Such terms should prevent a conflict between the duties required of a practitioner by their employer and by their professional registration body. This was a recommendation of the Report of the Inquiry into the Bristol Royal Infirmary children's heart surgery,[13] but was rejected by the Department of Health in respect of the contracts of medical practitioners.

DEFINITION OF JOB DESCRIPTION

The midwife must ensure that as her expected duties enlarge she has a clear agreement with the employer over what she is expected to undertake in relation to other staff, particularly medical staff. This is of particular importance in the development of midwife-managed units where there may not be 24-hour medical cover and where the midwife should identify the skills she requires in order to be able to care for the mother and baby appropriately. (This is further considered in Chapter 34.)

Areas of practice which not all midwives at present practice include:

- resuscitation of the new born

- suturing

- transfusion of blood

- IV administration of antibiotics and other medications not presently normally covered by the midwives' powers of prescribing and medication under Rule 41 (see Chapter 20)

- epidurals (midwives now top up epidurals in conjunction with medical staff but it may be that they can develop the skills for the complete administration of an epidural)

- forceps (this has been an activity normally carried out only by medical staff)

- vacuum extraction

- acting as first assistant in theatre (see Box 5.1 above)

- undertaking various complementary therapies such as acupuncture (see Chapter 34).

The suggestion was made in 1994 by Rupert Fawdry[14] that 'in ten years time, it may even be appropriate for 5-10 specially trained "obstetrician midwives" in each district to provide emergency and elective Caesarean section for mothers who need that particular method of delivery. The midwives could truly be called "practitioners in their own right", with the needs of women rather than any traditional role as the fundamental guide to their conduct.' At the present time there has been little progress in this direction and many midwives would not consider that this was the right direction in which to move.

All employers have the right in law to define the job description of the employee. The employee has an implied duty to obey the reasonable orders of the employer and to undertake all duties with all reasonable care and skill. What is 'reasonable' may lead to some discussions. For example, is it 'reasonable' to ask a midwife to work on the gynaecology wards when the midwifery unit is not busy? What is reasonable would depend upon the duration of that work, and the capacity in which the midwife is required to work. It would, for example, be unreasonable to ask a direct entry midwife to be a staff nurse, if she does not have the competence; it may be reasonable to ask the midwife to help out for an afternoon, in the appropriate capacity, but unreasonable to ask her to work there for three months which would deskill her as a midwife. 'Reasonableness' must therefore be defined in the context of what is lawful, what would be the recommendations of the professional registration body, and what would be within the job description of the midwife. Where instructions of the employer are unreasonable, then it would be lawful for the midwife to refuse to obey them.

Where the midwife is aware that a policy of the trust appears to conflict with the rights of clients/mothers, or with the regulations and guidance of the UKCC and its replacement the NMC, and with her own right to use her professional judgement, she should ensure that this is brought to the attention of her Supervisor of Midwives and the senior managers so that the dispute can be resolved before it gives rise to problems in practice. If necessary, the internal procedure set up under the Public Interest Disclosure Act 1998 could be used to ensure that she is not victimised as a result of bringing the concern to the attention of managers.

WATER BIRTHS

The development of skills in handling births in water can be used as an example of the application of the principles set out in The Scope of Professional Practice.

Much publicity was given in 1993 to the tragic deaths of two babies delivered in water, one in Sweden, the other in Bristol. The baby in Sweden died after being delivered with the help of two midwives, but not in a hospital.[15] In Bristol, a baby died after the mother spent part of the labour in a birthing pool at St Michael's hospital. A second baby was born with brain damage 18 months later. Professor Stirrat said that in both cases the children appear to have been deprived of oxygen: 'We think that something happened during the first stage of labour. We speculate that it might have been the temperature of the water. We think that the fetal temperature might have gone up, and that stressed the baby.'[16] As a result of the publicity given to these events, several trusts decided to inform their midwives that they should not participate in water births either in the community or in trust hospitals.

In Hertfordshire, two midwives were disciplined when they assisted in a home confinement when the mother refused to get out of the bath. The trust had a policy of allowing women to labour in water, but not to give birth in water.[17] One midwife received a final written warning which meant that she would be dismissed if she committed another transgression in the next two years, the other received a final written warning and was required to undergo three months' updating. The Chief Executive of the trust made it clear that:

– the technique of delivering in water is still not fully evaluated

– the contract between purchaser and provider does not include the provision of water births

– no staff are trained in water births

– the trust would have no defence if a medical catastrophe were to occur

– any patient wishing to have a water birth may book at other hospitals

– if evidence becomes available to confirm the safe and effective nature of the technique then the trust will revise its policies.

Research has now been conducted by the National Perinatal Epidemiology Unit in

Oxford, commissioned by the Department of Health, into the safety of water births. The survey was initiated in response to a recommendation of the Commons Select Committee that all hospitals should provide the pools where practicable.[18] In September 2000 a set of evidence-based practical guidelines for midwives on using water in labour and birth was prepared by Ethel Burns and Sheila Kitzinger[19] with the intention that they will be regularly updated. The guidelines are based upon advice from midwives experienced in using birth pools and upon a wide range of published studies and can be used in any care setting. Ethel Burns has also published an analysis of the data on the use of water births taken from 1,300 women and shows that water immersion can be a safe and satisfying choice for women in childbirth who have experienced an uncomplicated pregnancy.[20] Garland and Jones[21] showed, using a five-centre audit, how audit data was able to make a useful contribution to evidence-based practice.

Where there is a simple direction from the employer forbidding certain activities within the course of employment, several issues emerge from the point of view of The Scope of Professional Practice:

– How is the standard of care determined in a water birth case?

– How is competence on the part of the midwife determined?

– To what extent is the midwife bound to obey the policies of the trust?

HOW IS THE STANDARD OF CARE DETERMINED?

In Chapter 13, the Bolam Test is discussed. This is the test used by judges to determine the standard of care which can be expected of the defendant in a case.

'The standard of care expected is the standard of the ordinary skilled man exercising and professing to have that special skill.' [22]

Evidence would be given in court by experts as to the practice which they would have expected to see followed in the case of such a method of delivery and birth. Yet this is difficult in an area which is still the subject of research and innovation. Initially it may have been difficult to define a set standard. However, over the past years many centres have developed the use of birthing pools, and skills and standards have developed as seen above. Any midwife who wished to take part in water births must ensure that she kept up-to-date with recent developments and constantly improved her practice. In any dispute over the standard of care which should have been followed in a water birth, expert evidence would be given to the court by specialists over what standard the client could have expected according to the Bolam Test.

The Royal College of Midwives has recently published guidelines on water births.[23]

Increasingly, guidance and recommended practice from the National Institute for Clinical Excellence (NICE) will be referred to in defining standards of practice across most clinical areas. Their guidance will create a presumption that that advice should be followed, and the clinical practitioner will have to show reasonable grounds why the guidance did not apply for that particular patient (see Chapter 21 on NICE).

HOW IS COMPETENCE DETERMINED?

In a field which is constantly developing, it is very difficult for the midwife to pinpoint the moment at which she is competent to assist in a water birth delivery. Attendance at a recognised centre, with assessment, is obviously desirable. However, this is a field which shows clearly the value of the principles laid down by the UKCC in The Scope of Professional Practice.[24] The midwife has to check out her own competence by assisting at water births under the control of more experienced midwives, learning as much as she can from what has been written, and delivering her first water birth baby under supervision. As with all other skills it will need constant updating in the light of research findings.

OBEDIENCE TO THE POLICIES OF THE TRUST

It is hoped that policies of trusts relating to midwifery services and practice will comply with the NMC (formerly UKCC) guidance and with the policies established by the Local Supervising Authority (see Chapter 3) in conjunction with the Supervisor of Midwives. Where there is a clash then clearly the midwife must take the advice of her senior manager and supervisor. The midwife has a contractual duty to obey the reasonable instructions of her employer. It is not possible to say that there will never be a clash between the instructions of her employer and her Professional Code of Conduct. However, it is extremely unlikely. The midwife is bound by the Rules: the trust must accept that and many trusts now incorporate the UKCC Codes within the contracts of employment of their registered practitioners. The NHS Trust as the provider of services must ensure through its risk management policies that precautions are taken to prevent any possibility of claims through litigation. One way of safeguarding this is through ensuring that staff are trained and competent.

If, however, a trust is to attempt to define in detail what a midwife can and cannot do, it raises questions as to the midwife's professional clinical judgement and the role it plays in her contract of employment. Rule 40, on the definition of the responsibility and sphere of practice of the practising midwife, would appear to leave little scope for trusts to define what is or is not in the competence of the midwife.

HIGHER LEVEL AND ADVANCED MIDWIFERY PRACTICE

Initially, it was not the intention of the UKCC to include advanced midwifery practice in its standards for specialist practice as part of the post-registration education and practice proposals. The UKCC stated:

'The Council recognises that many practitioners will undertake additional studies in pursuit of advanced midwifery practice and such studies are likely to be at Masters level. The Council does not, however, at this stage, propose a formal preparation and qualification with explicit links with the Council's Register. Many midwives hope that this is only for the immediate short term and that eventually there will be formal recognition for the skills to be acquired through advanced midwifery practice by Council itself.' [25]

The UKCC considered that advanced practice was not about specific tasks but involves a broader concept of nursing, midwifery and health visiting, an important part of which is advancing the practice of others. In 1998 and 1999 the UKCC carried out a series of consultations about higher level practice and launched pilot studies. There was a general feeling amongst many midwives, reflected in RCM reports, that midwives already practised at a 'higher level'.[26] In 2000, the UKCC received a report on the possibility of measuring higher level practice,[27] which the Midwifery Committee of the UKCC felt was not entirely appropriate to midwifery practice. The UKCC found a survey of maternity service users supported the idea of higher level practice for midwives.[28]

The concept of advanced midwifery practice[29] is analysed by Maureen L Sookhoo and Margaret S Butler. The authors emphasise that advanced practice in midwifery is not synonymous with extending the role of the midwife, but about developing midwifery practice in order to enhance quality of care. They suggest from their study that advanced midwifery practice requires an expertise associated with skills and knowledge to enable the provision of holistic client-orientated care, and any programmes leading to advanced midwifery practitioner status should be client-centred as opposed to organisation-centred. Following their definition, it would appear that it should be part of the professional development of every midwife to secure advanced practice. Undoubtedly the new status of Consultant midwife is linked to the concept of advanced practice.

CONSULTANT MIDWIVES

One of the recommendations of Making A Difference,[30] a report from the Department of Health published in 1999 with the aim of improving recruitment, strengthening education, improving working lives and enhancing the quality of care, was that Consultant nurses and midwives should be appointed. The key features of the Consultant midwife as envisaged in the Making a Difference,[31] are shown in Box 5.5.

Box 5.5 Key features of the Consultant midwife

– Expert practice

– Professional leadership and consultancy

– Education and development

– Practice and service development linked to research and evaluation.

It is envisaged that Consultant midwives will spend at least 50% of their time on clinical work with career opportunities. NHS trusts are required to agree the posts with regional offices of the DoH. It is perhaps too early to determine the effectiveness of the role of the Consultant midwife and the likely impact of this role on advanced midwifery practice.

CONCLUSIONS

It is essential that midwifery should be a research-based profession (see Chapter 31). Water births are just one example of changing practices and techniques in childbirth with which the effects and implications of The Scope of Professional Practice can be seen.

The training and development of the midwife ventouse practitioner in community maternity units is considered by V Tinsley.[32] She emphasises that any expansion of the midwife's role cannot be undertaken lightly and considers the extensive preparation and training, supervised practice, clear protocols, on-going clinical audit and appropriate equipment which must be made available, together with support from management, GPs and obstetricians. This would apply to every other area of potential role expansion which midwives might consider.

In Chapter 6, we consider the conflict which can arise when the mother is requesting a home birth and the trust states that it does not have the resources to provide a home birth service, and the problems that this presents to the midwife. The UKCC guidance attempts to ensure that the mother's wishes are supported but it also recognises that the midwife has a contractual duty to obey the reasonable instructions of her employer.

QUESTIONS AND EXERCISES

1. Identify activities which you do not at present undertake as part of your role as a midwife and consider how you could develop the expertise to undertake those activities within the principles laid down by The Scope of Professional Practice.

2. What limits do you consider should be placed by Act of Parliament on the functions and role of the midwife?

3. Consider whether there are any potential conflicts between your job description and the policies relating to midwifery laid down by your employer.

4. Obtain a copy of the procedure set up by your employer as a result of the Public Interest Disclosure Act 1998 and analyse how it would apply in the event of your being aware of a major health and safety concern.

5. What role do you consider that the Consultant midwife plays, and what is its likely impact upon advanced midwifery practice?

References

1 Nurses, Midwives and Health Visitors (Midwives Amendment) Rules Approval Order. SI 1998 No 2649

2 Nurses, Midwives and Health Visitors Rules 1983 SI 1983 No 873 and Nurses, Midwives and Health Visitors (Amendment) Rules Approval Order 1986 SI 1986 No 786

3 UKCC 1997. *Scope in Practice*. London: UKCC

4 Proud J. 1997. *Understanding Obstetric Ultrasound*. 2nd edition. Oxford: Books for Midwives Press

5 Tinsley V. 1998. Ventouse extraction- a midwifery skill? *Changing Childbirth Update*, 11, 15

6 Hayes S. 1997. Ventouse deliveries by midwives. *MIDIRS Midwifery Digest*, 7(2), 197-200

7 Parslow L. 1997. Reflections on becoming a midwife ventouse practitioner. *Midwives*, 110(1314), 175-7

8 News item. 1998. Midwife ventouse practitioners. *Practising Midwife*, 1(12), 7

9 Lomax A. 2001. Expanding the midwife's role in examining the newborn. *British Journal of Midwifery*, 9(2), 100-2

10 News item. 2000. Midwives could provide medical abortions. *Practising Midwife*, 3(4), 6

11 Read M. 1998. Night vision. *Health Service Journal*, 108(5587), 24-5; Ramsay B, 1997. When midwives perform obstetric tasks at night, trainees can spend more supervised time in clinics. *BMJ*, 314(7096), 1830

12 *Health Service Circular* 1999/198

13 Bristol Royal Infirmary. 2001. *Learning from Bristol: the report of the public inquiry into children's heart surgery at the Bristol Royal Infirmary 1984-1995. Command Paper CM 5207*; www.bristol-inquiry.org.uk/

14 Fawdry R. 1994. Midwives and the care of 'normal' childbirth. *British Journal of Midwifery*, 2(7), 302-3

15 George N. 16 October 1993. *The Times*

16 Laurance J and Berrington L. 16 October 1993. *The Times*

17 Lewison H. 1994. *British Journal of Midwifery*, 2(4), 146-7

18 Royal College of Obstetricians and Gynaecologists. *Guidelines: birth under water*.

www.rcog.org.uk/guidelines/birthwater.html

19 Burns Eand Kitzinger S. 2000. *Midwifery guidelines for use of water in labour.* Oxford: Oxford Centres for Health Care Research and Development, Oxford Brookes University; www.sheilakitzinger.com/WaterBirth.htm

20 Burns E. 2001. Waterbirth. *MIDIRS Midwifery Digest,* 11(s2), s10-13

21 Garland D and Jones K. 2000. Waterbirths – supporting practice with clinical audit. *MIDIRS Midwifery Digest,* 10(3), 333-6

22 Bolam v. Friern Hospital Management Committee QBD [1957] 2 All ER 118

23 Royal College of Midwives. 2000. The use of water in labour and birth: Position Paper 1a. *RCM Midwives Journal,* 3(12), 374-5

24 UKCC. 1992. *The Scope of Professional Practice.* London: UKCC

25 UKCC 1997. *Registrar's Letter: The Council's decision on PREP and advanced practice.* London: UKCC

26 Royal College of Midwives. 1999. *Midwives already practice at a higher level;* Anderson T. 1999. Higher Level Midwives- who needs them? *Practising Midwife,* 2(3), 4-5

27 UKCC. 2001. *Future work on a higher level of practice to be part of the wider post-registration framework: UKCC Council Report.* London: UKCC

28 UKCC. 2000. *Users of midwifery services support the idea of higher level practice for midwives.* London: UKCC

29 Sookhoo ML and Butler MS. 1999. An analysis of the concept of advanced midwifery practice. *British Journal of Midwifery,* 7(11)

30 Department of Health. 1999. *Making A Difference: strengthening the nursing, midwifery and health visiting contribution to healthcare.* London: HMSO

31 Department of Health. 1999. *Making a Difference: The new NHS.* London: HMSO

32 Tinsley V. 2001. Rethinking the role of the midwife. MIDIRS Midwifery Digest, 11(s2), s6-9

CLIENT RIGHTS

This Section considers the legal issues relating to a woman and her legal rights in childbirth. It begins by considering the implications of the Human Rights Act 1998 and then looks at the changing background to the provision of maternity services and the legal implications of this. Specific topics such as the right to give consent, confidentiality, access, and the rights of the fetus are considered in subsequent chapters in this section.

Chapter 6
WOMAN-CENTRED CARE
THE HUMAN RIGHTS ACT 1998

Following the Second World War, this country, together with many other European countries, was a signatory to the European Convention on Human Rights. People who considered that their rights had been infringed could take a case to the European Court of Human Rights which was based in Strasbourg. (This is entirely separate from the European Economic Community which has its European Court of Justice in Luxembourg.) In 1998 the Human Rights Act was passed. This was brought into force for England and Wales on 2 October 2000 and for Scotland on devolution. Its main effect was to place a duty upon public authorities and those organisations exercising functions of a public nature to implement the articles of the Convention. In addition, those people who considered that their rights as set out in the European Convention on Human Rights had been infringed could take public authorities to court in this country, instead of going to Strasbourg. These Articles are set out in Schedule 1 to the Act and can be found in Appendix 1 of this book.

Articles 2, 3, 5, 6, 8, 9,10 and 14 are likely to be of particular concern to midwifery practice.

ARTICLE 2

Everyone's right to life shall be protected by law. No one shall be deprived of his life intentionally save in the execution of a sentence of a court following his conviction of a crime for which this penalty is provided by law.

Recent decisions of the courts show how this right is interpreted. For example in a recent case,[1] parents lost their attempt to ensure that a severely handicapped baby born prematurely was resuscitated if necessary. The judge ruled that the hospital should provide him with palliative care to ease his suffering, but should not try to revive him as that would cause unnecessary pain. (The case is considered in Chapter 9.)

In another case, the President of the Family Division, Dame Elizabeth Butler-Sloss, held that withdrawal of life-sustaining medical treatment was not contrary to Article 2 of the Human Rights Convention and the right to life, where the patient was in a persistent vegetative state. The ruling was made on 25th October 2000 in cases involving Mrs M, 49, who suffered brain damage during an operation abroad in 1997 and was diagnosed as being in a persistent vegetative state (PVS) in October 1998 and Mrs H, 36, who fell ill in America as a result of pancreatitis at Christmas 1999.[2]

Article 2 was also invoked in the case involving the separation of Siamese twins, in which the Court of Appeal decided on 22nd September 2000 that they could be separated even though this would undoubtedly lead to the death of the one who depended upon the heart and the lungs of the other. The Court of Appeal defended its decision on the grounds that the baby who had a chance of survival was having its lifeblood drained away by the other who had no chance of survival if she were to be separated, and therefore doctors were acting on behalf of that one in self-defence. Acting in self-defence can be a justification for depriving another of the right to life. The parents, who had refused to give consent to the operation of separation, decided against appealing to the House of Lords. At the inquest a unique finding of death was made, the coroner resorting to a 'narrative verdict':

'Mary died after surgery to separate her from her conjoined twin, and that the surgery was permitted by order of the High Court, confirmed by the Court of Appeal'.[3]

There could be more cases heard where patients and relatives urge the courts to accept that there has been an infringement of Article 2 of the European Convention of Human Rights. For example, it may be used if a person is marked down as Not for Resuscitation (NFR) and the relatives disagree with the clinicians. In addition, the Article may also be relied upon where a patient alleges that failure to provide health services is infringing her right to life. It seems unlikely that judges will wish to give it this dimension.

In the case where a woman suffering the terminal stages of motor neurone disease applied to the High Court for a declaration that it would be lawful for her husband to assist her in ending her life,[4] the High Court held that Articles 2 and 3 of the European Convention on Human Rights did not protect the right to procure one's own death or confer a right to die. The right to the dignity of life was not a right to die with dignity but the right to live with as much dignity as could possibly be afforded until that life reached its natural end (see also Chapter 9).

The High Court held that the Director of Public Prosecutions had no power under the Suicide Act to give an undertaking not to consent to the prosecution of a person for aiding and abetting, counselling or procuring of a suicide of another, where the acts which might constitute such an offence had not yet occurred or been investigated. The House of Lords dismissed Diane Pretty's appeal holding that there was no conflict between the Articles of the European Convention of Human Rights and Section 2(1) of the Suicide Act 1961 which made it a criminal offence to aid and abet a suicide.

ARTICLE 3

No one shall be subjected to torture or to inhuman or degrading treatment or punishment.

Whilst it is hoped that torture does not take place in healthcare, there are evident examples of degrading and inhuman treatment. Most midwives would probably agree that a recent case where a pregnant prisoner was handcuffed to the bed during her labour would appear to be a prima facie breach of this right (see below). The European Court of Human Rights has ruled that corporal punishment by parents to discipline their children was a breach of Article 3 of the European Convention on Human Rights.[5] A step-father had on several occasions beaten a 9-year-old boy with a garden cane. The step-father had been prosecuted for assault occasioning actual bodily harm, but had been acquitted by the jury who accepted his defence that the caning had been necessary and reasonable to discipline the boy. The European Court of Human Rights held that ill-treatment must attain a minimum level of severity if it is to fall within the scope of Article 3. It depended on all the circumstances of the case, such as the nature and context of the treatment, its duration, its physical and mental effects and in some instances, the sex, age, and state of health of the victim. In finding that there had been a breach of Article 3 the court awarded the boy £10,000 against the UK government, and costs. The UK government acknowledged that UK law failed to provide adequate protection to children and should be amended. Subsequently, guidance was issued by the government on the use of corporal punishment against children. Midwives should analyse their practice and the way in which the mothers are treated right through antenatal, intrapartum and postnatal care and decide if there are grounds for believing that this Article is not respected. Action should then be taken to remedy the situation in order to prevent possible litigation.

ARTICLE 3 AND WOMEN PRISONERS

It was reported in 1994[6] that a prisoner who was transferred to Wythenshawe hospital for the delivery of her child was handcuffed during the confinement.[7] It appeared that she had absconded three times before and therefore staff kept her handcuffed at all times including during the birth.

A prison service spokesman stated that guidelines had been issued to cover such a situation and the Director General of the Prison Service, at that time Derek Lewis, issued an official apology to the mother. The RCM welcomed the apology given by the Director General of the Prison Service to Susan Edwards who had been moved from Styal prison to Wythenshawe hospital for the delivery.[8] Hansard reported that a letter from the Director General read out in Parliament confirmed that

'Handcuffs must be removed in any case if the doctor treating the patient so requests.'

It might have been thought that with these promises of new guidelines and apologies, a situation of handcuffing a woman during labour would not recur. Yet in 1996 it was reported that Annette Walker was taken from Holloway prison to the Whittington Hospital in handcuffs, where she spent 10 hours in labour chained to a bed, in the presence of a male and a female officer.[10] Ann Widdecombe, the Home Office Minister, defended the action initially, saying that Whittington Hospital had not been concerned about the handcuffing of women prisoners while in labour at their hospital. However she subsequently apologised for this inaccurate statement.[11] It was later reported that the Home Office, following discussions with the RCM, was dropping the policy of keeping pregnant women in handcuffs during labour and delivery.[12] Subsequently, supported by AIMS, Annette Walker sued the prison service and accepted £19,000 compensation.[13] For further information on mothers in prison see article by Christine Cading-Paull.[14] Sally Price and Helen Ridge also consider the implications for pregnant women in prison.[15]

Yet shackling of pregnant women continued: Theresa McDonagh, a pregnant woman, was shackled to a radiator for five hours when she appeared in court on a £27 theft charge.[16] Many individuals and organisations have fought valiantly to ensure that the rules are changed: Sheila Kitzinger and the National Childbirth Trust, Beverley Beech and AIMS, the Maternity Alliance, the Royal College of Midwives, and the Howard League for Penal Reform to name only a few. Their campaigning has ensured that such gross breaches of human rights are brought to public attention and promises secured over improvements.

ARTICLE 5

Everyone has the right to liberty and security of person. No one shall be deprived of his liberty save in the following cases and in accordance with a procedure prescribed by law.

Many exceptions are then given, including:

(f) the lawful detention of persons for the prevention of the spreading of infectious diseases, or persons of unsound mind, alcoholics or drug addicts or vagrants.

It could be argued that the House of Lords decision in the Bournewood[17] case, which held that a person who lacked the mental capacity to consent to admission to psychiatric hospital could be detained there in his best interests without being detained under the Mental Health Act 1983, was in breach of this Article. Although such detention is justified under common law (i.e. judge-made law), the common law, unlike the Mental Health Act 1983, does not lay down a procedure for such detention. Such persons are at present outside the jurisdiction of the Mental Health Act Commission, and there are no provisions for bringing in a second doctor to provide an opinion on treatment. There are considerable differences between the legal position of these people and those who are detained under the Mental Health Act. Legislation is awaited on both decision-making on behalf of mentally incapacitated adults (see Chapter 7) and also on a new Mental Health Act which is considered in Chapter 33. The Court of Appeal has held that in the absence of statutory provision for mentally incapacitated adults, the court did have an inherent power to hear issues involved in the day-to-day care of such persons and to grant declarations in the best interests of mentally incapable persons.[18]

ARTICLE 6: THE RIGHT TO A FAIR TRIAL

This right will have significant implications since it applies not just to criminal charges but also to the determination of civil rights and obligations. It would therefore apply to disciplinary actions and other such forums, where at present employees may not have representation and they may be in a very weak situation compared with the employer. A challenge that the proceedings of the UKCC failed to comply with Article 6[19] led to the UKCC reviewing its procedures.[20] The arrangements for the new Nursing and Midwifery Council have taken account of the provisions of the Human Rights Act 1998 by establishing an appeal process to a Nursing and Midwifery Independent Appeals Tribunal (Articles 35-37). This is considered in Chapter 4.

ARTICLE 8

1. Everyone has the right to respect for private and family life, his home and his correspondence.

2. There shall be no interference by a public authority with the exercise of the right except such as is in accordance with the law and is necessary in a democratic society in the interests of national security, public safety or the economic wellbeing of the country, for the prevention of disorder or crime, for the protection of health or morals, or for the protection of the rights and freedoms of others.

This right will require greater sensitivity about patient privacy than has been shown in the past within healthcare. The traditional ward round, where a curtain is seen as a sound-proof barrier but in fact all those on the ward can hear the intimate details of a patient's diagnosis, prognosis and treatment, will have to be reviewed. Many other actions may have to be taken in order to ensure that this right of the patient is recognised and protected. The Caldicott Guardians, whose role is considered in Chapter 10, will have to take on the responsibility for ensuring that there is no breach of Article 8.

The respect for family life did not enable a prisoner to obtain artificial insemination[21] and it was held that high security restrictions on child visits were valid and not a breach of Article 8.[22] In contrast, a woman in Holloway prison won her appeal against the decision that her baby would be taken away from her at birth.[23] This was held to be a breach of Article 8 of the Human Rights Convention and the United Nations Convention on the Rights of the Child. Article 8 of the European Convention could be interpreted as giving a baby a right to be breast-fed if the mother so wished, and of continuing contact with the mother, irrespective of her being in custody. In contrast, the High Court has ruled in two cases (brought by P and by Q) that the policy of the prison service that children should cease to live with their mothers in prison at 18 months old was lawful and not contrary to Article 8.[24] Article 8 gave a right to respect for family life and the qualifications contained in Article 8.2 were in play by reason of the legality, recognised by Article 5, of the prisoner's imprisonment. The Court of Appeal held[25] that the prison service was entitled to have a policy that children aged 18 months should cease to stay with their mothers in prison, but such a policy should not be operated rigidly. The reasons for the need for flexibility were firstly the aim of promoting the welfare of the child (which had to be related to the circumstances of the prison) and secondly the interference with the child's family life had to be justified under Article 8.2 of the Human Rights Convention. The Court dismissed the appeal of P but allowed the appeal of Q.

A patient at Ashworth High Security Hospital lost his application for judicial review on the grounds that the provisions relating to the discretionary power of the Special Hospitals to record and listen to a random 10% of telephone calls infringed his right to respect for privacy under Article 8. The court held that the recording was a justified infringement of Article 8 since it was a proportionate measure and necessary to achieve security for high risk patients.[26]

Article 8 has to be interpreted in relation to Article 10 which recognises a right to freedom of expression. Both Articles 8 and 10 are qualified by specified circumstances in which the right is limited, and the courts will balance one against the other in determining whether there has been a breach of either Article.

OTHER SIGNIFICANT ARTICLES

Whilst these Articles have been looked at in detail there are others which have considerable significance for healthcare. Article 14, for example, prohibits discrimination and this is considered in Chapter 22 on employment. Article 2 of the First Protocol recognises a right to education, which may be significant for staff who are caring for children with long-term illnesses. Parents also have the right to ensure that such education and teaching is in conformity with their own religious and philosophical convictions.

THE DATA PROTECTION ACT 1998
AND THE FREEDOM OF INFORMATION ACT 2000

This legislation also recognises many rights of the patient in the protection of confidential information and in the right of access to information held by public authorities. The Data Protection Act is considered in Chapter 10 and the Freedom of Information Act is considered in the next chapter.

STATUTORY DUTY TO PROVIDE MATERNITY SERVICES

In Chapter 21 the statutory authorities within the NHS are considered, along with the duty placed upon the Secretary of State to provide services for expectant and nursing mothers and young children 'as he considers are appropriate as part of the health service'. Whilst this is not an absolute duty, it is impossible to have a waiting list in maternity care: nature does not wait. Therefore minimum standards for antenatal, intrapartum and postnatal care must be provided. In other fields of healthcare court actions against the Secretary of State for the provision of services have usually failed. Thus patients who had been waiting several years for hip replacement operations in the West Midlands failed in their action against the Secretary of State[27] and a mother who was concerned at the delay in providing her child with heart surgery lost her case.[28] The court held that it was not for the court to substitute its own judgement for that of those responsible for the allocation of resources. It would only interfere if there had been a failure to allocate funds in a way which was reasonable or where there had been breaches of public duties. The same principle was followed in the much-publicised case of Jamie Bowen, a 10-year-old girl who suffered from leukaemia. She needed another course of chemotherapy and a bone marrow transplant, after the first one failed. The Health Authority took medical advice that there was a very low chance of success and therefore would not allocate the funds for this additional treatment. Her father brought a court action and the High Court judge suggested that the Health Authority should review its decision. The Court of Appeal upheld the decision of the Health Authority.[29] The Court of Appeal were unable to fault the process of reasoning of the Health Authority and allowed its appeal. The Master of the Rolls (Sir Thomas Bingham) stated:

'while I have every sympathy with B, I feel bound to regard this as an attempt – wholly understandable, but nevertheless misguided – to involve the court in a field of activity where it is not fitted to make any decision favourable to the patient'.

An anonymous donor then came forward and paid for further treatment for the child, but she died a year later.

There have, however, been some recent cases which suggest that the court may be taking a more interventionalist role. Thus, where a Health Authority had a blanket policy not to fund transsexual operations, the court held that any policy of funding by a health authority must have genuine regard for the clinical needs of the individual and recognise the possibility of exceptional circumstances.[30] The court did not, however, consider that there had been a breach of Articles 3 or 8 of the European Convention. In a second case, the court held that failure by a Health Authority to permit the prescribing of Beta Interferon for multiple sclerosis patients in its area, was not in accordance with guidance issued by the Department of Health.[31] A declaration was granted that the policy adopted by the Health Authority was unlawful and an 'order of mandamus' was made, requiring the defendants to formulate and implement a policy which took full and proper account of national policy as stated in the circular.

Failure by an NHS trust or Health Authority to provide reasonable services for the care of pregnant women, mothers and babies could therefore lead to action against the Authority and the Secretary of State for breach of a statutory duty. Such a case may be supported by an allegation of failure to comply with the Articles of Human Rights (especially Articles 2 and 3 – see above). It does not follow, however, that a woman would be successful in suing for failure to provide a specific form of care, such as a water birth. There is built into the statutory provisions a discretion over the services to be provided. Once the National Service Framework in child and maternity services is published, then women will be able to bring a complaint if their local services fall below the minimum outlined in these standards. (See Chapter 21.)

MATERNITY SERVICES DEVELOPMENTS AND STANDARDS

The Health Committee of the House of Commons reported on Maternity Services in February 1992.[32] Its main recommendations are shown in Box 6.1. These are culled from nine pages of recommendations and it is difficult to give credit to the wide-ranging and comprehensive scope of the report in this short account.

Box 6.1 Main recommendations of the House of Commons report

- The relationship between the woman and the care-givers is recognised as being of fundamental importance.

- Schemes should be set up enabling women to get to know one or two health professionals during pregnancy who will be with them during labour and delivery whether at home or in hospital, and who will continue the care of the mother and baby after birth.

- The majority of maternity care should be community based and near to the woman's home, and obstetric and other specialist care should be readily available by referral from midwives or GPs.

- Those GPs who wish to provide a continuum of care throughout pregnancy, labour and the puerperium should be able to do so; and their training should equip them to do so.

- Women needing intensive obstetric care within the NHS should also be able to enjoy continuity of care and carer, so far as is possible.

▶

▶

– Within a hospital women should be able to exercise choice as to the personnel who will be responsible for their care.

– The woman having a baby should be seen as the focus of care; and professionals providing that care should identify their needs and develop arrangements to meet them which are based on full and equal co-operation between all those charged with her care.

– Proper attention should be paid to the needs of the baby, with particular regard to skilled resuscitation at birth, examination for abnormalities, and the encouragement of breastfeeding.

The Secretary of State responded by setting up an expert panel under the chairmanship of Baroness Cumberlege to consider the recommendations and make proposals for implementation.[33] A consensus conference was held in March 1993, arranged by the King's Fund Centre for the Department of Health. Following the consensus conference a statement drawn up by an independent panel was submitted as evidence to the Expert Committee on Maternity Services.[34]

Changing Childbirth, the report of the expert committee, was published in August 1993[35] The recommendations are given under four main headings:

– Woman-centred care

– Professional support

– Accessible maternity services

– Effective and efficient services.

Box 6.2 shows the indicators of success as set out in Chapter 5 of the Cumberlege recommendations.

Box 6.2 Indicators of success

Within five years:

1 All women should be entitled to carry their own notes.

2 Every woman should know one midwife who ensures continuity of her midwifery care – the named midwife.

3 At least 30% of women should have the midwife as the lead professional

▶

4 Every woman should know the lead professional who has a key role in the planning and provision of her care.

5 At least 75% of women should know the person who cares for them during their delivery.

6 Midwives should have direct access to some beds in all maternity units.

7 At least 30% of women delivered in a maternity unit should be admitted under the management of the midwife.

8 The total number of antenatal visits for women with uncomplicated pregnancies should have been reviewed in the light of the available evidence and the RCOG guidelines.

9 All front-line ambulances should have a paramedic able to support the midwife who needs to transfer a woman to hospital in an emergency.

10 All women should have access to information about the services available in their locality.

The government responded warmly to the report of the expert advisory committee and NHS authorities were required to review maternity services in the light of the report's recommendations and develop a strategy for implementing these within the resources available.

The NHS Management Executive (EL(94)9) instructed NHS authorities to reflect the Expert Maternity Group's recommendations in NHS contracts for 1995-96. The guidance required purchasers to draw up implementation plans for Changing Childbirth and ensure that its recommendations were reflected in both their 3-5 year purchasing strategy and their 1995/6 purchasing plans. Purchasers were also requested to set a date by which they expected to be able to offer a Changing Childbirth service, as defined in Annex A of the circular. Regional strategies were also to be prepared. An advisory group was established to support the NHS in implementing Changing Childbirth. A Patient's Charter leaflet was to be issued to set out what the current Patient's Charter rights and standards mean for pregnant women.

RECENT INITIATIVES

The NHS Plan[36] envisages major changes and initiatives in the NHS including maternity services. In addition, following the NHS White Paper[37] and the Health Act 1999, the National Institute for Clinical Excellence and the Commission for Health

Improvement have been established. These organisations and their significance are considered in Chapter 21. A National Service Framework for maternity and child health is, at the time of writing, awaited. In the meantime, an All-Party Parliamentary Group on Maternity has been set up, chaired by Julia Brown MP,[38] which is discussed in Chapter 21. A Maternity and Neonatal Workforce Group (MNWG) has been set up under the Chairmanship of Dr Sheila Adam, the Deputy Chief Medical Officer of Health. Increasingly therefore over future years, there will be greater emphasis on nationally set standards for maternity provision based on researched evidence. In addition, the NHS Plan places greater emphasis on the involvement and representation of the patient in healthcare. This may also have a major impact upon the running of midwifery and obstetric departments.

THE PATIENT'S CHARTER AND MATERNITY SERVICES

As part of the Patient's Charter initiative, the government's Citizen's Charter Unit published a leaflet explaining the special standards for maternity services. This set out the following rights:

- To be told the name of the midwife who will be responsible for the care

- To have the opportunity to see a Consultant obstetrician at least once during the pregnancy

- To have the opportunity to see a Consultant paediatrician if the obstetrician anticipates problems with the baby

- To have a right to see the maternity records and have the confidentiality respected

- To be given information on local maternity services

- To have an appointment system for antenatal clinics and to be seen within 30 minutes of the time fixed

- To have the choice of whether a partner or other friend or relative should be present during the confinement

- To have the baby identified for security reasons

- To have information on feeding the baby

- To have respect for privacy, dignity, religious and cultural beliefs

- To be able to have visitors at all reasonable times

- To have access to hospital and community services according to any special needs.

These rights are not legally enforceable by the individual client, unless there are separate rights recognised by statute or by the common law. Thus, as will be seen in

Chapter 10, the mother has a statutory right of access to her health records unless certain exemption conditions exist. Similarly, if the baby requires specialist input from a paediatrician and the GP, midwife or obstetrician fails to refer the baby to a paediatrician and the baby suffers harm as a result then there would be a breach of the duty recognised by the common law to take care of the client.

Where, however, such legal rights do not already exist to support those standards identified in the Charter, the only remedy for the client is to use the complaints system (see Chapter 11) and bring to the attention of the trust or Health Authority failures in the standards prescribed by the Charter. For example, the Charter standard for waiting in an antenatal clinic is a maximum of 30 minutes after the appointment time. If a woman waits two hours for her examination, she has the right to complain, but it is unlikely that she can enforce this standard personally through action in the courts. The NHS Plan envisages that a new Citizen's Charter is to be published.

DEVELOPMENT OF MATERNITY SERVICES

In May 2001[39] the Government announced that £100 million was being made available to transform maternity services: an extra 2,000 midwives would be appointed by 2005 (former midwives would be offered £1,500 to help them through a retraining period and also help with childcare worth up to £150 per week); there would be a wholesale refurbishment of maternity wards so that they became a home away from home, rather than a clinical environment and there would be greater freedom for women to choose a home birth. A further allocation of £100 million was made in October 2001[40] (see Chapter 21). It was anticipated that the National Service Framework (NSF) being prepared for child and maternity services (see above) will set out how the target of ensuring that every woman will have access to a dedicated midwife when in established labour 100% of the time can be achieved. This target was described as the 'gold standard'. In June 2001[41] the Department of Health gave further details of these plans, including improving facilities for fathers and for bereaved parents in maternity units. It is intended that women who lose their babies are not placed in postnatal wards with new mothers.

THE RIGHT TO A HOME BIRTH

As an example of the weakness of rights which are legally enforceable in the area of midwifery and child care we will take the example of a woman who wishes to have a home birth. It is clear that government policy as set out in the Cumberlege Report and in the NHS Plan favours the right of patient decision-making and maximum involvement of the patient in the care they obtain. If, however, a woman was to request that she had a home birth, it appears that there are considerable pressures against her. The report of the National Birthday Trust confidential enquiry in 1994 showed that there was considerable anecdotal evidence that GPs refused to allow women to book for home birth. Other evidence showed that some women have been struck off the GP practice for insisting on home birth.[42] Obstacles are placed in the way of a home birth. It takes a very assertive and strong woman to overcome these obstacles and insist upon a home confinement. The National Birthday Trust Report[43] quoted earlier showed that 'women booking home births were of a higher social class, had continued in education for longer and were more likely to breastfeed.' The vast majority of women would probably be defeated by the first refusal and accept hospital confinement even if the stay is only a few hours.

There is evidence that the average uncomplicated vaginal birth costs 68% less in a home than in a hospital.[44] There is also some evidence that, following careful selection for home birth, the risks are lower.[45] It will be noted from the discussion above that the courts in the past have been reluctant to become involved in decisions against the Secretary of State where resource issues arise. If a woman were to bring a court action against the trust to compel provision for a home birth the court may be reluctant to issue an order for specific performance requiring arrangements to be made for her home confinement, since there is a general reluctance for the court to order persons to carry out particular activities when the court cannot itself supervise them. However, payment of compensation may be seen as an alternative for not having a home birth. In theory, there may well be a legal right for the woman to insist upon a home confinement, if she can show that it is in her best interests and that the resource implications benefit the NHS, but in practice it may be very difficult for her to secure this.

Many organisations have worked strenuously to support the woman's right to have a home birth, if clinical conditions permit. The National Childbirth Trust, the Association for the Improvement in Maternity Services, the Association of Radical Midwives, the Association of Community Based Maternity Care and the International Home Birth Movement have all promoted the provision of information to women so that they have clear choices over the place of birth. Seven years have passed since the publication of Changing Childbirth and there is little evidence that the situation for women has significantly altered.

The UKCC published a position statement on supporting women who wish to have a home birth[46] and updated this on 31st August 2001.[47] This clarified the situation where an employer says that it is unable to provide a planned home birth service, because there are insufficient midwives available to support both the hospital and the home birth services. The UKCC stated its position as follows:

'It is the Council's expectation that a practising midwife will be competent to provide midwifery care in any setting and that women who wish to have their baby at home can be supported to achieve this by a midwife who is able to practise within the home environment. The Council supports women having choice in the method and place of birth... While the employed midwife has a contractual duty to her employer, she also has a professional duty *to provide midwifery care for women and would not wish to leave a woman in labour at home unattended, thus placing her at risk at a time when competent midwifery care is essential.'*

The UKCC noted that across the four countries of the UK there is no statutory duty to provide any specific aspect of the maternity services. It also recognises that an employed midwife has a primary contractual duty to carry out the wishes of her employer, although the employer would not expect an employee to do anything illegal, including anything which contravenes the Midwives Rules. It states:

'A midwife would not be in breach of her professional duty if unable to attend a woman requesting a home birth by reason of her employer's decision not to provide such a service. In an emergency situation, the midwife has a professional responsibility to provide midwifery care to the best of her ability.'

The UKCC emphasises that a midwife should not refuse to continue to provide care for woman on the basis of where the woman intends the birth to take place.

The midwife must ensure that her supervisor is brought in if there are such difficulties.

'The Supervisor of Midwives must be mindful of the woman's right to choose and so has a key role to play in providing professional support for the midwife.'

In the future, the National Institute for Clinical Excellence may publish recommendations on research-based practice and the clinical effectiveness of home confinements. The establishment of primary healthcare trusts may assist women in having a real choice and may encourage home confinements. However, to secure these changes general practitioners will have to become convinced that home births are, where clinically possible, the preferred option, and midwives will have to have the confidence that they will not be penalised as a result of supporting the woman's choice.

THE RIGHT TO A CAESAREAN

Of considerable controversy at the time of writing is whether a woman has a right to insist on having a Caesarean even when there are no clinical grounds to support such a decision. Almost 1 in 4 births are now by Caesarean section and this increase is due partly to the result of increasingly defensive practice by obstetricians but also because of pressure from women. The author has argued that there is no legal right for a patient to demand care when there is no clinical justification.[48] However, a midwife may come across a situation where a Consultant, although he or she does not personally see a clinical need for a Caesarean section to take place, is prepared to support the woman's request. In such circumstances the midwife has no alternative other than to provide the woman with all the appropriate care which she would have if the Caesarean was clinically indicated.

A warning about the dangers of believing too easily that the figures showing an increase in the rate of caesarean sections result from pressure of patients' choice is given by Tricia Anderson.[49] Anderson comments on an article[50] which suggested that maternal choice accounts for 49% of the decision-making process when deciding whether to opt for an elective Caesarean section. She warns of the danger of obstetricians creating a view that Caesarean section is best and urges the importance of women being given full information about the risks inherent in a Caesarean section. She sees the increase in the rate of Caesarean section as the result of 30 years of hospitalised, medicalised birth as recommended in the Peel Report of 1970.[51]

A National Sentinel Caesarean Section Audit was carried out by the RCOG, the RCM, the Royal College of Anaesthetists and the National Childbirth Trust funded by the Department of Health through NICE.[52] The results were presented at a launch meeting in October 2001[53] and showed that the Caesarean section rate overall in England was 21% and 24% in Wales and Northern Ireland. (This compares with the 10-15% range recommended by the World Health Organisation in its consensus statement in 1985.[54]) The Sentinel Report was discussed by the All-Party Parliamentary Group on Maternity on 6th November, 2001 and a conference was held in January 2002. The NICE guidelines on Caesarean section are to be published in 2002.

CONCLUSIONS

In this chapter we have looked at the rights set out in the European Convention of Human Rights, the statutory duty to provide maternity services, the Cumberlege Report and changes in the establishing of standards within the NHS, including clinical governance, CHI, NICE and the National Standards Frameworks. The Cumberlege Report concluded that the mother should have a major role in the determination of the care she receives. The House of Commons Report (Paragraph 52) stated:

'We conclude that there is a widespread demand among women for greater choice in the type of maternity care they receive; and that the present structure of the maternity services frustrates, rather than facilitates, those who wish to exercise this choice'.

As we noted, however, the legal entitlement of the woman to receive services and to be involved in the choices relating to her care depends upon the existing laws relating to the provision of statutory services, trespass to the person, consent to treatment, the duty in negligence to provide information and the Articles of the European Convention of Human Rights as set out in the Human Rights Act 1998.

As we shall see in subsequent chapters there are many deficiencies and weakness in the law in relation to the pregnant woman, and cases show that there is no clear legal basis at present to the concept of woman-centred care. Nor would there appear to have been comprehensive implementation of the 'know your midwife concept'.[55] The proposals in the NHS Plan to strengthen patient representation and advocacy are considered in Chapter 11. The Report of the Bristol Inquiry[56] into children's heart surgery recommended that the patient should be at the centre of healthcare and that there should be an equal partnership between patient and healthcare professional. The implementation of its recommendations could have significant consequences for woman-centred care. The Report is considered in Chapter 21. In September 2001 the Department of Health published plans to give patients suffering from chronic conditions more control over managing their own illness.[57] There is no reason why the philosophy and principles behind this initiative should not become incorporated into midwifery practice, since that was at the heart of the Changing Childbirth proposals.

The next two chapters explore the law relating to consent and to receiving information.

QUESTIONS AND EXERCISES

1 Consider the targets set out in Box 6.2 in the light of your own practice and determine what steps would be needed to implement them.

2 Do you consider that a woman should have a legally enforceable right to receive the kind of care which she wants?

3 What effect would a National Standards Framework for maternity care have on your practice and the rights of your clients?

References

1 A National Health Service Trust v. D. Times Law Report 19 July 2000; [2000] Lloyds Rep Med 411

2 NHS Trust A v. Mrs M and NHS Trust B v. Mrs H. Family Division 25 October 2000; [2001] 1 All ER 801

3 Re A(Minors)(Conjoined Twins: Separation) [2000] Lloyd's Rep Med 425

4 R (Pretty) v. Director of Public Prosecutions and another, Medical Ethics Alliance and others, interveners. Times Law Report 23 October 2001

5 A v. The United Kingdom (100/1997/884/1096) judgement on 23 September 1998

6 News item. 28 April 1994. *The Times*

7 See also Dimond B. 1997. Dilemma: The prisoner. *Accident and Emergency Nursing Journal*, 5(4), 219-20

8 News item. 1994. RCM response to prison service apology. *Midwives Chronicle*, 107(1277), 219

9 News item. 1994. Handcuffing pregnant prisoners. *Bulletin of Medical Ethics*, 98, 9

10 Walker A. 1996. The shame I felt in chains. 11 January 1996. *The Guardian*

11 Home Office. 1996. *Health Service Journal*, 106(5486), 6

12 News item. 1996. Manacles policy loosened. 16 January 1996. *The Guardian*; Travis A. 1996. End to

chains for pregnant prisoners.16 January 1996. *The Guardian*

13 Beech BAL. 1998. Shackled prisoner wins compensation. *AIMS journal*, 10(2), 13

14 Cading-Paull C. 1994. Mothers in prison. *Modern Midwife*, 4(6), 26

15 Price S and Ridge H. 2001. MIDIRS Midwifery Digest, 11(3), 325-8

16 News item. 1998. Pregnant women shackled to radiator for five hours. *RCM Midwives Journal*, March 1998, 2

17 R v. Bournewood Community and Mental Health NHS Trust ex parte L [1998] 3 All ER 289

18 Re F (Adult: Court's Jurisdiction) [2000] 2 FLR 512 Court of Appeal; [2000] Lloyds Rep Med 381

19 Tehrani v. UKCC [2001] IRLR 208

20 Nurses, Midwives and Health Visitors (Professional Conduct)(Amendment) Rules 2001 Approval Order 2001. SI 2001 No 536

21 R v. Secretary of State for the Home Department ex parte Mellor. Times Law Report 31 July 2000

22 R v Secretary of State for Health ex parte Lally. Times Law Report 11 October 2000

23 Kitzinger S. 1999. Birth in prison: the rights of the baby. *Practising Midwife*, 2(1), 16-18

24 R (P) v. Secretary of State for the Home Department; R (Q) v. the same. Times Law Report 1 June 2001

25 R (P) v. Secretary of State for the Home Department; R (Q) v. the same. Times Law Report 1 August 2001

26 R (on the application of N) v. Ashworth Special Hospital Authority [2001] EWHC Admin 339; The Times 26 June 2001

27 R v. Secretary of State for Social Services ex parte Hincks and others. 29 June 1979 [1979] 123 Solicitors Journal 436

28 R v. Central Birmingham Health Authority ex parte Walker [1987] 3 BMLR 32; The Times 26 November 1987

29 R v. Cambridge HA ex parte B [1995] 2 All ER 129

30 R v North West Lancashire HS ex parte A, D, and G [1999] Lloyds Law Reports Medical 399; [1999] 53 BMLR 148 CA

31 NHS Executive Letter: EL (95)97

32 House of Commons. Second report of Health Committee Session 1992/92 on maternity services: Winterton Report

33 Expert Committee on Maternity Services set up by Baroness Cumberlege

34 King's Fund Centre for Health Services Development. *Consensus statement on maternity care: choice, continuity and change.* London: King's Fund Centre

35 Department of Health. 1993. Changing Childbirth. London: HMSO

36 Department of Health. 2000. The NHS Plan: A plan for investment, a plan for reform. London: HMSO

37 Department of Health. 1997. The New NHS: Modern, dependable. London: HMSO

38 Contact Catherine Eden at the National Childbirth Trust 020 8992 2616; c_eden@national-childbirth-trust.co.uk

39 Department of Health. 2 May 2001. Press release 2001/0212. Milburn announces £100 million boost for maternity units and 2000 extra midwives by 2005

40 Department of Health. 10 October 2001. Press release 2001/0470 Maternity units receive £100 million to modernise and improve facilities

41 Department of Health. 14 June 2001. Press Release 2001/0262 Health Minister sets out plans to modernise maternity services

42 Carlisle D. 1995. Laboured relations. *Nursing Times*, 91(50), 16

43 National Childbirth Trust. 1995. GPs block home births. *Health Visitor*, 68(3), 87

44 Andeson RE and Anderson DA. 1999. The cost effectiveness of home birth. *Journal of Nurse-Midwifery*, 44(1), 30-5

45 Chamberlain G, Wraight A, Crowley P (eds). 1997. *Home Births: the report of the 1994 confidential enquiry by the National Birthday Trust Fund.* Carnforth: Partheon Publishing Group; MIDIRS abstract in *MIDIRS Midwifery Digest*, March 1997, 109

46 UKCC. 2000. Position Statement: Registrar's Letter 20/2000

47 UKCC. 2001. Position Statement: Registrar's Letter 21/2001

48 Dimond B. 1999. Is there a legal right to choose a Caesarean? *British Journal of Midwifery*, 7(8), 515-8

49 Anderson T. 2001. Commentary. *MIDIRS Midwifery Digest*, 11(3), 368-70

50 Marx H, Wiener J and Davies N. 2001. A survey of the influence of patients' choice on the increase in the Caesarean section rate. Journal of Obstetrics and Gynaecology, 21(2), 124-7

51 Central Health Services Council. 1970. Standing Maternity and Midwifery Advisory Committee. *Domiciliary midwifery and maternity bed needs*. Chairman Sir John Peel. London: HMSO

52 Thomas J and Paranjothy S. 2001. Royal College of Obstetricians and Gynaecologists Clinical Effectiveness Support Unit. The National Sentinel Caesarean Section Audit Report. London: RCOG Press; www.rcog.org.uk

53 Royal College of Midwives and National Childbirth Trust. 2001. The rising Caesarean rate: causes and effects for public health. Conference Report November 2000; London: RCM and NCT

54 World Health Organisation. 1985. Appropriate technology for birth. *Lancet*, 2(8452): 436-7

55 Flint C and Poulengeris P. 1987. *The Know Your Midwifery Report 1987*. Obtainable from 49 Peckarmans Wood, Sydenham Hill, London SE26 6RZ

56 Bristol Royal Infirmary. 2001. *Learning from Bristol: the report of the public inquiry into children's heart surgery at the Bristol Royal Infirmary 1984-1995*. Command Paper CM 5207; www.bristol-inquiry.org.uk

57 Department of Health. 14 September 2001. Press release 2001/0421 Patients to become the key decisions-makers in their own care

Chapter 7
CONSENT

In the main, two legal actions can arise in relation to consent. The first is an action for trespass to the person, where there is no consent to the touching of another person or other legal justification, or there has been fraud or duress. In this action, harm need not be proved: merely the touching or apprehension of touching. The other action is one for negligence where the person has not been informed of significant information. In this action the claimant would have to prove that harm has been suffered which would not have been suffered if the information had been given. This chapter considers the action for trespass to the person and the defences including the defence of consent. The next chapter looks at the information which must be given and the duty of care which includes the duty to inform.

Guidance has been provided by the Department of Health on consent, which can be accessed via the Internet and is intended to be updated on a regular basis.[1] There are separate guidelines for use by adults, children and young persons, those with learning disabilities, parents and relatives and carers. The Department of Health identifies 12 key points on consent which are expanded upon in the Reference guide. These cover the following areas:

– When is consent needed?

– Can children consent for themselves?

– Who is the right person to seek consent?

– What information should be provided?

– Is the patient's consent voluntary?

– Does it matter how the patient gives consent?

– Refusals of treatment.

– Adults who are not competent to give consent.

MIDWIFERY INTERVENTIONS

Firstly, what are the various kinds of treatment and diagnostic procedures over which the woman might wish to exercise choice?

Box 7.1 sets out a few of the decisions which may be made during the course of a pregnancy.

Box 7.1 Decisions during pregnancy

*Caesarean section	Vitamin K injections
*Episiotomies	Syntometrine
*Epidurals	*Anaesthetic
*Admission to obstetric unit	Tubal ligation
Home confinement	Seeing the doctor
*Fetal monitoring	*Blood transfusion
Induction	Screening for syphilis and HIV
*Artificial rupture of membranes	Anti-D injections
Water birth	Examination by students
Catheterisation	Fetal blood sampling
*Blood tests	Suppositories
*Forceps	Enemas
*Intravenous infusion/treatment	*Intrauterine monitoring
*Suturing	*Fetal scalp electrodes
Vaginal examination	Rectal examinations
Removal of jewellery	Ultrasound scanning

The list shown in Box 7.1 is not exhaustive but it shows the many decisions which may have to be made during the pregnancy. Most, however, are not of a life-saving necessity, either for the mother or baby, and the mother could refuse most of these procedures without any major disadvantages healthwise. However, to carry out any of these tasks or procedures without consent would, in the absence of lawful justification, be regarded as a trespass to the person. Those procedures marked * are ones which could lead to serious harm to the mother or baby, if the mother refused to give consent for them.

TRESPASS TO THE PERSON

The definition of trespass to the person is shown in Box 7.2.

Box 7.2 Trespass to the person

An act of the defendant which directly and intentionally causes either some physical contact with the person of the claimant without the claimant's consent (this is known as a battery) or causes the claimant immediately to apprehend a contact with his person (this is known as an assault).

The claimant is the person suing for compensation in the civil courts, formerly known as the plaintiff. Like its fellow causes of action, trespass to goods and trespass to land, no harm has to be proved. The action is known as 'actionable per se', i.e. actionable in its own right, and is unlike an action for negligence where harm must be established. The mere fact that there is a touching of a person's body without authorisation is sufficient to constitute a trespass. Social touching would not normally however constitute a trespass in the absence of unusual factors.

This means that, even where the midwife has acted out of good will and in the best interests of the mother, if she has failed to obtain consent and in the absence of any of the other defences mentioned below, she could be liable to an action for trespass to the person. (In practice, the claimant would sue the midwife's employer who is vicariously liable for the actions of an employee who is acting in the course of employment (see Chapter 13), unless of course the midwife was self-employed.)

DEFENCES TO AN ACTION FOR TRESPASS TO THE PERSON

These are set out in Box 7.3.

Box 7.3 Defences to an action for trespass to the person

- Consent to treatment by patient (and/or in the case of a person under 18 by the parent or guardian)

- Necessity

- Statutory authorisation eg. Mental Health Act 1983

- Declaration of the court

CONSENT

This is the main defence to an action for trespass to the person, i.e. that the individual who was touched, or feared a touching, gave consent to that action.

What, however, is meant by consent? Are there any factors which could invalidate an apparently valid consent? What capacity is required of the person in order to give a valid consent? Does the law require it to be given in any specific form?

REQUIREMENTS OF A VALID CONSENT

ABSENCE OF DURESS OR FRAUD

To be valid as a defence to an action of trespass to the person, the consent which the defendant is relying upon must be given freely and without duress and without fraud, by a mentally competent person. Evidence of compulsion or fraud would invalidate the consent. However, where prisoners claimed that the very nature of their confinement in a prison institution made consent invalid, they failed in their action for trespass to the person.[2] The Court of Appeal stated that they were not incapable in law of giving a valid consent by reason of the fact they were in prison and that refusal might adversely affect prison privileges or even parole.

RELEVANT TO THE DEFENDANT'S ACTION

Clearly the consent must be relevant to the act of the defendant. Consent to a Caesarean would not be a defence to carrying out a hysterectomy, though other defences (eg. necessity) might be relevant. This is an important area for the midwife since it must be clear whether or not the mother has given consent to an intimate examination and the midwife must protect the mother against any unauthorised intimate examinations.[3] When consent is given, the person should have a general idea as to the purpose of the contact proposed. However, absence of sufficiently detailed information is more likely to be grounds for an action for negligence, for failure on the defendant's part to fulfil the duty of care in informing the patient, and would not invalidate the consent for the purpose of defending an action of trespass. This was explained clearly by the High Court in the case of Chatterton v. Gerson.[4]

The claimant ran kennels with her twin sister. When her sister became a nurse, she worked as a universal aunt. In 1973 she went into hospital for treatment of varicose veins and she was advised at that time that a hernia repair operation should be carried out. Unfortunately afterwards she suffered intractable and chronic pain as the result of the ilco-linguinal nerve being trapped. After various unsuccessful treatments, she was referred to Dr Gerson, a pain specialist, and was given treatment which unfortunately resulted in her right leg becoming completely numb, considerably impairing her mobility. She claimed damages against the defendant, alleging that he had not given her an explanation of the operations and their implications so that she could make an informed decision about whether to risk them, and that

(a) he had committed a trespass to the person since her consent to the operation was vitiated by the lack of prior explanation, and

(b) he had been negligent in not giving an explanation as he was required to do as part of his duty to treat a patient with the degree of professional skill and care expected of a reasonably skilled medical practitioner.

She failed on both counts: point (a) is considered here; point (b) is discussed in the next chapter.

In deciding that her action for trespass to the person failed, Judge Bristow said:

'In my judgement once the patient is informed in broad terms of the nature of the procedure which is intended, and gives her consent, that consent is real, and the course of action on which to base a claim for failure to go into risks and implications is negligence, not trespass... In this case Miss Chatterton was under no illusion as to the general nature of what an intrathecal injection of phenol solution nerve block would be, and in the case of each injection her consent was not unreal.'

MENTAL COMPETENCE OF THE PERSON GIVING CONSENT

This is considered below.

FORMS OF EVIDENCING CONSENT

The agreement of the person that the touching may take place can occur in various ways as shown in Box 7.4.

Box 7.4 Forms of consent

- In writing (this may or may not be on a specially designed consent form)

- By word of mouth

- By implication.

WRITTEN CONSENT

Forms have been issued by the Department of Health[1] as part of its Good Practice in Consent implementation guide, replacing those issued by the NHS Management Executive in 1990 and updated in 1992. Box 7.5 shows more details about the new forms.

Box 7.5 Consent forms issued in the Department of Health's Good Practice in Consent implementation guide[5]

Consent Form 1: Patient agreement to investigation or treatment

– Name of treatment and brief explanation

– Health Professional's Statement

   Intended benefits

   Serious/frequently occurring risks

   Any extra procedures which may become necessary during the procedure

   Leaflets/tapes provided

   Anaesthesia/sedation required

   Health Professional's name, signature and contact details

– Statement of interpreter (where appropriate)

– Statement of patient

   I agree to the procedure.

   I understand that you cannot give me a guarantee that a particular person will perform the procedure. The person will, however, have appropriate experience.

   I understand that I will have the opportunity to discuss the details of anaesthesia with an anaesthetist before the procedure, unless the urgency of my situation prevents this. (Only applies to patients having general or regional anaesthesia)

   I understand that any procedure in addition to those described on this form will only be carried out if it is necessary to save my life or prevent serious harm to my health.

   I have been told about additional procedures which may become necessary during my treatment. I have listed below any procedures which I do not wish to be carried out without further discussion.

There are also provisions made for a witness to sign where an adult is unable to do so but has indicated his consent, and for a person with parental responsibility to

▶

▶ sign. Consent Form 4 is for adults who are unable to consent to investigation or treatment, and includes

- Details of the procedure or course of treatment proposed

- Assessment of the patient's capacity

- Assessment of the patient's best interests

- Details of the involvement of the patient's family and significant others.

Only on rare occasions is there a statutory requirement for consent to be given in writing or for consent to be evidenced in writing. Box 7.6 lists such circumstances.

Box 7.6 Statutory requirements relating to the giving of consent

- The Abortion Act 1967 requires forms to be completed by the doctors who confirm that the statutory requirements are met (except in an emergency).

- The Mental Health Act 1983 Part IV covers the giving of treatment for mental disorder. The responsible medical officer has to confirm, in specified circumstances, that the patient is capable of understanding the nature, purpose and likely effects of the treatment and has given consent.

- The Human Fertilisation and Embryology Act 1990 sets out specific requirements on consent, preceded by counselling in relation to the use of gametes and embryos (see Chapter 27).

Where special forms are not required, written consent which is not on one of the recommended forms will not be invalid, provided that it clearly indicates the object of the consent and gives the signature of the person consenting. It must be remembered that the form is not the actual consent, but evidence that consent was given.

The forms may incorporate a phrase such as 'I also give consent to any other procedure deemed necessary'. This would be interpreted in the light of the treatment or procedure for which consent has been given. It would not cover a procedure unrelated to the treatment. For example, if a mother has signed such a statement in relation to a Caesarean, it would not necessarily cover a sterilisation. If such a procedure was considered to be life-saving, it would be better for the professionals to rely on the defence of the necessity (see below) than assume that actual consent has been obtained for this.[6] Diana Brahams, a medical lawyer, stated that in her view when the consent form included permission for such surgery as the surgeon thinks necessary, there should have been a discussion with the patient over those further options that might arise during the agreed procedure.

'Otherwise a catch-all form may not constitute consent, and a dissatisfied patient may seek remedy via the police or by civil proceedings against the surgeon for compensation.'

In certain circumstances failure by the surgeon to obtain consent to a procedure could be treated as a criminal offence of battery and assault.

The legal significance of birth plans is considered below.

CONSENT BY WORD OF MOUTH

This consent may be just as valid as consent in writing, but in the event of dispute it is very much more difficult for the fact that consent was given to be proved. Unless witnesses were present, it may be a case of the mother's word against that of the midwife. It is therefore recommended that for cases where the procedure is risky or hazardous, and where there could be a controversy as to whether consent was ever given, the midwife should attempt to obtain consent in writing.

IMPLIED CONSENT

The view has been taken that simply coming into hospital or seeing a midwife, automatically implies that the woman agrees to all the treatments and procedures which they recommend. In the light of the variety of treatments and procedures now available and the emphasis upon the involvement of the mother in decision making, it would be better to confine the term 'implied consent' to those circumstances where the mother indicates by her non-verbal behaviour that she agrees that certain treatment can be given. For example, she raises her sleeve for blood pressure readings to be taken or for an injection to be given, she lies on the couch for a physical examination; such actions denote an agreement for the midwife or other professional to proceed.

Care however must be taken that the action carried out is that to which the implied consent refers. This shows the weakness of relying upon the implied consent of the mother, and the problems of misinterpretation. Where any risky procedure is contemplated, written consent (preferably) or consent by word of mouth should be obtained.

WHO CAN GIVE CONSENT?

MENTALLY COMPETENT PERSONS OVER 18 YEARS

Each mentally competent adult has the right to give or withhold consent. The courts respect the autonomy of the individual. This was clearly stated by the Court of Appeal in the case of Re T[7] (see below). Competence would be defined in relation to the procedure/treatment which is proposed. Thus, in relation to a woman with learning disabilities, she might have the competence to give consent to having stitches for a wound, but not to give consent for an abortion or Caesarean section. The determination of capacity is considered below.

THE 16 AND 17-YEAR-OLD

These young persons have a statutory right to give consent under the Family Law Reform Act 1969 Section 8. Consent can be given for surgical, medical and dental treatment and the definition of treatment covers any procedure undertaken for the purposes of diagnosis and any ancillary procedures such as administration of anaesthetic.

The parents also have the right to give consent on behalf of the 16 and 17-year-old. This is preserved by Section 8(3) of the Family Law Reform Act 1969. Where there is a clash between the parent and the minor, the professional would normally follow the wishes of the minor. However, much depends upon the circumstances. In the case of Re W 1992[8] a 16-year-old who suffered from anorexia refused to go to a specialist unit for treatment and the courts decided that she could be compelled to go against her wishes since it was in her best interests to receive treatment. The case is important to the midwife who is caring for pregnant minors of 16 and 17 since although they have a statutory right to give consent to treatment (including ancillary and diagnostic procedures), their refusal can in certain circumstances be overruled. The case would usually be referred to the court.

The following is a decision by the House of Lords over the sterilisation of a 17-year-old girl.

RE B (1987)[9]

A 17-year-old girl (who became later known as Jeanette) who had a mental age of five or six years was in the care of the local authority. It was established that she would have no understanding of sexual intercourse, pregnancy, and birth. The local authority applied for her to be made a ward of court and for leave to be given for the operation of sterilisation to be carried out.

The House of Lords held that the paramount consideration for the exercise of its wardship jurisdiction was the welfare and best interests of the child. The Court held that it was in the best interests of the minor for the sterilisation to proceed and permission was given to the operation.

THE CHILD UNDER 16 YEARS

Whilst children under 16 years of age do not have a statutory right to consent to treatment, the right to give consent at common law (i.e. judge-made law) was recognised by the House of Lords in the Gillick case.[10]

If a child has the maturity to understand the nature, purpose, and likely effects of any proposed treatment, then she could give a valid consent without the involvement of the parents. Whilst the Gillick case itself was concerned with family planning and treatment, the principle applies to other forms of treatment, including abortion. The principle that the ascertainable wishes and feelings of the child concerned (considered in the light of his age and understanding) should also be taken into account is also stated in the Children Act 1989 Section 1(3)(a) as one of the factors to which the court shall have regard in determining what if any orders should be made or varied. Again this right of the child is paralleled by a right and even duty of the parent to give consent. In addition, Section 3(5) of the Children Act 1989 enables a person who

(a) does not have parental responsibility for a particular child; but

(b) has care of the child

to do what is reasonable in all the circumstances of the case for the purposes of safeguarding or promoting the child's welfare.

Thus if the midwife were caring for a pregnant minor, and if the patient did not have the competence to give consent herself, a person caring for her could do so.

If the parent or guardian of a minor under the age of 16 refused to give consent to treatment which was necessary in the best interests of the minor, the doctor could act out of necessity in the best interests of the minor according to the principle set out in Re F (see below). Alternatively the authority of the court could be sought for treatment to proceed against the parents' wishes. Should the parents fail to give consent to essential treatment or arrange for the treatment to take place, they can face prosecution in the event of harm befalling the child. For example, a Rastafarian couple who had refused on religious grounds to allow their diabetic daughter who was nine years old to be given insulin were convicted of manslaughter on October 28th 1993 in Nottingham. The father was given a sentence of imprisonment and the mother a suspended sentence.[11]

An example of a clash between parents and under-age daughter is seen in the following case which related to abortion.

RE P (1982)[12]

A girl of 15 who had already given birth to a boy, and was in the care of the local authority, became pregnant again. Her parents wished to prevent her having an abortion and refused to give consent. The girl herself wished to have an abortion and the requirements of the Abortion Act 1967 were satisfied. The judge, Mrs Justice Butler-Sloss, using the test that the welfare of the girl was of paramount importance, decided that the termination should proceed.

THE MENTALLY INCOMPETENT ADULT

Where an adult is mentally incompetent there is at present no person who is authorised to give consent on her behalf. Her parents cannot give consent once the minor has attained the age of majority (i.e. 18 years). An example of the problem of consent to abortion and sterilisation arose in the following case of T v. T.

T V. T (1988)[13]

T was 19 years old and pregnant. She was doubly incontinent, had a mental age of two-and-a-half years and could barely communicate. Her mother and doctors applied for a declaration that it would be lawful to abort the baby and then sterilise her. The judge granted the declaration stating that the doctor was justified in taking such steps as good medical practice demands and that in her case, her mental abnormality was such that she would never be able to give a valid consent. It should be noted that the court did not itself give permission for the operation to proceed.

There is at present no statutory provision covering decision-making on behalf of mentally incapacitated adults. Health professionals and others have the power to act in the best interests of the mentally incapacitated adult. The problems created by this vacuum have been considered by the Law Commission in a series of consultation papers on decision-making and the mentally incapacitated adult.[14]

The Law Commission issued its final report on Mental Incapacity in 1995.[15] It included draft legislation for a Mental Incapacity Bill, which envisaged that there should be new courts which would have the jurisdiction for decision-making on behalf of mentally incapacitated adults. In 1997 the Lord Chancellor issued a consultation paper[16] which led to the publication of a white paper.[17] The white paper proposed the establishment of courts to hear significant decisions about mentally incapacitated adults, a statutory power to make decisions in the best interests of the mentally incapacitated adult and the recognition of a continuing power of attorney by which persons could make treatment decisions on behalf of a mentally incapacitated adult. At the time of writing, legislation is awaited.

THE MIDWIFE AND THE MOTHER WITH LEARNING DISABILITIES

The midwife may become involved in such judicial hearings to make decisions where she is caring for a mentally impaired adult or a person who becomes unconscious. For example, it is likely that one of the special category procedures for which the judicial forum would have to make a decision would be whether a mentally impaired woman should be sterilised following a pregnancy. If a pregnant woman becomes unconscious following a road accident, decisions on whether the mother should be kept alive on a ventilation machine during the pregnancy might also be considered by the judicial forum. Other decisions which may be left to the professional might be the decision to induce a mentally incompetent person and the management of her confinement.

COMMON LAW POWERS

Until the white paper's recommendations are embodied in legislation, decisions on the care and treatment of the mentally incapacitated adult must be on the basis of the decision in Re F,[18] with reference to the court where necessary.

In Re F the House of Lords held that if a patient is incapable of giving a valid consent, the professional must act in the patient's best interests and follow the approved accepted practice of the reasonable professional, i.e. the Bolam Test.[19] (See Chapter 13 for discussion of this Test.) Acting in the best interests of a mentally incapacitated adult is known as the 'defence of necessity' and this is discussed below. In a more recent case, also known as Re F, the Court of Appeal held that the Court had the inherent power to make day-to-day decisions on behalf of the mentally incapacitated adult.[20]

VALIDITY OF A REFUSAL

Where the patient refuses life-saving treatment, the Court of Appeal has emphasised that the professional has a duty to ensure that the refusal is valid.

RE T (1992)[21]

The patient was a 20-year-old pregnant woman who had been brought up by her mother who was a Jehovah's Witness. She was injured in a road accident and when admitted to hospital told the nurse that she would not wish to have a blood transfusion. At that stage it seemed highly improbable that one would be required. However her condition deteriorated and she went into labour. She was transferred to the maternity unit and told the midwife that she was a Jehovah's Witness and would not accept a blood transfusion. The midwife got her to put her name on a form which she had not read and of which she probably did not understand the significance. Her condition worsened until it was realised that a blood transfusion was essential. At this stage the father and the cohabitee referred the case to court.

The judge hearing all the facts decided that her refusal was not valid and the transfusion should proceed. His decision was upheld shortly afterwards by the Court of Appeal which, whilst it stated that the adult mentally competent person has a right to refuse treatment, emphasised that professionals must ensure that a refusal of life-saving treatment is given by a person who is mentally competent and who is not overborne by the views of another or under the influence of drink or drugs.

WITHDRAWAL OF CONSENT

It is a necessary corollary that where treatment is being given on the basis of consent, then that consent can be withdrawn at any time. This could of course pose problems. For example, a woman who may initially have given agreement to an epidural, might change her mind as it is being done and it may not be possible to stop the procedure part-way through. Where however it is possible to stop the procedure without causing harm to the woman, then this should happen if consent is withdrawn. If it is not possible, presumably the professional must continue to give the treatment and rely upon one of the other defences to an action for trespass to the person, such as necessity.

NECESSITY

It has long been recognised at common law (i.e. judge-made law) that there may be circumstances where urgent action needs to be taken in the interest of a person, where his/her consent is lacking. It may be for example in a situation where the person is unconscious. It may be because the person lacks the mental capacity to give consent. In such circumstances the House of Lords has laid down the following principle:

'A doctor may lawfully operate on or give treatment to a person who lacks capacity to give consent provided that it is in the best interests of the patient, being necessary to save life, or to prevent a deterioration, or ensure an improvement, in his physical or mental health.'

RE F (1989)[18]

A severely mentally impaired woman had formed an attachment with a fellow patient in a hospital for the mentally handicapped. It was clear that she did not have the capacity to understand or cope with a pregnancy and it was considered that it would be advisable if she were sterilised. However since she was over 17, no one had in law the right to give consent on her behalf. A declaration was therefore sought from the courts that she could be sterilised. In giving the required declaration, the court recommended that whilst most day-to-day activities by professionals on behalf of mentally incapacitated adults could take place under the doctrine of necessity, it wished applications in relation to sterilisations to come before the courts and a Practice Direction covering this has subsequently been published.

Two points should be emphasised about the decision in Re F (1989). One is that the court stated that in acting in the best interests of the patient, the professional should follow the Bolam Test (see Chapter 13). The other is that the decision refers to the patient who lacks capacity or for some reason is unable to give consent. Where the patient has the capacity to give consent but refuses, Re F does not justify compulsory treatment.

THE DETERMINATION OF MENTAL CAPACITY

In order to give a valid consent, a person must have the requisite mental capacity. How is the capacity of the patient determined? This was the issue before the court in a case involving a Broadmoor patient who obtained a court injunction prohibiting doctors from amputating his leg.

RE C (1994)[22]

C, a 68-year-old patient suffering from paranoid schizophrenia, developed gangrene in a foot during his confinement in a secure hospital while serving a seven year term of imprisonment. He was removed to a general hospital where the Consultant surgeon diagnosed that he was likely to die imminently if the leg was not amputated below the knee. The prognosis was that he had a 15% chance of surviving without amputation. He refused to consent. The hospital authorities considered whether the operation could be performed without C's consent and made arrangements for a solicitor to see him concerning his competence to give a reasoned decision. Treatment with antibiotics and conservative surgery averted the immediate threat of imminent death but the hospital refused to give an undertaking to the solicitor that in recognition of his repeated refusals it would not amputate in any future circumstances. An application was made to the High Court for an injunction restraining the hospital from carrying out an amputation without his express written consent. The hospital contended that C's capacity to give a definitive decision had been impaired by his mental illness and that he had failed to appreciate the risk of death if the operation was not performed.

The High Court, exercising its inherent jurisdiction, granted the declaration sought by C. It held that although C's general capacity to make a decision had been impaired by schizophrenia, the evidence failed to establish that he lacked sufficient understanding of the nature, purpose, and effects of the proposed treatment, but instead showed that he had understood and retained the relevant information, believed it and had arrived at a clear choice. It followed that the presumption in favour of his right to self-determination had not been displaced.

There were three tests of capacity laid down by the court:

1 Could the patient comprehend and retain the necessary information?

2 Was he able to believe it?

3 Was he able to weigh the information, balancing risks and needs, so as to arrive at a choice?

Applying these tests to the patient, the court decided that he did have the necessary capacity to refuse the amputation and issued the injunction to stop any doctor operating without his consent.

REFUSAL OF TREATMENT IN A CAESAREAN CASE

In a much disputed case, Re S,[23] a woman who refused to give consent to a Caesarean on religious grounds was compelled by the Family Division court to have one (see below). This decision is difficult to reconcile with the case of the Broadmoor patient and is now discredited.

RE S (1992)[23]

The Health Authority applied for a declaration to authorise the surgeons and staff of a hospital to carry out an emergency Caesarean operation upon a patient, referred to as Mrs S. She was 30 years old and was in labour with her third pregnancy. She was admitted to hospital on Saturday 10th October 1992 with ruptured membranes and in spontaneous labour and continued in labour. She was 6 days overdue beyond the expected date of birth, which was 6th October, and she refused, on religious grounds, to submit herself to a Caesarean section operation. She was supported in this by her husband and they were described as 'born-again Christians' and were considered quite sincere in their beliefs.

The obstetrician in charge of the patient gave evidence of the condition of the patient, which was described by the President of the Family division as follows:

'Her situation is desperately serious, as is also the situation of the as yet unborn child, The child is in what is described as a position of "transverse lie", with the elbow projecting through the cervix and the head being on the right side. There is the gravest risk of a rupture of the uterus if the section is not carried out and the natural labour process is permitted to continue. The evidence of the obstetrician is that we are concerned with "minutes rather than hours" and it is a "life and death" situation.'

The obstetrician and other staff had done their best to persuade the mother that the only means of saving her life, and also the life of her unborn child, was to carry out a Caesarean section operation. The obstetrician stated that it was absolutely the case that the baby could not be born alive if a Caesarean operation was not carried out.

The President of the Family Division made the declaration in the knowledge that there was no English legal authority directly in point. The timing shows the speed of the decision. The application came to the notice of court officials at 1.30pm. It came on for hearing just before 2.00pm and at 2.18pm the declaration was made. No appeal was brought against the decision and it is understood that the mother accepted the ruling and the Caesarean section was performed. The baby died but the mother survived.

Had the reasoning for this decision been supported in subsequent cases, there would have been major implications in terms of the rights of the mother, and the possibility that a slippery slope would commence, where interventions could be made against the will of a competent mother, in the interests of the baby, thus treating the pregnant woman as lacking the ability to make decisions.

One of the implications of the decision in Re S was that the mother could be forced to recognise the potential harm and action could be taken against her. Drugs, smoking, alcohol, eating unwisely, dangerous sporting and leisure activities have all been shown to have the potential to cause underweight or premature babies. On the basis of Re S, action could have been taken to restrict a mother's activities in the interests of the unborn child.

CASES AFTER RE S

There was considerable outcry as a result of the Re S decision. The Ethics Committee of the Royal College of Obstetricians and Gynaecologists published guidelines which commented adversely on the decision and made the conclusions set out in Box 7.7.

Box 7.7 Conclusions of the RCOG ethics committee on Re S

1 The aim of those who care for pregnant women is to foster the greatest benefit to both mother and fetus with the least risk.

2 Occasionally problems arise when a pregnant woman and her doctor fundamentally disagree over action believed to be in the best interest of mother and fetus or when advice is in conflict with her religious scruples.

3 Although obligations to the fetus in utero increase as it develops, UK law does not grant it personal legal status. This comes from the moment of birth.

4 The law provides no restriction on a woman's freedom on account of her pregnancy. Any medical action requires her informed consent.

5 A pregnant woman has a natural duty and moral obligation to the welfare of her fetus as a future person and member of society.

6 Society should provide all the necessary services and incentives to help the pregnant woman to fulfil her obligation.

7 It is rare for a doctor to be faced with a conflict where judicial intervention on behalf of the fetus might be considered.

8 Such circumstances are usually unexpected and the requirement of haste leaves little time for the case to be properly prepared and decided.

9 Doctors must recognise that medical advice is based on evidence that is seldom infallible. It is the doctor's duty to provide appropriate information so that the pregnant woman can make an informed and thoughtful decision.

10 Where conflict arises the doctor should seek help and advice from other professional colleagues and, with the patient's agreement, it may be appropriate to involve other members or friends of her family.

11 A doctor must respect the competent pregnant woman's right to choose or refuse any particular recommended course of action whilst optimising care for both mother and fetus to the best of his or her ability. A doctor would not then be culpable if these endeavours were unsuccessful.

12 We conclude that it is inappropriate, and unlikely to be helpful or necessary, to invoke judicial intervention to overrule an informed and competent woman's refusal of a proposed medical treatment, even though her refusal might place her life and that of her fetus at risk.

SUBSEQUENT DECISIONS SINCE RE S

Re S was followed by several other cases where compulsory Caesarean operations were carried out, without the consent of the woman. In one case[24] the patient suffered from paranoid schizophrenia, was detained in a psychiatric hospital under Section 3 and was refusing to have a Caesarean operation. The consultant psychiatrist gave evidence that if there were a stillbirth, that would lead to a profound deterioration of the patient's mental health and once the pregnancy was over, the woman could have the anti-psychotic medication which had been discontinued during the pregnancy because of dangers to the fetus. The judge declared that the operation could proceed under Section 63 of the Mental Health Act 1983 as being treatment for mental disorder. (Section 63 enables treatment (not coming under 57 brain surgery for mental disorder or 58 medication after three months or electro convulsive therapy) to be given without the consent of the patient as being treatment for mental disorder, if the treatment is given by or under the direction of the responsible medical officer.) This decision could be criticised on the grounds that treatment for mental disorder was given too wide a definition: if a Caesarean section is considered to be treatment for mental disorder, it would be difficult to find any treatment which by reason of some benefits to the mental state, would not come within the definition of treatment for mental disorder.

In a second case,[25] a pregnant woman had a history of psychiatric treatment and had had three previous children who were delivered by Caesarean section. A Consultant psychiatrist examined her and declared that she was not suffering from mental disorder at the time, but she was unable to balance the information given to her. The application was made to the court for a forceps delivery to take place, and if necessary a Caesarean section. The judge decided that in the light of the evidence, she lacked the mental competence to make a decision about treatment. A declaration was made on the lines sought.

After these decisions, which received much adverse publicity in the press, there was a need for clarification by the Court of Appeal and this came in the case of Re MB.

RE MB (1997)[26]

Miss MB required a Caesarean Section in order to save her fetus. However, whilst she gave consent to the operation, she suffered from a needle phobia which caused her to panic and refuse the preliminary anaesthetic. The trust applied for a declaration that the Caesarean could take place on the grounds that the needle phobia rendered her mentally incapacitated and therefore the operation should proceed in her best interests.

The judge held that the woman was mentally incapacitated as a result of the phobia and the operation could therefore proceed in her best interests.

The same day the Court of Appeal upheld that decision. In a reserved judgement it set out how capacity was to be determined (see Box 7.8) and the general principles which apply to the refusal of treatment (see Box 7.9).

The Court of Appeal emphasised that every person is presumed to have the capacity to consent to or to refuse medical treatment unless and until that presumption is rebutted. A competent woman who has the capacity to decide may, for religious reasons, other reasons, for rational or irrational reasons or for no reason at all, choose not to have medical intervention, even though the consequence may be the death or serious handicap of the child she bears, or her own death. In that event, the courts do not have the jurisdiction to declare medical intervention lawful and the question of her own best interests, objectively considered, does not arise.

Box 7.8 Determining capacity: Re MB

A person lacks the capacity if some impairment or disturbance of mental functioning renders him unable to make a decision on whether to consent to or to refuse treatment. That inability to make a decision will occur when:

(a) The patient is unable to comprehend and retain the information which is material to the decision, especially as to the likely consequences of having or not having the treatment in question

(b) The patient is unable to use the information and weigh it in the balance as part of the process of arriving at the decision.

Box 7.9 Principles laid down in Re MB and incorporated in guidance issued by the Department of Health[27]

1 The court is unlikely to entertain an application for a declaration unless the capacity of the patient to consent to or refuse the medical treatment is in issue.

2 For the time being, at least, the doctors ought to seek a ruling from the High Court on the issue of competence.

3 Those in charge should identify a potential problem as early as possible so that both the hospital and the patient can obtain legal advice.

4 It is highly desirable that, in any case where it is not an emergency, steps are taken to bring it before the court, before it becomes an emergency, to remove the extra pressure from the parties and the court and to enable proper

▶

instructions to be taken, particularly from the patient and where possible give the opportunity for the court to hear oral evidence, if appropriate.

5 The hearing should be inter parties.

6 The mother should be represented in all cases, unless, exceptionally, she does not wish to be. If she is unconscious she should have a guardian ad litem.

7 The Official Solicitor should be notified of all applications to the High Court...

8 There should in general be some evidence, preferably but not necessarily from a psychiatrist, as to the competence of the patient, if competence is in issue.

9 Where time permits, the person identified to give the evidence as to capacity to consent to or refuse treatment should be made aware of the observations made by the Court of Appeal in this judgement.

10 In order to be in a position to assess a patient's best interests the judge should be provided, where possible and if time allows, with information about the circumstances of and relevant background material about the patient.

ST GEORGE'S HEALTHCARE NHS TRUST V. S[28]

This case reaffirmed the principles set out by the Court of Appeal in the case of Re MB. A woman who was about 36 weeks pregnant was diagnosed as suffering from severe pre-eclampsia, severe oedema and proteinuria. She was advised to have early induction of labour as a life-saving necessity. She refused, on the grounds that she would prefer to let nature take its course. She was then examined by an approved social worker and two doctors and was detained in hospital under Section 2 of the Mental Health Act 1983. From there she was transferred to St George's Hospital for obstetric treatment. She was advised by a solicitor that she had the right to refuse treatment. The hospital applied in an ex parte application to the High Court judge stating that it was a life and death situation and the patient had gone into labour. This latter information was incorrect, and the judge was not informed that the patient had instructed solicitors. The judge made the declaration that S's consent could be dispensed with. S was then given a Caesarean section. She was transferred back to the psychiatric hospital where a doctor decided that she was not suffering from mental disorder and ended the detention under Section 2, following which she took her own discharge.

The case eventually came before the Court of Appeal which emphasised the pregnant woman's right of self-determination, that the Mental Health Act should not have been used when a person was refusing treatment for hypertension, and that an unborn child is not a separate person from its mother.

Lord Justice Judge held that:

'(A pregnant woman) is entitled not to be forced to submit to an invasion of her body against her will, whether her own life or that of her unborn child depends on it. Her right is not reduced or diminished merely because her decision to exercise it may appear morally repugnant. The declaration in this case involved the removal of the baby from within the body of her mother under physical compulsion. Unless lawfully justified, this constituted an infringement of the mother's autonomy. Of themselves, the perceived needs of the fetus did not provide the necessary justification.'

STATUTORY AUTHORISATION

Certain Acts of Parliament justify actions which would otherwise be regarded as a trespass to the person. Thus the Mental Health Act 1983 has provisions which enable treatment for mental disorder to be given to a detained patient under specific conditions without the person's consent. The care of those with a mental disorder is considered in Chapter 33.

The Police and Criminal Evidence Act enables a citizen to carry out a lawful arrest in certain circumstances, and if the specified circumstances exist, an action for trespass to the person would not succeed.

DECLARATION OF THE COURT

If there is doubt over the capacity of the woman to give consent, and life-saving action is required, a declaration can be sought from the court. The issue before the court will be whether or not the person has the mental capacity to make their own decisions. If the person is deemed to lack the appropriate mental capacity (and evidence would have to be given of the incapacity) then a declaration could be issued, where appropriate, that treatment could proceed in the person's best interests. In the case of Re D (the Broadmoor patient – see above) the patient succeeded in obtaining an injunction preventing the doctors from operating upon him.

BIRTH PLANS

It would be wrong to see birth plans as written consent to treatment. Rather they result from discussions between midwife and mother over the options available and reflect the mother's wishes at a given moment in time. Where the philosophy behind Changing Childbirth is implemented, then there is likely to be far greater usage of birth plans as the outcome of the discussions. Where, however, consent is required to specific procedures, it is preferable to obtain this consent in writing, and the usual consent form should then be completed.

WHAT IS THE LEGAL SIGNIFICANCE OF BIRTH PLANS?

If the above view of the birth plan is taken, then it is seen not as a legal document binding upon the midwife but rather as the expression of the mother's wishes if all goes according to plan.

If the mother and midwife agree at the beginning of the pregnancy on the preferred choices for the mother, but in the event it is not clinically possible for these preferences to be followed without harm to mother or child, what is the midwife's position? Could she still carry out those procedures to which the mother has not consented?

Ideally, of course, in obtaining the mother's involvement in the treatment and confinement agreement it should be made clear that the plan is subject to the clinical situation. In some situations the clinical needs of the mother may conflict with her original wishes and the preferences she expressed. For example the mother might have expressed a wish to have a natural birth but after protracted labour and fetal distress it might be essential for her own life and that of the child for her to have a Caesarean. Should problems arise then it is highly recommended that the midwife should have the freedom to act in the mother's best interests at the time. It is preferable that a restraint is not placed upon the professional judgement of the midwife and obstetrician. If the mother accepts this, then there is every justification for the midwife in departing from the birth plan should this be clinically necessary. If the mother refuses to accept the possibility of variations from the birth plan, and she is mentally competent, she has the right to refuse any recommended procedure. However, the mother should be given the opportunity to change her mind at a later stage. Care should be taken to ensure that the mother is fully informed about all the risks which could occur if the proposed treatment does not go ahead. Where there is reason to believe the woman lacks the necessary mental competence to make a valid refusal, then the fact of that incompetence and the issue of what is in the mother's best interests would be referred to court.

The Maternity Alliance has published a booklet, *Your Baby, Your Choice*, as a guide to planning labour. It makes it clear that 'the birth plan is best used in an antenatal class, as a trigger for discussion'. It thus gives information on various procedures before confinement, positions for labour and delivery, checking the baby's heartbeat, pain relief, induction and acceleration, cuts and tears after the birth, Caesarean sections, special care and breastfeeding. The birth plan form it provides enables the mother to consider which options she would prefer. However there is no legal status to the document and it recognises that what the mother wants is not always possible.

'Many of us will plan one kind of birth and end up with another, either because the labour proved more difficult than we had hoped or possibly because some forms of pain relief are not available locally.'

IMPLICATIONS OF THE EUROPEAN CONVENTION ON HUMAN RIGHTS

The articles of the Convention are discussed in Chapter 6 and can be found in Appendix 1. Whilst there is no explicit right to give consent recognised in the Convention, failure to obtain consent would be a breach of Article 3, 'Not to be subjected to inhuman or degrading treatment'. There may also be a breach of Article 5 and the right to liberty and security of person if a woman is held against her will without lawful authority.

CONCLUSIONS

The decisions of the Court of Appeal in the case of Re MB and St George's are to be welcomed, since they have clarified the legal situation where a pregnant woman is refusing life-saving treatment. They have emphasised that a mentally competent pregnant woman, like any other mentally competent adult, can validly refuse life-saving treatment. If the refusal of a mentally competent adult were overruled, this would constitute a trespass to the person, as well as possibly a criminal act.

In the next chapter we consider the information which must be given to a woman to fulfil the duty of care to inform.

QUESTIONS AND EXERCISES

1 The mental capacity of a woman to refuse life-saving treatment is central to the question of whether action can be taken in the best interests of the woman and the baby. What arrangements do you have for determining the mental capacity of a mother?

2 Do you consider there are any dangers or advantages in making birth plans legally enforceable?

3 Analyse your practice and during a week of work consider the different ways in which you obtain the consent of the mother to treatments proceeding. What proportion of the total number are obtained in writing?

References

1 Department of Health. 2001. Reference Guide to Consent for Examination or Treatment. London: HMSO; www. doh.gov.uk/consent

2 Freeman v. Home Office [1984] 1 All ER 1036

3 Caswell A. 1992. Medical Rape. *Medical Journal of Australia*, 157(8), 561-2. Reprinted in *MIDIRS Midwifery Digest*, March 1993, 3(1)

4 Chatterton v. Gerson [1981] 1 All ER 257

5 Department of Health. 2001. Good practice in consent: implementation guide. London: HMSO

6 Brahams D. 1993. *Medico-Legal Journal*, 62(1), 225-6 (Reprinted from the Lancet)

7 Re T. [1992] 4 All ER 649; [1992] 3 WLR 782.

8 Re W (a minor)(medical treatment) [1992] 4 All ER 627

9 Re B (a minor)(wardship: sterilisation) [1987] 2 All ER 206

10 Gillick v. W. Norfolk and Wisbech Area Health Authority [1986] 1 AC 112

11 *The Times*. 29 October 1993

12 Re P (a minor) [1982] 80 Local Government Reports 301

13 T v. T [1988] 1 All ER 613

14 Law Commission. Paper 119 (1991), and papers 128, 129 and 130 (1993). London: HMSO

15 Law Commission. 1995. *Mental Incapacity*. London: HMSO

16 Lord Chancellor. 1997. *Who Decides? Making decisions on behalf of mentally incapacitated adults*. London: Lord Chancellor's Office

17 Lord Chancellor. 1999. *Making Decisions*. London: Lord Chancellor's Office

18 Re F v. West Berkshire HA [1989] 2 All ER 545

19 Bolam v. Friern HMC QBD [1957] 2 All ER 118

20 Re F (adult: court's jurisdiction) [2000] 2 FLR 512 Court of Appeal

21 Re T [1992] 4 All ER 649; [1992] 3 WLR 782

22 Re C (adult: refusal of medical treatment) Family Division [1994] 1 All ER 819

23 Re S (adult: refusal of medical treatment) [1992] 9 BMLR 69; [1993] FAM 123

24 Tameside and Glossop Acute Services Trust v. CH [1996] 31 BMLR 93

25 Norfolk and Norwich Healthcare (NHS) Trust v. W [1996] 2 FLR 613

26 Re MB (an adult: medical treatment) [1997] 2 FLR 426

27 Department of Health Circular EL (97)32 1997

28 St George's Healthcare NHS Trust v. S; R v. Collins ex parte S [1998] 44 BMLR 160 CA

Chapter 8
THE DUTY TO INFORM

In the last chapter we considered an action of trespass and the defences available if an apparent trespass has been committed. Of increasing importance in the field of consent is, however, the extent and nature of the information which should be given to the mother before she decides to go ahead with certain procedures. It will be recalled that in the case of Chatterton v. Gerson the distinction was made between the action for trespass, which will not succeed if a valid consent has been given, and an action in negligence on the basis that insufficient information has been given. See the statement of the judge in Box 8.1.

Box 8.1 Chatterton v. Gerson: Judge's statement

'The court has to ask, was there real consent? I think justice requires that in order to vitiate the reality of consent there must be a greater failure of communication between doctor and patient than that involved in a breach of duty if the claim is based on negligence. When the claim is based on negligence the plaintiff must prove not only the breach of duty to inform but that had the duty not been broken she would not have chosen to have the operation. Where the claim is based on trespass to the person, once it is shown that the consent is unreal, then what the plaintiff would have decided if she had been given the information which would have prevented vitiation of the reality of her consent is irrelevant.'

What standard is applied to the giving of information to the patient? Is there a difference where the patient asks questions compared to situations where the patient does not ask for further information? Is it ever lawful to withhold information from the patient?

These questions will be considered in the light of the cases of Sidaway v. Bethlem Royal Hospital Governors and others, and Blythe v. Bloomsbury Health Authority.

SIDAWAY V. BETHLEM ROYAL HOSPITAL GOVERNORS AND OTHERS[1]

In this case the plaintiff suffered chronic and intractable pain following an operation for a hernia repair. She was eventually referred to a specialist in pain relief who warned her of the possibility of disturbing a nerve root and the possible consequences of so doing, but did not mention the possibility of damage to the spinal cord. The risk of spinal cord damage was less than 1%.

She consented to the operation which was carried out by the surgeon with due care and skill. However, in the course of the operation she suffered injury to her spinal cord which resulted in her being severely disabled. She sued the surgeon for breach of his duty of care to warn her of all possible risks inherent in the operation.

The different judges in the House of Lords all had different bases for their views, but they agreed that in general she had failed in her action. Lord Diplock applied the Bolam principle to the duty of care to inform. Lord Bridge distinguished between two extremes: warning the patient of all possible risks and, once the treatment has been decided upon in the patient's best interests, not warning the patient of any risks, in order not to alarm the patient. Between these two extremes, Lord Bridge suggested that the Bolam Test should be applied, but this did not mean handing over to the medical profession the entire question of the scope of the duty of disclosure. There will be circumstances where the judge could come to the conclusion that disclosure of a particular risk was so obviously necessary to an informed choice on the part of the patient that no reasonably prudent medical man would fail to make it. Lord Templeman stated:

'In my opinion, if a patient knows that a major operation may entail serious consequences, the patient cannot complain of lack of information unless the patient asks in vain for more information or unless there is some danger which by its nature or magnitude or for some other reason required to be separately taken into account by the patient in order to reach a balanced judgement in deciding whether or not to submit to the operation.'

Lord Scarman supported a 'prudent patient test', a concept derived from an American case, Canterbury v. Spence.[2] In this case it was recognised that there were four principles:

1 Every human being of adult years and of sound mind has a right to determine what shall be done with his own body.

2 The consent is the informed exercise of a choice and that entails an opportunity to evaluate knowledgeably the options available and the risks attendant on each.

3 The doctor must therefore disclose all 'material risks'; what risks are 'material' is determined by the 'prudent patient' test, which is as follows:
A risk is... material when a reasonable person, in what the physician knows or should know to be the patient's position, would be likely to attach significance to the risk or cluster of risks in deciding whether or not to forgo the proposed therapy.

4 The doctor has, however, a therapeutic privilege. This exception is that a reasonable medical assessment of the patient would have indicated to the doctor

that disclosure would have posed a serious threat of psychological detriment to the patient.

The House of Lords accepted that English law did not recognise the doctrine of informed consent. Risks should be disclosed to enable the patient to make a rational choice whether to undergo the particular treatment recommended by a doctor. This duty was subject to the doctor's overriding duty to have regard to the best interests of the patient. Accordingly it was for the doctor to decide what information should be given to the patient and the terms in which that information should be couched.

The claimant therefore lost her appeal.

HOW MUCH INFORMATION SHOULD BE GIVEN?

The ruling in the Sidaway case was followed in a subsequent case by the Court of Appeal, where the issue arose as to how much information should be given to a patient.

BLYTHE V. BLOOMSBURY HEALTH AUTHORITY AND ANOTHER[3]

Mrs Blythe, a nurse, became pregnant in May 1978 and was referred to University College Hospital for antenatal care. She saw a Consultant who diagnosed that she had no or insufficient immunity to rubella. She could not be vaccinated against rubella because she was at a late stage of her pregnancy and the vaccine, if given, could have had an adverse effect on a fetus if she became pregnant again within three months. However, it was necessary that steps be taken to provide her with contraceptive protection. The general practice at the hospital was to use Depo-Provera (a progesterone-only contraceptive) unless countervailing factors existed or the patient did not want it.

In December 1978 she was admitted to the hospital for the birth of her baby where she received

a. a rubella vaccination, and

b. an injection of Depo-Provera.

She did not object to the prescription or the administration of Depo-Provera.

On December 18th she was admitted to the labour ward where she subsequently gave birth to a healthy son.

On December 19th the rubella vaccine was prescribed by a senior house officer (the vaccination being administered on December 23rd by a nursing sister).

On December 23rd she was seen by a senior house officer who discussed the Depo-Provera drug with the plaintiff (a dose was subsequently administered by injection on the following morning December 24th.) On her discharge from hospital she was given a leaflet detailing the drug's effects on the human body, how long the injection lasted, and advised that she should consult her GP.

On January 31th 1979 she saw two doctors at the hospital's baby clinic.

On March 27th 1979 she saw her GP who prescribed 'Micronor'.

In June 1979 a further dose of Depo-Provera was prescribed.

In April 1980 she had a miscarriage.

In July 1980 she sought the advice of a professor of medicine, who was strongly opposed to the use of Depo-Provera; shortly afterwards she had a miscarriage.

In April 1981 she gave birth to a second child.

She initiated an action for negligence on December 16th 1981 on the grounds shown in Box 8.2.

Box 8.2 Grounds for Mrs Blythe bringing an action

1 The assurances that she had received from the senior house officer concerning Depo-Provera were wrong and inaccurate.

2 She would not have agreed to the injection if she had been told of all the drug's side effects.

3 She had suffered damages as a consequence.

Subsequent amendments were added:

4 The Health Authority was negligent in failing to adopt a system or practice which enabled patients to receive skilled counselling, warning, or advice regarding the drug's side effects.

5 Alternatively, if there was a system, that such a system or practice was not adhered to in the plaintiff's case.

The High Court dismissed Mrs Blythe's allegations against the senior house officer, but ruled that there was a case against the Health Authority on the grounds that although it had a system or practice whereby patients who received the Depo-Provera drug could receive skilled counselling, warning and/or advice in relation to the drug's side effects, the Health Authority had failed to put its system into operation in relation to the plaintiff. She was awarded £3,600.

The Health Authority appealed to the Court of Appeal against the findings of negligence.

The Court of Appeal allowed the appeal because:

1 There was no obligation to pass on to the plaintiff all the information available to the hospital, i.e. all the information contained in the senior house officer's files.

2 What a claimant should be told in answer to a general enquiry could not be divorced from the Bolam Test any more than when no such enquiry was made.

3 Answers given must depend upon the circumstances, the nature of the enquiry, the nature of the information which was available, its reliability, relevance, and the condition of the patient.

4 The extent of the duty to give information was to be judged in the light of the state of medical knowledge in December 1978.

5 There was no rule of law that, where questions were asked or doubts expressed by a patient, a doctor was under an obligation to put the patient in possession of all the information on the subject which may be available in the files of a Consultant, who may have made a special study of the subject.

6 The amount of information to be given must depend on the circumstances – it must be governed by the Bolam Test.

INFORMATION TO PATIENT

From the House of Lords decision in the Sidaway case, although the different appeal judges had different bases for their reasoning, the basic ruling was that the amount of information which should be given to the patient would be judged according to reasonable professional practice, i.e. the Bolam Test (see Chapter 13). In the Sidaway case, the House of Lords also recognised that there could be exceptional circumstances, where a doctor could exercise a right of therapeutic privilege and withhold information from the patient because it would have an undue influence upon the decision-making of the patient. The Blythe decision shows that there is no legal expectation that a person can receive all the information which a hospital or doctor has about a particular treatment. However, the fact that the mother cannot necessarily enforce through a court of law the right to receive all relevant information should not be seen as relieving the midwife of the duty to give as full information as possible to the mother.

PEARCE V. UNITED BRISTOL HEALTHCARE NHS TRUST[4]

Mrs Pearce was expecting her sixth child. The expected date of delivery was 13th November 1991. On 27th November the baby had still not arrived, when she saw the Consultant. She begged the doctor to induce her or carry out a Caesarean. He preferred to let nature take its course, and explained to her the risks from induction and a Caesarean section. The baby died in utero sometime between 2nd and 3rd December. The delivery of a stillborn baby was induced on 4th December. Mrs Pearce brought an action alleging that the Consultant should have advised her of the increased risk of stillbirth as a result of the delay in delivery between 13th November and 27th November.

The trial judge dismissed her claim, holding that there had been no negligence on the part of the Consultant in not advising Mrs Pearce of the small risk attached to waiting for natural labour to begin. The Court of Appeal held that the experts had agreed that the risk of the child being stillborn was not a significant risk – possibly 0.1- 0.2%. The Court of Appeal stated that it would not interfere with the clinical opinion of the expert medical man responsible for treating Mrs Pearce. It accepted that there would be occasions in which the courts could decide that the expert opinion is not acceptable to the court.

In this decision, the Court of Appeal was following the ruling in the Bolitho case,[5] where the House of Lords held that there would be occasions where the courts could find that the expert opinion presented to it was not acceptable. The House of Lords held that:

'The use of the adjectives "responsible, reasonable and respectable" (in the Bolam case) all showed that the court had to be satisfied that the exponents of the body of opinion relied upon could demonstrate that such opinion had a logical basis.'

Overruling experts was seen, however, as an extreme situation.

'It would seldom be right for a judge to reach the conclusion that views held by a competent medical expert were unreasonable.'

INFORMATION ABOUT SPECIFIC RISKS

Where certain procedures are being contemplated, such as ultrasound, other screening procedures and other high technology investigations and treatment, the midwife needs to be aware of current knowledge relating to any significant risks from such procedures. Her duty is to give to the woman the information which any reasonable midwife following approved accepted practice would give, or to refer her to a person who did have the necessary information. Giving information in relation to Vitamin K is discussed in Chapter 14.

WITHHOLDING INFORMATION

The House of Lords in the Sidaway case recognised the right, in exceptional circumstances, to withhold information from a patient. These exceptional circumstances would include when the information would constitute a serious threat of psychological detriment to the patient. There is therefore no recognition at common law (i.e. judge-made law) that a patient has an absolute right to obtain all information from health professionals. This is comparable to the situation under the Data Protection Act 1998 and the statutory instruments under that Act, which permits access to health records to be refused if there is a reasonable fear that serious harm would be caused to the physical or mental health or condition of the applicant or of another patient. (This is considered in Chapter 10.) Clearly any midwife, who, in exceptional circumstances, deliberately withheld information from a patient, should have very clear justification for this decision and should ensure that there is full documentation of her actions and their justification.

Information about services available

One of the key themes in Changing Childbirth (see Chapter 6) is the importance of ensuring that the mother has full information about the range of local services and her options in relation to antenatal care, delivery and postnatal care. The specific midwife allocated to the mother (the named midwife) should ensure that she herself is conversant with the local facilities and services and gives this information to the mother. The midwife might also be involved in talking to local groups such as the National Childbirth Trust and others about the choices available, and obtaining their feedback on the services provided.

The right of the woman to access information about public services is strengthened by the Freedom of Information Act 2000 which is to be brought in over the next five years. Under Section 1 of this Act, there is a general right of access to information held by public authorities. There are many exceptions to this right, including access to personal information which comes under the Data Protection Act 1998. Section 40 of the Freedom of Information Act 2000 exempts access to personal information from the Act and the provisions of the Data Protection Act would then apply (see Chapter 10).

WRITTEN INFORMATION AND LEAFLETS

There are considerable benefits in putting in writing information which is given to the mother. This has several advantages:

- It can be useful evidence that the information was given.
- It supports information given by word of mouth and enables the woman to read through more complex information at her leisure.

– It enables the woman to follow up the information with questions on points about which she is unsure.

The midwife should have an input into the information which is provided to the mother at different stages of pregnancy. A study carried out by Brighton Health Authority into the written material provided for patients[6] showed that many of the leaflets and general information were considered unacceptable (of 356 in-house publications produced by the Department concerned, 246 items were unacceptable). They cited as a particularly poor example a leaflet for women going home after a hysterectomy, which featured on the front cover an inappropriate tasteless cartoon of a chicken wearing an apron and a chef's hat stirring a pot with the title 'Your recipe for home'. Vital information was missing and there were many misprints. As a result of the research, a code of good practice was prepared and advice from a public relations officer made available. The Code recommended the guidelines shown in Box 8.3.

Box 8.3 Brighton Health Authority. Information for patients should:

1 Have the department heading, the date and the Health Authority logo

2 Have an introduction and a list of contents with page numbers if appropriate

3 Have all text in sentences, without abbreviations, jargon, or complicated medical terms

4 Be professionally printed or at least produced on a word processor

5 Have short paragraphs with double spacing between them. Numbering of paragraphs may be helpful

6 Be photocopied from the original material

7 Be assessed by as many medical and non-medical people as possible before reproduction.

THE MOTHER IN CUSTODY

Some pregnant women receive custodial sentences and therefore may give birth whilst still in custody. The midwife may find that her professional practice is circumscribed by the conditions of the custodial arrangements. However, she should ensure through discussions with her supervisor during the antenatal period that the welfare of the mother and baby is not prejudiced by the security concerns. (The handcuffing of women prisoners during childbirth is discussed in chapter 6 in relation to Article 3 of the European Convention on Human Rights.) The High Court has held that a woman in prison is entitled to the same standard of care in relation to her pregnancy as a woman at liberty.[7]

CONCLUSION

The midwife has a responsibility as part of her duty of care to the mother to ensure that she provides to her the information which any reasonable midwife following the approved standard of care would give. She must answer the woman's questions honestly and as fully as possible and ensure that she keeps up-to-date with the information which is available. She must also be aware of her ignorance and ensure that where she does not have sufficient information to answer a woman's questions, she can refer the woman to someone who does.

QUESTIONS AND EXERCISES

1 Look at three procedures or treatments which may have to be carried out during pregnancy and confinement in the light of any possible side effects, and look carefully at the information which is given to the mother before consent is obtained.

2 Consider the information which your unit provides for the mother when pregnancy is first diagnosed. Do you consider that it is clear and sufficiently informative? Is there any additional information which you consider should be given?

3 It was held in the Sidaway case that there may be exceptional circumstances where there exists a therapeutic privilege to withhold information from a patient before consent is obtained. What circumstances do you consider relevant in the case where a Caesarean operation is being discussed?

References

1 Sidaway v. Bethlem Royal Hospital Governors and others [1985] 1 All ER 643

2 Canterbury v. Spence 464 F 2d 772 (DC, 1972)

3 Blythe v. Bloomsbury Health Authority and another Court of Appeal [1993] 4 Medical Law Report 151

4 Pearce v. United Bristol Healthcare NHS Trust [1998] n48 MLR 118 CA

5 Bolitho v. City and Hackney HA [1997] 4 All ER 771

6 Bennett J, Bridger P. 1992. *British Medical Journal*, 305(6864), 1294. Reported in *MIDIRS Midwifery Digest* March 1993 3(1)

7 Brooks v. Home Office. Times Law Report 17 February 1999

Chapter 9
LETTING DIE AND EUTHANASIA

In the last two chapters we looked at different aspects of consent. In this chapter we look at the law relating to the letting die of another individual, in relation to both the mother and the baby.

The care of neonates can give rise to legal issues or sometimes present midwives with the problem of whether there is a duty in law to carry out every possible procedure known to science in order to save the life of the baby, or whether the law allows a person to be allowed to die. In addition, the midwife needs to know what if any rights the parents have in such circumstances: if they wish the baby to be allowed to die, would the professionals be acting illegally to go against their wishes? This chapter also looks at the law relating to euthanasia and the duty of care in keeping a patient alive.

VOLUNTARY EUTHANASIA

Voluntary euthanasia means the killing of a person with that person's consent. This is unlawful. It could amount to murder which is punishable on conviction by life imprisonment. Alternatively, if the act amounts to assistance in a suicide bid, then it is illegal under section 2(1) of the Suicide Act 1961 which is shown in Box 9.1.

Box 9.1 Assisting a person to commit suicide

A person who aids, abets, counsels or procures the suicide of another or an attempt by another to commit suicide, shall be liable on conviction on indictment to imprisonment (up to 14 years).

The High Court has stated in the Diane Pretty case that the Director of Public Prosecutions has no power to pardon in advance a person who wished to aid and abet the suicide of another.

Mrs Pretty was suffering from motor neurone disease and had very little movement left. She wanted her husband to be given permission to assist her in ending her life,[1] so that she would be spared the suffering and indignity that she would otherwise have to endure. She was unable to take her own life without assistance. The High Court held that Articles 2 and 3 of the European Convention on Human Rights did not give a right to procure one's own death or confer a right to die. In addition, Articles 8 and 9 were not absolute rights and did not give her a right to die. There was no incompatibility between the provisions of the Suicide Act 1961 and the articles of the European Convention of Human Rights in these circumstances. On 1 November 2001 she was given leave to appeal to the House of Lords. She lost her appeal. The House of Lords held that the refusal to grant immunity was not an infringement of Articles 2, 3, 8, 9 or 14 of the European Convention on Human Rights. Any change in the law relating to aiding and abetting a suicide must be enacted through Parliament.[2]

Even where the parents wish a grossly handicapped baby to die, any professional who intentionally speeded up the process of death could be guilty of causing the death of the child. In the case of R v. Arthur[3] a paediatrician was prosecuted for attempting to cause the death of a grossly handicapped baby who was suffering from Down's Syndrome and who had other disabilities when he prescribed dihydro-codeine and nursing care only. The judge stated that

'There is no special law in this country that places doctors in a separate category and gives them extra protection over the rest of us... Neither in law is there any special power, facility or license to kill children who are handicapped or seriously disadvantaged in an irreversible way.'

Dr Arthur was acquitted.

THE CASE OF DR NIGEL COX[4]

Dr Nigel Cox, a rheumatologist in Winchester, was convicted of causing the death of a patient to whom he had administered potassium chloride. He was given a suspended prison sentence. The patient was in crippling pain, and terminally ill, and her relatives were concerned at her condition. Dr Cox was also brought before his employers, the Wessex Regional Health Authority to face disciplinary proceedings, but retained his post. He was also brought before professional conduct proceedings of the General Medical Council, but stayed on the Register.

PAIN RELIEF AND CAUSING DEATH

THE CASE OF DR BODKIN ADAMS

In contrast to the case of Dr Cox, Dr Bodkin Adams was acquitted following a trial where it was alleged that he had caused the death of Mrs Morell, a resident in a nursing home in Eastbourne, by giving her excessive morphine.

The trial judge, Mr Justice Patrick Devlin, directed the jury that:

'There has been a good deal of discussion about the circumstances in which a doctor might be justified in giving drugs which would shorten life in cases of severe pain. It is my duty to tell you that the law knows of no special defence of this character. But that does not mean that a doctor aiding the sick or dying has to calculate in minutes or hours, or perhaps in days or weeks, the effect on a patient's life of the medicines which he administers. If the first purpose of medicine – the restoration of health – can no longer be achieved, there is still much for the doctor to do, and he is entitled to do all that is proper and necessary to relieve pain and suffering, even if the measures he takes may incidentally shorten life... It remains a law, that no doctor has the right to cut off life deliberately... What counsel for the defence was saying, was that the treatment that was given by the doctor was designed to promote comfort, and if it was the right and proper treatment of the case, the fact that incidentally it shortened life does not give any grounds for convicting him of murder.' [5]

This ruling still applies today. However, note would be taken of what is 'right and proper treatment'. It could be that a very high dose of morphine was justified for a patient who needed that level to achieve pain relief, whereas that dose for a person who had not become resistant to morphine would be lethal and grossly reckless, and justify a criminal conviction. 'Right and proper treatment' must also take into account current research on effective pain management.

Annie Lindsell, a sufferer from motor neurone disease, brought a court action for a declaration that her GP could administer palliative drugs which could have the effect of shortening her life. She was told that a responsible body of medical opinion supported her doctor's treatment plan and she then withdrew her application for the court's intervention.[6] She died a few months later.

DISTINCTION BETWEEN KILLING AND LETTING DIE

Do these cases mean that it is never lawful to permit a patient to die, whatever the circumstances of his/her condition? The answer is that the law does not expect constant medical intervention whatever the prognosis, and that in certain circumstances it is legally permissible to let die. A distinction is however drawn between letting die and killing. Examples from decided cases will illustrate the difference.

RE B (1981)[7]

A child was born suffering from Down's syndrome and an intestinal blockage. She required an operation to relieve the obstruction if she was to live more than a few days. If the operation were performed, the child might die within a few months, but it was probable that her life expectancy would be 20 to 30 years. Her parents, having decided that it would be kinder to allow her to die rather than live as a physically and mentally handicapped person, refused to consent to the operation. The local authority made the child a ward of court and, when a surgeon decided that the wishes of the parents should be respected, they sought an order authorising the operation to be performed by other named surgeons. The judge decided that the parents' wishes should be respected and refused to make the order. The local authority appealed to the Court of Appeal which allowed the appeal. It stated that

1. The question for the court was whether it was in the best interests of the child that she should have the operation and not whether the parents' wishes should be respected.

2. Since the effect of the operation might be that the child would have the normal span of life of a mongol, and

3. Since it had not been demonstrated that the life of a mongol was of such a nature that the child should be condemned to die,

4. The court would make an order that the operation be performed.

Crucial to the decision in this case was the prognosis of the child.

RE C (1989)[8]

In a contrasting case, a baby was born suffering from congenital hydrocephalus and had been made a ward of court for reasons unconnected with her medical condition. The local authority sought the court's determination as to the appropriate manner in which she should be treated, should she contract a serious infection, or her existing feeding regimes become unviable. A specialist paediatrician assessed C's condition as severely and irreversibly brain-damaged, the prognosis of which was hopeless. He recommended that the objective of any treatment should therefore be to ease suffering rather than prolong life. While not specifying the adoption or discontinuance of any particular procedures, he further advised consultation with C's carers as to the appropriate method of achieving that objective. The judge accepted this report and approved the recommendations as being in her best interests. Paragraph 3 of his order is shown in Box 9.2, but subsequently on reflection the judge amended it to that shown in Box 9.3.

Box 9.2 Judge's initial order in Re C

The hospital authority shall be at liberty to treat the minor to die and... shall administer such treatment to the minor as might relieve her from pain, suffering and distress inter alia by sedation... but it shall not be necessary either

(a) to prescribe and administer antibiotics to treat any serious infection which the minor might contract or

(b) to set up intravenous or nasal feeding regimes for the minor.

Box 9.3 Amendment to judge's order in Re C

For the words 'to die'

(To treat the minor) 'to allow her life to come to an end peacefully and with dignity.'

The official solicitor who had been appointed guardian ad litem of the child appealed to the Court of Appeal on the grounds that the judge had no jurisdiction and was plainly wrong in the exercise of his discretion to make an order that the hospital be at liberty to treat the minor to die. He also appealed on the grounds that by Paragraph 3 of his order the judge had seemed to provide that in no circumstances should certain treatments be undertaken, such direction being inconsistent with Paragraph 4.

The Court of Appeal changed the wording of the order by the deletion of Paragraph 3 but otherwise upheld the judge's decision (Box 9.4).

Box 9.4 Court of Appeal's decision in Re C

1. Whole of paragraph 3 to be deleted because it was inconsistent with Paragraph 4

4. Paragraph 4 to stand

'The hospital to continue to treat the minor within the parameters of the opinion expressed by [the specialist paediatrician] in his report of 13.4.1989 which report is not to be disclosed to any person other than the health authority.'

This case raised many issues:

1. What is meant by the best interests of the child?

2. What is the role of the doctor?

3. What is the role of the registered midwife/nurse?

4. What rights do the parents have?

5. What is the role of the courts?

1. The best interests of the child are determined by what the professionals, following the Bolam Test, would consider appropriate in the light of the specific circumstances of that individual child. It is clear that heroic surgery and medical intervention will not necessarily always be in the best interests of the child, and the court is unwilling to direct specialists over what should be done, preferring to leave the actual decisions to the clinical judgement. (See below the case of Re J 1992.)

2. The doctor has a duty to make a clinical assessment, following the reasonable standard of care.

3. The role of the midwife/neonatal nurse is to ensure that she provides all the relevant information to the doctor and takes a full part in the multi-disciplinary discussions relating to the future of the baby. She is likely to have greater contact with the parents and should ensure that they have support and if necessary counselling to cope with the decisions which are made.

4. The parents do not have the right to insist that treatment ends for the child, or even that treatment is commenced. Their participation in the clinical decisions which are made is however essential and the midwife/neonatal nurse will have an important role to play in this.

5. There has recently been a spate of referrals of decisions relating to neonates to the court. This is not always the most appropriate forum for such decisions to be made and the legislation which may follow the Law Commission's recommendations on decision making and the mentally incapacitated adult (see Chapter 33) may bring about changes in this respect.

RE J (1990)[9]

The baby was a ward of court. In contrast with the case of Re C, the baby was not at the point of death. However, the prognosis was not good and although he was expected to survive a few years he was likely to be blind, deaf, unable to speak and have serious spastic quadriplegia. The judge made an order that he should be treated with antibiotics if he developed a chest infection, but if he were to stop breathing he should not receive artificial ventilation. The official solicitor on behalf of the child appealed against the order on the grounds that unless the situation was one of terminal illness, or it was certain that the child's life would be intolerable, the court was not justified in approving the withholding of life-saving treatment. The court held that the court can never sanction positive steps to terminate the life of a person. However, the court could direct that treatment, without which death would ensue, need not be given to prolong life, even though he was neither on the point of death or dying. The Court had to undertake a balancing exercise in assessing the course to be adopted in the best interests of the child, looked at from his point of view and giving the fullest possible weight to his desire, if he were in a position to make a sound judgement to survive, and taking into account the pain and suffering and quality of life which he would experience if life was prolonged, and the pain and suffering involved in the proposed treatment.

CAN THE COURT ORDER DOCTORS TO TREAT?

RE J (1992)[10]

J was born in January 1991 and suffered an accidental fall when he was a month old, with the result that he was profoundly handicapped both mentally and physically. He was severely microcephalic, his brain not having grown sufficiently following the injury. He also had severe cerebral palsy, cortical blindness and severe epilepsy. He was in general fed by a nasal gastric tube. Medical opinion was unanimous that J was unlikely to develop much beyond his present functioning, that that level might deteriorate and that his expectation of life, although uncertain, would be short. The paediatrician's report stated that given J's condition it would not be medically appropriate to intervene with intensive procedures such as artificial ventilation if he were to suffer a life-threatening event. The baby was in the care of foster parents with whom the local authority shared responsibility. The local authority applied to the court under Section 100 of the Children Act 1989 to determine whether ventilation should be given to the child. The judge had regarded J's best interests as well as the interests of justice in preserving his life as both pointing in favour of the grant of an interim injunction requiring such treatment to take place. The mother supported the requirement that the hospital and doctors should be forced to put the baby on a life support machine.

Lord Donaldson, Master of the Rolls, stated that he could not at present conceive of any circumstances in which to require a medical practitioner, or Health Authority acting by a medical practitioner, to adopt a course of treatment which in the bona fide clinical judgement of the practitioner was contra-indicated as not being in the patient's best interests, that would be other than abuse of power as directly or indirectly requiring the practitioner to act contrary to the fundamental duty he owed to his patient.

Lord Donaldson said that the order of the judge, ordering specific treatment to take place, was wholly inconsistent with the law as stated in Re J and in Re R and could not be justified on the basis of any known authority. It was also erroneous on two other substantial grounds:

a. its lack of certainty as to what was required of the Health Authority, and

b. its failure adequately to take account of the sad fact of life that Health Authorities might on occasion find that they had too few resources, either human or material or both, to treat all the patients whom they would like to treat in the way they would like to treat them. It was their duty to make choices. The court would have no knowledge of competing claims to a Health Authority's resources and was in no position to express any view on their deployment.

The Court of Appeal thus held that where a paediatrician caring for a severely handicapped baby considered that mechanical ventilation procedures would not be appropriate, the court would not grant an injunction requiring such treatment to take place.

The effect of the Court's decision to set aside the judge's ruling, was to leave the Health Authority and its medical staff free, subject to consent not being withdrawn, to treat J in accordance with their best clinical judgement. That did not mean that in no circumstances should J be subjected to mechanical ventilation.

- The Court of Appeal affirmed the freedom of doctors to decide for themselves what is the best treatment.

- The Court showed its reluctance to interfere in medical practice.

LETTING DIE AND HUMAN RIGHTS

In a recent case it was argued that letting a baby die was contrary to Article 3 of the European Convention on Human Rights (see Chapter 6 and Appendix 1). The court, however, held that it was not contrary to the human rights of a severely handicapped baby to allow him to die.[11] Where parents disagree with the medical decision that it is in the interests of a grossly handicapped child to let him die, the case should be referred to the court.

In a case in Portsmouth, relatives of a severely disabled boy fought with staff over the treatment proposed, believing that the doctors had decided that the child should be allowed to die.[12] The Court of Appeal refused to give an advance order over what should be decided at a future time, but stated that in the event of a dispute between parents and doctors there should be an application to court to determine what was in the best interests of the child. Subsequently relatives were prosecuted for assault.

GUIDANCE ON LETTING DIE

The Royal College of Paediatrics and Child Health has published guidelines on when it is appropriate to withhold or withdraw medical treatment.[13] The guidelines distinguish between the following clinical situations:

– The brain dead child

– The persistent vegetative state

– The 'no chance' situation

– The 'no purpose' situation

– The 'unbearable' situation

In all these situations, the possibility of withholding or withdrawal of curative medical treatment might be considered. The guidance emphasises the importance of the fundamental principles of the duty of care and partnership of care and the respect for the rights of the child as set out in the United Nations Convention on the Rights of the Child.[14] The guidelines of the Royal College of Paediatrics and Child Health represent its interpretation of the law, but are not the law itself. Further advice has been published by the British Medical Association.[15] Reference could also be made to Chapter 6 in the BMA's recent book on consent and the rights of children and young people.[16]

AIREDALE NHS TRUST V. BLAND (1993)[17]

The House of Lords had to decide if it was lawful to permit artificial feeding to be discontinued in the case of a patient in a persistent vegetative state. The patient was a victim of the football stadium crush at Hillsborough and it was established that although he could breathe and digest food independently, he could not see, hear, taste, smell or communicate in any way and it appeared that there was no hope of recovery or improvement. The House of Lords decided that it would be in the best interests of the patient to discontinue the nasal gastric feed and he was later reported as having died. The House of Lords recommended that if any similar decisions were required to be made in the future, there should be application before the courts.

In two recent cases it was argued on behalf of women in a persistent vegetative state that it was contrary to their right to life under Article 2 of the European Convention of Human Rights for artificial feeding to be discontinued. The President of the

Family Division, Dame Elizabeth Butler-Sloss held that the withdrawal of life-sustaining medical treatment was not contrary to Article 2 of the Human Rights Convention and the right to life, where the patient was in a persistent vegetative state. The ruling was made on 25th October 2000 in cases involving Mrs M, aged 49 years, who suffered brain damage during an operation abroad in 1997 and was diagnosed as being in a persistent vegetative state (PVS) in October 1998 and Mrs H, 36, who fell ill in America as a result of pancreatitis at Christmas 1999.[18]

In 1994 the Select Committee of the House of Lords reported[19] that there should be no change in the law to permit euthanasia. The report's recommendations are shown in Box 9.5.

Box 9.5 Recommendations of Select Committee of House of Lords on Medical Ethics

1. No change in law to permit euthanasia.

2. Right of competent patient to refuse consent to any medical treatment is strongly endorsed.

3. Full reasons must be given if an individual refusal of treatment by a competent person is overruled by the courts.

4. Development and growth of palliative care services in hospitals and in the community strongly commended.

5. Withholding of treatment which would give relief is not justified, as long as the doctor acts in accordance with responsible medical practice with the objective of relieving pain or distress, and without the intention to kill.

6. Treatment-limiting decisions should be made jointly by all involved in the care of a patient.

7. Definition of PVS and the development of a code of practice relating to its management.

8. Development and acceptance of the idea that, in certain circumstances, some treatments may be inappropriate may make it unnecessary to consider the withdrawal of hydration and nutrition.

9. Treatment-limiting decisions should not be determined by considerations of resource availability.

10. Rejection of euthanasia as an option for the individual entails a compelling ▶

▶

social responsibility to care adequately for those who are elderly, dying or disabled.

11. Palliative care should be made more widely available.

12. Research into pain relief and symptom control should be adequately supported.

13. Training for healthcare professionals should prepare them for ethical responsibilities.

14. Long-term care of dependent people should have special regard to maintenance of individual dignity.

15. Proposal for the creation of a new judicial forum with power to make decisions about medical treatment for incompetent patients.

16. The creation of a new offence of mercy killing is not recommended.

17. Mandatory life sentence for murder should be abolished.

18. No change in the law on assisted suicide is recommended.

19. Commends the development of advance directives, but concludes that legislation for advance directives generally is unnecessary.

20. Code of practice on advance directives should be developed.

21. Do not favour the more widespread development of a system of proxy decision-making.

LIVING WILLS/ADVANCE REFUSAL OR DIRECTIVE

A mentally competent person can decide in advance that at a subsequent time he or she would not wish to have treatment. At present we do not have any statutory provision (i.e. Act of Parliament) recognising living wills. They would however be recognised at common law (i.e. judge-made law, or case law). This was stated by the House of Lords in the Tony Bland case.[20] Living wills, also known as advance refusals, or advance directives, are designed to convey the wishes of an adult, when mentally competent, to cover a future occasion when mental competence is lacking. The British Medical Association has published a Code of Practice for its members on advance statements about medical treatment.[21] It gives guidance on the law in relation to consent to medical treatment and advance statements and advice on the drafting and contents of an advance statement. It emphasises that there must be no pressure on patients. It also gives guidance about determining the patient's capacity to make decisions. The responsibility for storing an advance directive is upon the individual but it is suggested that a copy should be given to the general practitioner. Finally a checklist is provided for making an advance directive and this is shown in Box 9.6.

Box 9.6 British Medical Association checklist for writing an advance statement

In drawing up an advance statement you must ensure, as a minimum, that the following information is included:

– Full name

– Address

– Name and address of general practitioner

– Whether advice was sought from health professionals

– Signature

– Date drafted and reviewed

– Witness signature

– A clear statement of your wishes, either general or specific

– The name, address and telephone number of your nominated person, if you have one.

NOT FOR RESUSCITATION INSTRUCTIONS

It follows from what has been said that a competent adult patient can request that there should be no resuscitation. This can be made either by means of an advance refusal or by refusing resuscitation when admitted for that particular course of treatment. For example, a man of 19 years[22] who was suffering from motor neurone disease sought a declaration from the court that it would be lawful to comply with his request to discontinue, two weeks from the date that he lost the ability to communicate, the artificial ventilation and the artificial nutrition and hydration which was being provided to him. He was able to communicate solely by the movement of one eyelid but this movement would shortly cease. The judge granted the declaration, holding that a patient's refusal to consent to medical treatment had to be observed where that patient was an adult of full capacity. In this case the man was of full capacity and had clearly communicated his wishes. Such a decision was not contrary to the Human Rights Act.

However, where the patient is mentally incompetent and has made no advance refusal, then the professional has a duty to take all reasonable care of the patient, and in certain cases this may involve providing resuscitation. If the prognosis is good, and there is no valid refusal of treatment by the patient, failure to resuscitate could in certain circumstances be a criminal act. Where, however, the clinician is of the view that the prognosis is extremely poor, a Not For Resuscitation (NFR) or Do Not (Attempt) Resuscitate(ion) (DN(A)R) instruction is valid. Difficulties can arise, where such instructions are not given in writing by doctors to nursing staff or where nurses have not had an input into the decision-making and are not aware of, or disagree with, the basis of the NFR/DN(A)R instruction. A report has been issued by the Royal College of Nursing[23] which sets out the moral and legal issues and strongly endorses the involvement of the healthcare professional team as well as the patient, relatives and friends.[24] The views of relatives may be relevant to the decision and certainly any evidence they can give of the patient's wishes will be important, but the relatives do not have the right in law to give or withhold consent to resuscitation.

PROFESSIONAL ADVICE AND GUIDANCE ON NFR

Prior to the implementation of the Human Rights Act 1998 the Department of Health drew attention to guidance which had been drawn up by the Resuscitation Council, the Royal College of Nursing and the British Medical Association.[25] This guidance was commended to NHS Trusts in September 2000 by the NHS Executive[26] in an NHS Circular. By this circular, Chief Executives of NHS Trusts are required to ensure that appropriate resuscitation policies which respect patients' rights are in place, understood by all relevant staff, and accessible to those who need them and that such policies are subject to appropriate audit and monitoring arrangements. The action required to be taken by NHS trusts is shown in Box 9.7. The Commission for Health Improvement (CHI) has been asked by the Secretary of State to pay particular attention to resuscitation decision-making processes as part of its rolling programme of reviews of clinical governance arrangements put in place by NHS organisations. Guidance emphasises that there must be no blanket policies, each individual patient must be assessed personally and policy cannot depend solely on the age of the patient.

Box 9.7 Resuscitation policies: Action to be taken by NHS trusts

- Patients' rights are central to decision-making on resuscitation

- The trust has an agreed resuscitation policy in place which respects patients' rights

- The policy is published and readily available to those who may wish to consult it, including patients, families and carers

- Appropriate arrangements are in place for ensuring that all staff who may be involved in resuscitation decisions understand and implement the policy

- Appropriate supervision arrangements are in place to review the resuscitation decisions

- Induction and staff development programmes cover the resuscitation policy

- Clinical practice in this area is regularly audited

- Clinical audit outcomes are reported in the trust's annual clinical governance report

- A non-executive Director of the trust is given designated responsibility on behalf of the Trust Board to ensure that a resuscitation policy is agreed, implemented, and regularly reviewed within the clinical governance framework.

According to the guidelines, cardiopulmonary resuscitation (CPR) should only be withheld in the following four situations:

- The mentally competent patient has refused treatment.

- A valid living will covering such circumstances has been made by the patient.

- Effective cardiopulmonary resuscitation (CPR) is unlikely to be successful.

- Successful CPR is likely to be followed by a length and quality of life which would not be in the best interests of the patient to sustain.

The court considered the validity of a DNR instruction in the case of a seriously disabled boy with malformation of the brain and cerebral palsy who had developed severe epilepsy, was blind, incontinent, and had other major disabilities, who at the time of the hearing was 23 years old.[27] The court held that in the light of the medical evidence the overriding principle was that the boy's life was so afflicted as to be intolerable and that it was not in the best interests of the boy to be subjected to cardiopulmonary resuscitation in the event of his suffering a cardiac arrest. This view was supported by the boy's parents. The court held that the DNR instruction was justifiable since CPR was unlikely to be successful.

In March 2001 the BMA, the Resuscitation Council (UK) and the RCN issued a joint statement.[28] It emphasised the importance of each health organisation having a resuscitation policy according to the principles set out in the guidance.

The laws relating to the removal, retention and storage of body parts and tissue are considered in Chapter 25.

CONCLUSIONS

The difference between giving a patient potassium chloride, as Dr Cox did, which is declared unlawful, and doctors being permitted lawfully to disconnect the feeding tube of a patient such as Tony Bland, is not always easy to understand. In fact, to some philosophers there is no moral difference.

However, the House of Lords in enabling the tube-feeding to be discontinued allowed the natural situation of the patient to take over. In contrast, in the Cox case, the administration of the drug was an unlawful act.

Failure to act, or an omission, could be evidence of negligence or a crime when there is a recognised legal duty to act. In the Bland case, the House of Lords considered that, given the best interests of the patient, the duty to continue active treatment had ended. Any such decisions should be brought before the court to ensure that the best interests of the patient are identified and that the patient is represented.

QUESTIONS AND EXERCISES

1 In which circumstances do you consider that it should be lawful to let a baby die?

2 Do you consider that a lack of resources could be a justifiable reason for letting a baby die?

3 An abortion of a fetus suffering from congenital disabilities results in a live birth. Do you consider that there should be a duty to keep that baby alive? What is the law? (Refer also to Chapter 26)

4 A woman wishes to draw up an advanced refusal of clinical interventions during her pregnancy and labour. What should such a statement contain to be lawfully valid?

5 Women who have been injured whilst pregnant have been kept on life support systems in order that the baby can survive. Do you consider that this practise raises any legal issues?

References

1 R (Pretty) v. Director of Public Prosecutions and another, Medical Ethics Alliance and others, interveners. Times Law Report 23 October 2001

2 R (Pretty) v. Director of Public Prosecution, Secretary of State for the Home Department intervening. Times Law Report 5 December 2001

3 R v. Arthur. The Times 6 November 1981

4 R v. Cox. The Times 22 September 1992; [1992] 12 BMLR 38

5 Bedford S. 1961. *The Best We Can Do.* Harmondsworth: Penguin Books

6 Wilkins E. 1997. Dying woman granted wish for dignified death. *The Times,* October 29 1997

7 Re B (a minor)(wardship; medical treatment) [1981] 1 WLR 1421

8 Re C (a minor)(wardship; medical treatment) [1989] 2 All ER 782

9 Re J (a minor)(wardship; medical treatment) [1990] 3 All ER 930

10 Re J. Times Law Report June 12 1992

11 A National Health Service Trust v. D. Times Law Report 19 July 2000; [2000] Lloyds Rep Med 411

12. R v. Portsmouth Hospitals NHS Trust ex parte Glass [1999] 50 BMLR 269

13 Royal College of Paediatrics and Child Health. 1997. *Withholding or Withdrawing Life Saving Treatment in Children.* London: RCPCH

14 United Nations. 1989. Convention on the Rights of the Child

15 British Medical Association. 2000. *Withholding and Withdrawing Life-Prolonging Medical Treatment.* 2nd edition. London: BMJ Books

16 British Medical Association. 2001. *Consent, Rights and Choices in Health Care for Children and Young People.* London: BMJ Books

17. Airedale NHS Trust v. Bland [1993] 1 All ER 821

18 Gibb F. 2000. Rights Act does not bar mercy killing. *The Times,* 26 October 2000; NHS Trust A v. Mrs M and NHS Trust B v. Mrs H Family Division [2001] Lloyd's Rep Med 27

19 Report of the Select Committee on Medical Ethics: House of Lords Session 1993-4. London: HMSO

20 Airedale NHS Trust v. Bland House of Lords [1993] 1 All ER 821

21 British Medical Association. 1995. Advance Statements about medical treatment: Code of Practice

22 Re AK (adult patient)(medical treatment: consent) [2001] 1 FLR 129

23 Royal College of Nursing. 1992. *Resuscitation: Right or Wrong? The moral and legal issues faced by healthcare professionals.* London: RCN

24 Dimond B. 1992. Not for resuscitative treatment. *British Journal of Nursing,* 1(2), 93-4

25 British Medical Association, Resuscitation Council (UK) and the Royal College of Nursing. 1999. *Decisions Relating to Cardiopulmonary Resuscitation.* London: BMA

26 NHS Executive. 2000. Resuscitation Policy. HSC 2000/028

27 Re R (adult: medical treatment) [1996] 31 BMLR 127

28 British Medical Association, Resuscitation Council (UK) and the Royal College of Nursing. 2001. *Decisions relating to cardiopulmonary resuscitation: A joint statement from the BMA, Resuscitation Council (UK) and the RCN.* London: BMA

Chapter 10
CONFIDENTIALITY AND ACCESS TO RECORDS

This chapter deals with two aspects of record keeping: the duty to maintain the confidentiality of information obtained by and about the client; and the right of the client to access information held about her. They are both regulated by the Data Protection Act 1998 and statutory instruments made under that Act. Guidance is provided by the UKCC for its registered practitioners.[1]

DATA PROTECTION LEGISLATION

The European Directive on Data Protection[2] was implemented in this country by the Data Protection Act 1998. Member states were required to comply with its provisions by 24th October 1998 although the UK did not meet this target. Under the legislation members had to establish a set of principles with which users of personal information must comply. The legislation also gives individuals the right to gain access to information held about them and provides for a supervisory authority to oversee and enforce the law. NHS guidance on the Act was provided by a circular in March 2000[3] and the NHS Information Authority action plan for the NHS is available on its website to ensure the processing of personal data within the organisation is in compliance with the Act.[4]

The Data Protection Act 1998 made significant changes to the 1984 Act. The most important change is that the 1998 Act applies to certain manual records (if they form part of a relevant filing system) as well as to computerised records. Most health records would therefore come under Data Protection legislation provisions. A possible exception to manual records not coming under Data Protection provisions are the supervision records kept by the supervisor of records in which specific patients are named. These may not come under the provisions of the Data Protection Act since they may not form part of a relevant filing system. However, a court decision on the interpretation of 'relevant filing system' is required to clarify the point. In 2001 an Information Commissioner was appointed to fulfil duties under both the Freedom of Information Act 2000 (see below) and the Data Protection Act 1998.

HUMAN RIGHTS

The Data Protection Act 1998 must after 2nd October 2000 be read in conjunction with the Human Rights Act 1998 (see Chapter 6 and Appendix 1), since Article 8 of the European Convention of Human Rights, which is set out in Schedule 1 of the Act, recognises an individual's right to privacy, subject to specific qualifications. The right to respect for privacy is to be balanced against Article 10 and the right to freedom of expression.

DATA PROTECTION ACT 1998

The main provisions of the Act are shown in Box 10.1.

Box 10.1 Data Protection Act 1998

- Part 1 Preliminary: basic interpretative provisions; sensitive personal data; the special purposes; data protection principles; application of Act; Commissioner and Tribunal

- Part 2 Rights of data subjects and others:
  - Rights of access
  - Rights to prevent processing likely to cause damage or distress
  - Rights to prevent processing for direct marketing
  - Rights in relation to automated decision-taking
  - Compensation for failure to comply with certain requirements
  - Rectification, blocking, erasure and destruction

- Part 3 Notification to the Data Controller: duty to notify; register of notifications; offences; preliminary assessment by Commissioner; power to make provision for appointment of data protection supervisors; duty of certain data controllers to make certain information available; functions of Commissioner in relation to making of notification regulations; fees regulations.

- Part 4 Exemptions:
  - National security
  - Crime and taxation
  - Health, education and social work
  - Regulatory activity
  - Journalism, literature and art
  - Research, history and statistics
  - Information available to the public by or under enactment
  - Disclosure required by law or made in connection with legal proceedings
  - Domestic purposes
  - Powers to make further exemptions by order

▶

- Part 5 Enforcement

- Part 6 Miscellaneous and general: Functions of the Commissioner

- Schedule 1 Data protection principles

- Schedule 2 Conditions for processing any personal data

- Schedule 3 Conditions for processing sensitive personal data

- Schedule 4 Cases where the 8th principle does not apply

- Schedule 5 Data Protection Commissioner and Data Protection Tribunal

- Schedule 6 Appeal proceedings

- Schedule 7 Miscellaneous exemptions

- Schedule 8 Transitional relief

- Schedule 9 Powers of entry and inspection

- Schedule 10 Assistance under Section 53

- Schedule 11 Educational records

- Schedule 12 Accessible public records

- Schedule 13 Modifications of Act having effect pre 24 October 2007

TERMINOLOGY

The following are definitions of terms used in the Data Protection Act 1998.

- The 'data subject' is 'the individual who is the subject of personal data.' Under the 1998 provisions, the law applies only to living people and if the information is anonymous, then the person will not be considered to be identifiable, unless it is possible to link together separate items of information in order to identify an individual. If that is possible, the Act would then apply.

- 'Processing' under the 1998 Act includes any operation involving personal data including the holding of the information.

– The term 'data user' (from the 1984 Act) is replaced by the term 'controller' and is the person who determines the purposes for which and the manner in which any personal data are to be processed.

– 'Computer bureaux' is replaced by 'processor'.

– The 'Data Protection Registrar', who is the national officer responsible for the oversight of the implementation of the law, is now to be known as the Commissioner.

DATA PROTECTION PRINCIPLES

The 1998 Act slightly amends the Data Protection Principles and the new wording is shown in Box 10.2.

Box 10.2 Data Protection Principles 1998 Schedule 1 Part 1

1. Personal data shall be processed fairly and lawfully and, in particular, shall not be processed unless:

    (a) at least one of the conditions in Schedule 2 is met; and

    (b) in the case of sensitive personal data, at least one of the conditions in Schedule 3 is also met.

2. Personal data shall be obtained only for one or more specified and lawful purposes, and shall not be further processed in any manner incompatible with that purpose or those purposes.

3. Personal data shall be adequate, relevant and not excessive in relation to the purpose or purposes for which they are processed.

4. Personal data shall be accurate and, where necessary, kept up-to-date.

5. Personal data processed for any purpose or purposes shall not be kept for longer that is necessary for that purpose(s).

6. Personal data shall be processed in accordance with the rights of data subjects under this Act.

7. Appropriate technical and organisational measures shall be taken against unauthorised or unlawful processing of personal data and against accidental loss or destruction of, or damage to, personal data.

▶

▶
8. Personal data shall not be transferred to a country or territory outside the European Economic Area unless that country or territory ensures an adequate level of protection for the rights and freedoms of data subjects in relation to the processing of personal data.

Interpretation of these principles is provided in Part 2 of Schedule 1 of the 1998 Act.

Principle 1 refers to Schedule 2 conditions and these include:

– The consent of the data subject

– The processing is necessary:

    - for the performance of a contract to which the data subject is a party

    - for taking steps, at the request of the data subject, to enter a contract

– The processing is necessary for compliance with a legal obligation of the data subject

– The processing is necessary to protect the vital interests of the data subject

– The processing is necessary

    - for the administration of justice

    - for the exercise of functions conferred by any enactment

    - for the exercise of a function of the Crown, Minister or government department, or

    - for the exercise of other functions of a public nature

– The processing is necessary to meet the legitimate interests of the data controller or a third party.

Clearly patient records are covered by several of these conditions, only one of which is needed to legitimise the processing.

SENSITIVE PERSONAL DATA

Sensitive personal data is defined in Section 2. See Box 10.3.

Box 10.3 Section 2 of Data Protection Act 1998

Sensitive personal data means personal data consisting of information as to:

- The racial or ethnic origin of the data subject

- His political opinions

- His religious beliefs or other beliefs of a similar nature

- Whether he is a member of a Trade Union

- His physical or mental health or condition

- His sexual life

- The (alleged) commission of any offence by him, or

- Any proceedings for any (alleged) offence, disposal of such or sentence.

Records relating to physical or mental health come within the definition of sensitive personal data and Schedule 3, conditions for disclosure of such information, is shown in Box 10.4.

Box 10.4 Schedule 3 Conditions for disclosure of sensitive personal data

1. The data subject has given his explicit consent to the processing of personal data

2.   (1) The processing is necessary for the purposes of exercising or performing any right or obligation which is conferred or imposed on the data controller in connection with employment.

   (2) The Secretary of State may exclude the application of sub-paragraph 1 in such cases as may be specified, or specify further conditions for satisfaction.

3. The processing is necessary:

   (a) to protect the vital interests of the data subject or another person, in a case where:

      i.   consent cannot be given by or on behalf of the data subject, or

      ii.   the data controller cannot reasonably be expected to obtain the consent or the data subject, or

  (b) in order to protect the vital interests of another person, in a case where consent by or on behalf of the data subject has been unreasonably withheld.

4. The processing:

  (a) is carried out in the course of its legitimate activities by any body or association which:

      i.   is not established or conducted for profit, and

      ii.   exists for political, philosophical, religious or trade union purposes

  (b) is carried out with appropriate safeguards for the rights and freedoms of the data subject

  (c) relates only to individuals who either are members of the body or association or have regular contact with it in connection with its purposes, and

  (d) does not involve disclosure of the personal data to a third party without the consent of the data subject.

5. The information contained in the personal data has been made public as a result of steps deliberately taken by the data subject.

6. The processing:

  (a) is necessary for the purpose of, or in connection with, any legal proceedings (including prospective legal proceedings)

  (b) is necessary for the purpose of obtaining legal advice, or

  (c) is otherwise necessary for the purposes of establishing, exercising or defending legal rights.

7. (1) The processing is necessary:

  (a) for the administration of justice

(b) for the exercise of any functions conferred on any person by or under an enactment, or

(c) for the exercise of any functions of the Crown, Minister of the Crown or a government department

7. (2) The Secretary of State may by order:

(a) exclude the application of sub-paragraph (1) in such cases as may be specified, or

(b) provide that, in such cases as may be specified, the condition in sub-paragraph (1) is not to be regarded as satisfied unless such further conditions as may be specified in the order are also satisfied.

8. (1) The processing is for medical purposes and is undertaken by:

(a) a health professional, or

(b) a person who in the circumstances owes a duty of confidentiality which is equivalent to that which would arise if that person were a health professional.

8. (2) In this paragraph, 'medical purposes' includes the purposes of preventative medicine, medical diagnosis, medical research, the provision of care and treatment and the management of healthcare services.

9. (1) The processing:

(a) is of sensitive personal data consisting of information as to racial or ethnic origin.

(b) Is necessary for the purpose of identifying or keeping under review the existence or absence of equality of opportunity or treatment between persons of different racial or ethnic origins, with a view to enabling such equality to be promoted or maintained, and

(c) Is carried out with appropriate safeguards for the rights and freedoms of data subjects.

9. (2) The Secretary of State may by order specify circumstances in which processing falling within subparagraphs (1)(a) and (b) is, or is not, to be taken for the purposes of sub-paragraph (1)(c) to be carried out with appropriate safeguards for the rights and freedoms of data subjects.

▶
> 10. The personal data are processed in circumstances specified in an order made
>   by the Secretary of State for the purposes of this paragraph.

CONSENT

Schedule 2 requires the consent of the data subject or one of the other conditions to be satisfied for processing to be carried on.

Schedule 3 requires the explicit consent of the data subject and the fact that processing is necessary to protect the data subject's vital interests, where consent cannot be given by or on behalf of the data subject or the data controller cannot be reasonably expected to obtain the consent of the data subject. This latter situation would obviously cover records relating to the mentally incapacitated adult and children. Another condition of Schedule 3 is that the processing is necessary for medical purposes (defined as including the purposes of preventative medicine, medical diagnosis, medical research, the provision of care and treatment and the management of healthcare services) and is undertaken by a health professional or a person who owes a duty of confidentiality which is equivalent to that which would arise if that person were a health professional. Satisfaction of this condition would obviate the need to obtain the explicit consent of every patient, in order for their health records to be processed.

RIGHTS OF THE DATA SUBJECT

The rights of the individual under the Data Protection Act 1998 are shown in Box 10.5.

Box 10.5 Rights of the data subject under the 1998 Act

1. Right of subject access (Sections 7 to 9)

2. Right to prevent processing likely to cause damage or distress (Section 10)

3. Right to prevent processing for the purposes of direct marketing (Section 11)

4. Right in relation to automated decision-taking (Section 12)

5. Right to take action for compensation if the individual suffers damage by any contravention of the Act by the data controller (Section 13)

6. Right to take action to rectify, block, erase or destroy inaccurate data (Section 14)

▶

▶ 7. Right to make a request to the Commissioner for an assessment to be made as to whether any provision of the Act has been contravened (Section 42).

INFORMATION COMMISSIONER

The Information Commissioner has the responsibility for promoting good practice and observance of the laws, providing an information service and encouraging the development of Codes of Practice. She has considerable powers of enforcement under Parts 3 and 5 of the Act. These include the power to serve enforcement notices and powers of entry and inspection. Information is available from the Commissioner's office free of charge.[5] An explanatory guide to the new legislation was issued in 1998 and has been updated to provide legal guidance[6] on the Act.

Offences under the Act are shown in Box 10.6.

Box 10.6 Offences under the Data Protection Act 1998

1. Offences relating to failure to notify the Commissioner or comply with his requests

2. Unlawfully obtaining personal data

3. Unlawful selling of personal data

4. Forcing a person to compel access

5. Unlawful disclosure of information by the commissioner/staff or agent.

GUIDANCE FROM THE NHS EXECUTIVE

The NHS Executive has published guidelines on the protection and use of patient information to support the implementation of the Data Protection Act.[7] It states that a Working Group at the Department of Health is developing national guidance to assist NHS bodies and local authorities on the principles and practical issues involved in sharing client/patient records for service delivery and of using such aggregated data for planning, commissioning, managing and monitoring.

CALDICOTT GUARDIANS

The Government appointed a Committee chaired by Dame Fiona Caldicott to make recommendations on how to improve the way in which the NHS managed patient confidentiality. It reported in December 1997 and included in its recommendations the need to raise awareness of confidentiality requirements, and specifically recommended the establishment of a network of Caldicott Guardians of patient information throughout the NHS. Subsequently a Steering Group was set up to oversee the implementation of the Report's recommendations. Following a consultation period the NHS Executive issued a circular on the establishment of Caldicott Guardians,[8] giving advice on the appointment of the Guardians, the programme of work for the first year for improving the way each organisation handles confidential patient information and identifying the resources, training and other support for the Guardians.

THE GUARDIAN

Each Health Authority, Special Health Authority, NHS trust and primary care group was required to appoint a Caldicott Guardian by 31st March 1999. Ideally the Guardian should be at Board level, be a senior health professional and have responsibility for promoting clinical governance within the organisation. The name and address of the Guardian is to be notified to the NHS Executive.[9] The Guardian is expected to liaise closely with others involved in patient information such as IM&T security officers and Data Protection Officers. In making the appointment and defining the role of the Guardian, the duties which are not to be delegated should be clarified. Guardians are responsible for agreeing and reviewing internal protocols governing the protection and use of patient-identifiable information by the staff of their organisation and must be satisfied that these proposals address the requirements for national guidance/policy and law. The operation of these policies must also be monitored. Policies for inter-agency disclosure of patient information must also be agreed and reviewed, to facilitate cross-boundary working.

In 2000 the Department of Health issued guidance to Caldicott Guardians on the method by which information flows should be reviewed in NHS organisations.[10] It provided a manual which covers the mapping of information flows, the prioritising of mapped flows for review purposes and a rolling programme of review. The specific areas which are considered include commissioning flows, clinical audit and coding, medical records and patient care services.

If issues on confidentiality arise a healthcare practitioner can raise these with the Caldicott Guardian, who in turn can access the legal advisers to the trust.

The Department of Health is currently working on policies for Caldicott Guardians in local authorities.[11]

THE HEALTH AND SOCIAL CARE ACT 2001

Sections 60 and 61 of the Health and Social Care Act 2001 enable the Secretary of State to draw up regulations for the control of patient information in the interests of improving patient care or in the public interest and to establish a Patient Information Advisory Group. Powers exercised under this Section must, of course, be compatible with the Articles of the European Convention of Human Rights. Regulations for the establishment of the Patient Information Advisory Group were published in August 2001.[12] The Advisory Group is to have between 12 and 20 members with one of them chosen by the Secretary of State as Chairman. The Group is to meet at least four times a year.

SOURCES OF THE DUTY OF CONFIDENTIALITY

The duty to respect confidentiality arises from a variety of sources which are set out in Box 10.7. Should the health professional be in breach of the duty of confidentiality, then the patient could bring an action in the civil courts and have the usual remedies for breach of trust.

Box 10.7 Sources of the obligation to respect the confidentiality of patient information

(a) Duty set out in Clause 10 of the UKCC Code of Professional Conduct

(b) Duty in the contract of employment

(c) Duty as part of the duty of care owed to the patient in the law of negligence

(d) Duty set out in specific statutes, especially the Data Protection Act 1998 and Human Rights Act 1998

(e) Duty as part of the trust obligation between health professional and patient.

DUTY SET OUT IN CLAUSE 10 OF THE UKCC CODE OF PROFESSIONAL CONDUCT

Clause 10 of the UKCC Code of Professional Conduct requires the UKCC practitioner to

'Protect all confidential information concerning patients and clients obtained in the course

of professional practice and make disclosures only with consent, where required by the order of a court or where you can justify disclosure in the wider public interest.'

Further advice is provided in the Guidelines for Professional Practice.[13]

DUTY IN THE CONTRACT OF EMPLOYMENT

Employed midwives also have a duty implied in the contract of employment that they will respect the confidentiality of information which they hear of in the course of their employment. This duty would be implied by the courts and failure to respect this duty could lead to disciplinary action being taken by the employer, with the ultimate sanction being dismissal.

DUTY AS PART OF THE DUTY OF CARE OWED TO THE PATIENT IN THE LAW OF NEGLIGENCE

There is some evidence to suggest that the duty of care owed to the patient may include a duty to respect the confidentiality of information which is learnt about the patient.[14]

DUTY SET OUT IN SPECIFIC STATUTES, ESPECIALLY THE DATA PROTECTION ACT 1998 AND HUMAN RIGHTS ACT 1998

It is clear from the principles of the Data Protection Act 1998 set out above that strict rules apply to the security of information from which a person can be identified. Other legislation also created a statutory obligation to respect confidentiality. One of the strictest rules on disclosure was the Human Fertilisation and Embryology Act 1990 which proved to be so exacting, that it was necessary to pass an amending Act in 1992 (see Chapter 27).

DUTY AS PART OF THE TRUST OBLIGATION BETWEEN HEALTH PROFESSIONAL AND PATIENT

The law would recognise that a relationship of trust is created between patient and health professional, which would give the right of action to the patient if there is evidence that the health professional intends to breach confidentiality without consent or other lawful justification. Those who have given information in the expectation that its confidentiality will be respected can enforce this obligation.[15]

EXCEPTIONS TO THE DUTY OF CONFIDENTIALITY

The main exceptions to the duty of confidentiality are shown in Box 10.8.

Box 10.8 Exceptions to the duty of confidentiality

(a) Consent of the client

(b) Information to the Supervisor

(c) Information given to other professionals in the interests of the client

(d) Order from the Court before or during legal proceedings

(e) Statutory justification eg.

    – Notification of registration of births and stillbirths

    – Infectious Disease Regulations

    – Police and Criminal Evidence Act

(f) Public interest.

CONSENT OF THE CLIENT

The duty of confidentiality exists to protect the client and the client can therefore agree to any disclosure. Such an agreement would be a defence against any action for breach. Care must however be taken to ensure that the client is fully aware of the implications of the consent and has the mental competence to give a valid consent.

This might be of importance if it were planned to video a delivery. If this is not at the client's instigation, eg. where a television company wish to televise or a recording is suggested as a training document, written consent should be obtained from the client and her capacity to consent should be certified by an appropriate professional not involved in the filming. In addition there should be a clear understanding as to what rights of distribution there are over any material obtained and the right, if any, of the client to withhold permission at a later stage.

The consent of the client is also important where the press are anxious to obtain details of the childbirth of a client who is a well-known person, or a multiple pregnancy which would attract media interest. The client is entitled to anonymity if she so wishes and only with her consent should any information be given to the press. Agreement on this could be obtained before the admission, but the client would of course be entitled to withdraw that consent at any time.

DISCLOSURE TO THE SUPERVISOR

Midwives are the only professionals who are required by statute to have a Supervisor. As can be seen from Chapter 3, the relationship between Supervisor and midwife should be a close one with the midwife informing the Supervisor immediately she is concerned about the care of the mother. If the mother gives confidential information to the midwife, it should be made clear to the mother that the midwife must inform her Supervisor of any relevant information likely to affect her practise and the safety of the mother, and advise the mother that this disclosure would be made. The midwife is obliged under Rule 43 to give her Supervisor, the Local Supervising Authority and the Council every facility to inspect her records. She could not refuse on grounds of a breach of confidentiality. The UKCC in Paragraph 34 of the Midwife's Code of Practice advises that the midwife should contact her Supervisor on all matters as required by the Midwives Rules.

'You and your Supervisor of Midwives, through your respective roles, should work towards a common aim of providing the best possible care for mothers and babies. You and your Supervisor of Midwives have a mutual responsibility for effective communication between yourselves in order that any problems can be shared and resolved.'

This advice clearly envisages the discussion of individual cases between midwife and Supervisor, and would be a defence against any allegation of breach of client confidentiality. The Supervisor of Midwives would clearly be bound to respect the duty of confidentiality in respect of information which she learnt from the midwife, unless one of the recognised lawful exceptions discussed here existed.

INFORMATION TO OTHER PROFESSIONALS
IN THE INTERESTS OF THE CLIENT

Clearly the midwife works as part of a multi-disciplinary team and therefore she must ensure that relevant information is given to those who are also caring for the mother and baby. This would in particular include the General Practitioner if s/he is involved in the care of the mother and also the obstetric team. The definition of 'relevant' might cause some difficulties. The midwife should be able justify any disclosure she makes in the interests of the mother and baby. Her records should reflect the basis of her decision where this is likely to be challenged.

Confidential information used for research purposes is considered in Chapter 31.

Midwives should ensure that the interests of the client are protected in any use of patient records whether the stated purpose be for audit or research or for the clinical care of the individual client.

COURT ORDER BEFORE OR DURING LEGAL PROCEEDINGS

If litigation is contemplated, the court has the right to make an order requiring disclosure of information relevant to an issue arising in a case.

Before litigation

Under Section 33 of the Supreme Court Act 1981, disclosure can be ordered against a person likely to be a party in a personal injury case before the writ is issued. Disclosure can be ordered to the applicant's legal advisers and any medical or other professional advisers of the applicants, or, if the applicant has no legal advisers, to any medical or other professional adviser of the applicant.

Thus if a client is suing in relation to an incident during the confinement, the records of the midwife could be ordered to be disclosed to the legal advisers or professional advisers of the client. Since the reforms of civil procedure as a result of the Woolf recommendations (see Chapter 14), a pre-action protocol exists which parties in civil litigation must follow and this enables early disclosure of information to be required.

After litigation has commenced

Under Section 34 of the Supreme Court Act 1981 disclosure can be ordered against a person who is not likely to be a party to a case, after the writ has been issued, if that person has information likely to be relevant.

This could cover a situation where the client who was pregnant and involved in a road traffic accident was suing the driver of the vehicle which caused the accident and he wished to have access to information about the client held by the midwife relating to the pregnancy. If, for example, there was a fear that the baby was harmed as a result of the road accident this could affect both liability and quantum. (See Congenital Disabilities (Civil Liability) Act 1976 in Chapter 17.)

Disclosure can also be ordered during any court proceedings where powers of subpoena exist to compel witnesses to attend court and bring relevant documents with them. The midwife has no defence of privileged information on the grounds that it was given to her in confidence if she is ordered by the judge to disclose the information. A refusal could be punished by imprisonment for contempt of court.

The reforms in civil court procedures have led to the adoption of a pre-action protocol which requires the parties to disclose information which is relevant to the dispute at an early stage and sanctions can be imposed for failure to conform to the protocol (see Chapter 14).

The only limitations on the powers of the court to order disclosure of information is where national security is at stake and a Minister of the Crown has signed a certificate to that effect, (the Scott enquiry recommended that this should not be done in criminal proceedings) and where the communication is one between lawyer and client for the purposes of litigation and is protected by the principle of legal professional privilege.

OTHER INVESTIGATIONS

In a recent case[16] a GP relied upon Article 8 of the European Convention of Human Rights in refusing to permit a health authority to access child protection records which the HA wished to see in connection with disciplinary investigations of the GP. The court permitted disclosure on the express condition that the confidentiality of the documents was preserved and that there would be effective and adequate safeguards of the patient's confidentiality and anonymity.

In the case of Junia Woolgar[17] the Court of Appeal held that a registered nurse and matron could not prevent the police disclosing to the UKCC details of their investigations into her activities as matron of a nursing home. Following their investigations the police did not charge her.

STATUTORY JUSTIFICATION

Certain Acts of Parliament require the midwife to pass on specified information and therefore would be a defence against an action for breach of confidentiality. In some situations the midwife would face legal proceedings herself if she failed to make the appropriate notifications.

The duty in relation to the notification of births and stillbirths is discussed in Chapter 25.

The duty in relation to the notification of infectious diseases can be found in Chapter 29.

PUBLIC INTEREST

This is the most difficult area and the advice provided in the UKCC guidance is invaluable.[18]

There have been two court cases which are not directly relevant to midwifery, but the rulings are of some assistance.

In W v. Egdell,[19] a detained psychiatric patient requested an independent report from a psychiatrist on his condition for the purposes of his application for discharge from the Section. The report was not favourable to him, and the doctor, against the wishes of the patient, sent a copy of the report to the Medical Director of the hospital and the Home Office. The patient lost his action against the doctor for breach of the duty of confidentiality since the doctor had a public duty to disclose this information.

In this case the patient had been convicted of killing five people ten years before and the possible dangers to the public from a premature release from detention were therefore clear. The case does not assist other than in providing a general statement as to when the public interest in the disclosure of information overrides the public interest in respecting the duty of confidentiality to an individual patient.

In X v. Y[20] the courts granted an injunction against a newspaper, preventing it publishing the names of two doctors working in the NHS who were suffering from AIDS. The court held that the information obtained from hospital records should be kept confidential and the public interest did not require the publication of the names (see also Chapter 29). The court did not order the disclosure by the press of their informant as the circumstances did not constitute one of the exceptional grounds on which the disclosure could be ordered against the press.

Midwives should ensure that they only disclose confidential information on the justification of the public interest if they can explain and record why the public interest arises. They should be able to respond to any challenge on the disclosure.

Some possible circumstances would include:

– A concern that a client was harming her existing child(ren).

> This should be reported to the Area Protection Committee through the procedure which should now exist in every area (see Chapter 32).

– A concern that a client may harm her baby when born.

> This should be reported to the Area Protection Committee. If there are fears for the mental health of the woman, reference should be made to Chapter 33.

– A concern that the client may harm herself.

> Action should be taken in the interests of the client, even against the client's will, to ensure that she is referred for the appropriate professional attention.

What, however, if the information which the midwife wishes to be made known relates not to the individual circumstances of the client but to fears concerning the environment of care and the possibility of dangers to the client. The Code of Professional Conduct requires the practitioner to make known her fears in relation to any possible danger to the patient/client.[21] This duty to 'whistle blow' is discussed further in Chapters 5 and 22. Midwives should make sure that they obtain copies of the circular and follow the procedure laid down by their employer.

CLIENT ACCESS TO RECORDS

The provisions for access to records are now covered by the Data Protection Act 1998, except for access to the records of those who have died, where the Access to Health Records Act 1990 still applies.

PATIENT-HELD RECORDS

Many midwifery units are now permitting mothers to hold their own records. Certainly during the antenatal stage, excellent results have been obtained by entrusting the records to the care of the patient. It has been found that patients are less likely to lose the records than a medical records department. Changing Childbirth set as one of the targets that all clients should hold their records (see Chapter 6). One of the indicators of success identified in Changing Childbirth[22] was that within five years all women should be able to carry their own notes. Antenatal records were often the earliest to be disclosed to or even kept by patients and in general midwives are able to have a more open policy of disclosure to mothers and do not require formal applications to be made under the Data Protection Act 1998 before access will be permitted.

Statutory entitlement by the patient to access health records is given by the statutory instrument enacted under Data Protection legislation. Access is also permitted to Medical Reports obtained for employment or insurance purposes under the Access to Medical Reports Act 1988.

RIGHT OF ACCESS TO PERSONAL DATA

Section 7 of the Data Protection Act 1998 enables an individual to be informed of data held about him and to access that data. Special provisions exist in relation to health, education and social work.

HEALTH EDUCATION AND SOCIAL WORK

Section 30 of the Data Protection Act enables the Secretary of State to draw up specific provisions setting exemptions from the statutory rights of access in relation to health, education and social work records. Statutory Instruments have been enacted setting out details of the restrictions on access to these records.[23]

RIGHT TO WITHHOLD ACCESS

Access can be withheld under the Data Protection Act 1998 in the following circumstances:

– where in the opinion of the holder of the record, serious harm would be caused to the mental or physical health or condition of the applicant or of any other individual

– where the identity of a third person would be made known and this person has not consented to access. (This does not apply where the other person is the health professional caring for the patient.)

– where the reports are confidential under a statutory provision such as information supplied in a report or other evidence given to the court by a local authority, Health or Social Services Board, Health and Social Services Trust or probation officer.

IMPLICATIONS FOR MIDWIVES

Voluntary system
Before any statutory provisions for access were in place many midwives and obstetric units permitted wide access to records, with many mothers being responsible for the antenatal records. The legislation does not replace this system, and open access can be permitted on a much wider basis than is required statutorily.

Standard of record keeping
Since the midwife knows that the mother has a statutory right of access, there is even more reason to ensure a high standard of record keeping. The fact that the mother can ask for corrections if she considers that the records are incomplete, misleading or inaccurate should encourage the midwife to maintain high standards to prevent possible criticisms (see Chapter 15).

PROBLEMS OF OPEN ACCESS

UNWANTED DISCLOSURE

One problem which openness can bring is shown in Box 10.9.

Box 10.9 Situation: unwanted information

Frances Davies had not told her husband that she had had a child when she was 15 years old, which was adopted, or that she had had a subsequent miscarriage. She was asked for details of the earlier gestation history when she booked into the antenatal clinic for her present pregnancy. In this clinic a system was operated whereby mothers took their antenatal records home, and Frances was concerned about her husband reading the previous obstetric history. She asked if these details could be omitted from her records.

The danger of agreeing with Frances's request and editing medical history is that at a subsequent time those events may become significant and to rely upon the patient being conscious or on there being a midwife present who remembered the missing details is clearly unsatisfactory. One possibility in such a case is to arrange for these records to be kept at the hospital and not to be taken home. Alternatively, it may be possible to devise a formula for detailing this information which would not be understood by the spouse. This cannot be done where the patient is requesting statutory right of access under the legislation since the holder of the records would have a duty to translate any jargon and decipher any illegible parts or find any missing parts so that the records are comprehensible to the applicant. Another possibility is to mark on the form that other information is held at the hospital. It would then be important for any midwife to ensure that she had both sets of records. There are obvious inherent dangers in a two-set record system. Another possibility is for the woman to be told to exercise her right of keeping the record confidential to herself and therefore secret from her husband. However, in the circumstances, this may not be a realistic possibility. Nor may the possibility of the woman making a full disclosure to the husband be realistic.

It is recognised by some midwives that some clients book late for antenatal clinic for the initial booking because their partner does not know of a previous pregnancy and they are afraid that it will become general knowledge. The midwife should reassure the client that this will be kept strictly confidential. Some midwives take the view that in order to preserve this confidentiality, there is no reason to record the fact of the previous history in the records, especially where the first birth or miscarriage was normal. There are, however, dangers in this approach, especially if the client is rhesus negative or if subsequent events make the earlier history significant.

FEAR OF LOST RECORDS

Another concern is the possibility that the records could be lost whilst being cared for by the mother and in the event of later litigation the midwife could suffer considerable disadvantages.

The loss of records may well be less when the mother has responsibility than when they are cared for by a medical records department. The absence of records would probably work more against the mother in litigation than in her favour, since the burden is on the claimant to show on a balance of probabilities that there has been negligence.

COMPUTERISED RECORDS

In March 2001 the government announced its intention to introduce by March 2005 a system whereby every patient would have an electronic health record. The electronic health record is defined by the Department of Health as a record holding summarised key data about patients, such as name, address, NHS number, registered GP and contact details, previous treatments, ongoing conditions, current medication, allergies and the date of any next appointments. The stated intention is that it will be securely protected, created with patient consent, with individual changes made only by authorised staff. Pilot schemes are in operation at the time of writing. Clearly, any system will have to comply with data protection legislation requirements over security and control over patient access. The scheme will also have implications for record keeping, which are discussed in Chapter 15.

FREEDOM OF INFORMATION ACT 2000

Over the next five years the Freedom of Information Act 2000 will be brought into force. It gives a right to people to obtain information from public authorities. An Information Commissioner (combining both Data Protection and Freedom of Information statutory duties) has been appointed and an Information Tribunal will adjudicate on grievances under the Act. Part 2 of the Act lists many areas of information which are exempt from the access provisions. Under Section 40, access to personal information will come under the Data Protection Act 1998.

CONCLUSIONS

Significant changes are taking place both in relation to the protection of personal information and also in relation to the access to information held by public authorities. The impact of the Articles of the European Convention on Human Rights in this area cannot at this early stage be evaluated. There will be significant court rulings as judges attempt to balance rights of freedom of expression and access to information with the rights of privacy. At the time of writing the Department of Health is drafting a strategy on confidential information and is hoping to publish a

Code of Practice for consultation in March 2002. It is hoped that the implementation of a strategy on the use of confidential information will secure the rights of patients in this complex field. Further reference may be made to the author's work.[24]

QUESTIONS AND EXERCISES

1. What measures do you think could be taken to ensure higher standards of confidentiality in midwifery units?

2. Disclosure in the public interest causes considerable difficulty. In the light of the UKCC guidance on confidentiality (as contained in the Guidelines for Professional Practice), draw up a protocol to be followed if disclosure in the public interest appeared to be justified.

3. There is no absolute right of access by the patient to her records. In what circumstances, if any do you consider that the right of the client to access should be withheld?

4. Consider the provisions of the Freedom of Information Act and decide how it could work for the benefit of pregnant women.

References

1 UKCC. 1996. *Guidelines for professional practice*. London: UKCC

2 European Directive on Data Protection, adopted by the Council of the European Union in October 1995

3 NHS Executive. 2000. Data Protection Act 1998. HSC 2000/009

4 www.standards.nhsia.nhs.uk/sdp

5 Information Commissioner, Wycliffe House, Water Lane, Wilmslow, Cheshire SK9 5AF. Information line: 01625 545745; Switchboard: 01625 545700; Fax 01625 524510

6 Information Commissioner. *Legal Guidance on Data Protection Act 1998*. www.dataprotection.gov.uk.

7 NHS Executive. 2000. Data Protection Act: Protection and Use of Patient Information. HSC 2000/009

8 NHS Executive. 1999. Caldicott Guardians. HSC 1999/012

9 Raj Kaur, NHS Executive, 3E58 Quarry House, Leeds LS2 7UE. Fax 0113 254 6114

10 Department of Health. 2000. Protection and using patient information: A Manual for Caldicott Guardians. London: HMSO

11 Department of Health contact: Carole Bell 0207 972 4978

12 Patient Information Advisory Group (Establishment) Regulations 2001 No 2836

13 UKCC. 1996. *Guidelines for Professional Practice*. London: UKCC

14 Furniss v. Fitchett [1958] NZLR 396

15 Stephens v. Avery and others [1988] 2 All ER 477

16 A Health Authority and another v. X and others. Lloyds Rep Med [2001] 349

17 Woolgar v. Chief Constable of Sussex Police and another [1999] 3 All ER 604 CA

18 UKCC. 1996. *Guidelines for Professional Practice*. London: UKCC

19 W v. Egdell [1990] 1 All ER 835

20 X v. Y [1988] 2 All ER 648

21 Clauses 11, 12, 13, UKCC Code of Professional Conduct June 1992

22 Cumberlege Report, 1993

23 Data Protection (Subject Access Modification)(Health) Order 2000 SI 2000 No 413; Data Protection (Subject Access Modification)(Education) Order 2000 SI 2000 No 414; Data Protection (Subject Access Modification)(Social Work) Order 2000 SI 2000 No 415

24 Dimond B. 2002. *The Legal Aspects of Confidentiality*. Wiltshire: Quay Books/Mark Allen Publishing

Chapter 11
COMPLAINTS

There is a statutory duty for all hospitals to have a complaints procedure (Hospital Complaints Procedure Act 1985). The Secretary of State has requested that this duty should be recognised also by NHS community health organisations. The duty was reinforced by the Patient's Charter, which expected all patients to have the opportunity to make known any concerns to the management. The NHS Plan published in 2000 also introduced new forms for participation and representation.

At present there are many ways in which complaints can be made, as shown in Box 11.1.

Box 11.1 Methods of making complaints

1. Health Authority or Primary Care Trust in respect of the services of General Practitioners, dentists and pharmacists

2. NHS trust in relation to hospital and community services

3. Health Authorities as the commissioners of healthcare services from trusts and from nursing homes

4. Local Authorities as the commissioners for community social services and residential accommodation

5. Professional registration bodies in respect of the conduct of individual practitioners

6. The Health Service Commissioner as the final stage in the NHS complaints procedure

7. Litigation via solicitors

8. Complaints via the Community Health Councils

9. Police

10. Members of Parliament, the media etc.

Midwives are increasingly likely to be involved in the hearing of a complaint, either in relation to their own practice or in being asked to give evidence about the practice of colleagues. Complaints may also be made about administrative procedures, property and other topics not directly the concern of the midwife. The midwife should, difficult though it may be, welcome complaints and regard them as an opportunity to monitor and improve the service to mothers. One of the advantages of the named midwife scheme is that some of the concerns and worries of mothers can be made known to the midwife and therefore addressed at an early stage informally so that they do not eventually become the subject of a formal complaint. However, for this to be so, the midwife must respond positively to the mother, making it easy for her to express her concerns and be vigilant in following up the anxieties.

INFORMAL COMPLAINTS

It is recommended that where concerns are expressed to the midwife, she should keep a brief note of the details shown in Box 11.2.

Box 11.2 Recording informal complaints/concerns

- Date and time

- Mother/client

- Brief description of concern

- Action taken by midwife

A note should also be made in the mother's records

Where the midwife has had to refer the issue to a senior manager or other professional, she should follow it up to ensure that action is taken where necessary. Her regular contact with the mother should also ensure that she discovers if the concerns are now allayed.

FORMAL COMPLAINTS

The midwife should always make it clear to the client that it is always open to the client to make a formal complaint. She must ensure that she knows the procedure and who is the designated Complaints Officer for the unit/hospital. Where necessary she should offer assistance to the complainant, particularly if the complainant has difficulty in expressing herself in writing. It should be made clear however that there is no requirement for the complaint to be put in writing by the complainant personally, and that someone else could do that on her behalf.

THE WILSON REVIEW

Because there were so many procedures and ways in which complaints could be made, and the existing systems were confusing and slow and could be bureaucratic, an expert committee was set up under the Chairmanship of Professor Alan Wilson to review NHS complaints procedures.[1] The report reviewed the current situation and set objectives for any effective complaints system. The principles it saw for any effective complaints system are set out in Box 11.3.

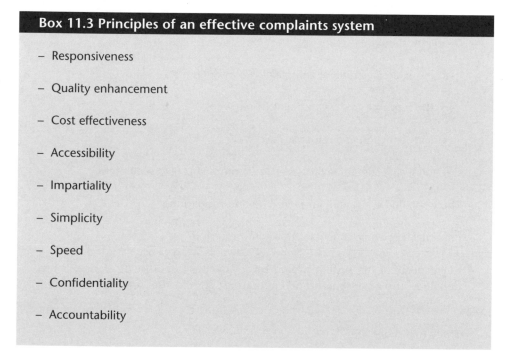

Box 11.3 Principles of an effective complaints system

- Responsiveness

- Quality enhancement

- Cost effectiveness

- Accessibility

- Impartiality

- Simplicity

- Speed

- Confidentiality

- Accountability

The report recommended that these principles should be incorporated into an NHS complaints system. The areas covered by its recommendations are shown in Box 11.4.

Box 11.4 Recommendations of the Wilson report on the review of complaints procedures

- There should be a common system for all NHS complaints

- The complaints procedure should not be concerned with disciplining staff

- Staff should be empowered to deal with complaints informally

- There should be training of staff

- Support should be provided for complainants and respondents

- The degree of investigation should relate to the complainant's required degree of response

- Conciliation should be made more widely available

- Time limits should be set

- Deadlines should be set for

    (a) the acknowledging of complaints (2 working days)

    (b) the response to the complaint (three weeks)

    (c) Further action and response (two weeks)

- Confidentiality should be preserved and complaints filed separately

- There should be a system for recording and monitoring

- Impartial lay people should take part in the system

- Key aspects of the system should be set by the Department of Health but detailed implementation and operation should be left to individual organisations

- Three fold procedures:

    - stage 1 immediate first line response

    - stage 2 investigation/ conciliation

    - stage 3 action by HA (formerly FHSA) officer or Chief Executive Officer for trusts. A panel should be set up to consider those complaints which cannot be resolved in the earlier stages.

- There should be training in communication skills

- Oral and written complaints should be treated with the same sensitive treatment

- Community service staff should have particular training in responding to complaints

- Purchasers should specify complaints requirements in their contracts with non-NHS providers

- Complaints about policy decisions should be referred to the Health Service Commissioner if they cannot be resolved locally by the purchasers

- Where more than one organisation is involved it should be the organisation which receives the complaint which makes sure that a full response is sent

- Community care: there should be close liaison with Local Authorities and the government should consider further integration of NHS and Local Authority complaints procedures

- Stage 2 procedures: there should be a screening officer

- The jurisdiction of the HSC should be extended to GPs and the operation of the FHSA service committees

- Recommendations on implementation.

The recommendations of the Wilson Committee were implemented in the NHS.

FIRST STAGE: LOCAL RESOLUTION

A complaint is initially heard at local level and should be responded to by the Chief Executive or General Practitioner concerned. There are guidelines on the times within which the complaint should be acknowledged and given a final reply.

SECOND STAGE: INDEPENDENT REVIEW PANEL (IRP)

In the event of the complainant being not satisfied by the response from the Chief Executive or General Practitioner following the first level of investigation, she can apply to the Non-Executive Director on the Board of the NHS trust or Health Authority, known as the complaints convenor. This person would then decide if the complaint should go to an independent review panel on which the convenor will sit. This system has been criticised since many consider that the involvement of a Director of the trust or Health Authority can be seen as lacking independence from those involved in the complaint.

THIRD STAGE: HEALTH SERVICE COMMISSIONER (HSC) (OMBUDSMAN)

If the complainant is not satisfied following the IRP or the complaints convenor has refused to agree to an IRP, then the complainant can refer the complaint to the Health Service Commissioner or Ombudsman. Legislation which came into force on 1st April 1996 widened its jurisdiction to include the investigation of matters concerned with the exercise of clinical judgement and the investigations of complaints about family practitioner services. The HSC has a duty to prepare a report which is submitted to Parliament, under Section 14(4) of the Health Service Commissioners Act 1993. The Select Committee of the House of Commons has the power to investigate further any complaint reported by the HSC, if necessary summoning witnesses to London for questioning. The HSC is completely independent of the NHS and the Government and has the jurisdiction to investigate complaints against any part of the NHS about:

– a failure in service, or

– a failure to purchase or provide a service one is entitled to receive, or

– maladministration (administrative affairs).

REVIEW OF COMPLAINTS PROCEDURE

Research was commissioned by the Department of Health on the effectiveness of the current complaints system. In the light of the results of that research the Department of Health published a document suggesting a number of ways to improve the current procedure.[2] It also issued a consultation document[3] on which feedback is invited at the time of writing. It is likely to lead to significant changes to the present complaints system in 2002. Midwives should keep alert to the changes to the complaints system which will eventually be made.

NHS PLAN[4]

Chapter 10 of the NHS Plan envisages giving patients more say in their own treatment and more influence over the way the NHS works. To achieve this the following initiatives are planned:

- Greater information to empower patients

- Greater patient choice

- Patient advocates and advisers in every hospital

- Redress over cancelled operations

- Patients' forums and citizens' panels in every area

- New national panel to advise on major reorganisations of hospitals

- Stronger regulation of professional standards.

These are considered briefly below.

GREATER INFORMATION TO EMPOWER PATIENTS

This will be provided through the publication of patient-friendly versions of NICE guidelines, the establishment of NHS Direct online, Digital TV and NHS Direct Information points in key public places. Better communication between clinicians and doctors will be secured by letters between clinicians about an individual patient being copied to the patients as of right; by smart cards for patients allowing easier access to health records. (See chapter 10 of this book on electronic patient records.)

GREATER PATIENT CHOICE

Patients have a choice of GP and this will be supported by more information being given to patients about the GP practices in their area. By 2005 it is envisaged that patients will be able to book hospital appointments and choose to be admitted at times which are convenient to them.

PATIENT ADVOCATES AND ADVISERS IN EVERY HOSPITAL

By 2002 an NHS-wide Patient Advocacy and Liaison Service (PALS) is to be set up in every trust. Patient advocates will act as independent facilitators to handle patient and family concerns.

REDRESS OVER CANCELLED OPERATIONS

If a hospital operation is cancelled on the day of surgery by the hospital for non-clinical reasons, the hospital must offer the patient an appointment within a maximum of 28 days or fund the patient's treatment at the time and hospital of the patients' choice.

PATIENTS' FORUMS AND CITIZENS' PANELS IN EVERY AREA

Patients' views will be sought by trusts which will have the responsibility of publishing an annual report covering the feedback. Financial rewards to trusts will be linked to the results of the annual National Patients' Survey. A new NHS Charter will replace the current Patients' Charter. Each Health Authority will be required to establish an independent local advisory forum chosen from residents of the area to provide a sounding board. Local government will be given the power to scrutinise NHS plans locally. Provision is made in the NHS Reform and Health Care Professions Bill 2002 for the establishment of Patients' Forums with powers to enter and inspect premises and the duty to provide an annual report. A corporate body known as the Commission for Patient and Public Involvement in Health is also to be established.

The Community Health Councils are to be abolished. (The Welsh Assembly decided in favour of the retention of CHCs.) Under the NHS Plan patients will be represented at all levels within the NHS.

NEW NATIONAL PANEL TO ADVISE ON MAJOR REORGANISATIONS OF HOSPITALS

The NHS Plan envisaged a new Independent Reconfiguration Panel to consider contested major service reconfigurations.

PATIENT REPRESENTATION

Involving patients and the public in healthcare[5] was issued by the Department of Health in September 2001 for consultation on proposals for greater public representation to replace the CHCs. In a press release on 3rd September 2001[6] the Department of Health announced that a new independent body, 'Voice', was to be established. There will be two levels: at national level a new national body called Voice – the Commission for Patient and Public Involvement in Health, and at local level local bodies called Voice which will report patients' concerns from PALS and Forums to the new Strategic Health Authorities. Voice will set national standards and monitor local services, helping to ensure communities have an effective say in their local NHS. Voice will work alongside the trust-based Patients' Forums and

Patient Advocacy and Liaison Services. These organisations will replace CHCs and legislation is contained in the NHS Reform and Health Care Professions Bill 2002.

STRONGER REGULATION OF PROFESSIONAL STANDARDS

New quality standards are being introduced into the NHS. There is now a mandatory national scheme for adverse incident reporting known as the National Patient Safety Agency (see Chapter 19) and the Chief Medical Officer's proposals[7] for improving standards of doctors, including annual appraisal and clinical audit, have been implemented. A National Clinical Assessment Authority has also been established with the role of reviewing an individual doctor's performance if concerns have arisen. The NHS Tribunal is to be abolished and new procedures introduced for the removal or suspension of doctors from practice. New regulatory machinery for registration bodies is being introduced. A Council for the Regulation of Health Care Professions is to be established under the NHS Reform and Health Care Professions Bill 2002 which will be responsible for the oversight of the workings of the regulatory bodies such as the NMC and the GMC. (See Chapter 3 of this book.)

CONCLUSIONS

Major innovations are taking place in healthcare as a result of the Health Act 1999 (see Chapter 21) and the NHS Plan. Part of these changes will be a new complaints system which at the time of writing is subject to consultation. The Bristol Royal Infirmary Inquiry[8] following the deaths of children during heart surgery recommended that patients must be given the opportunity to pass on views on the service which they have received, and emphasised there is a duty of candour, i.e. a duty to tell a patient if adverse events have occurred, which is owed by all those working in the NHS to patients. The Inquiry recommends:

'Complaints should be dealt with swiftly and thoroughly, keeping the patient (and carer) informed. There should be a strong independent element, not part of the trust's management or board, in any body considering serious complaints which require formal investigation. An independent advocacy service should be established to assist patients (and carers).'

The implementation of the many recommendations contained in the Inquiry Report should have significant implications for the standards of care of every midwifery patient including how complaints are handled. The Government has published its response to the Kennedy Report which is considered by the author.[9]

QUESTIONS AND EXERCISES

1. Consider the complaints relating to midwifery services over the past year and discuss the extent to which these could be used to improve the services provided.

2. Obtain a copy of the Department of Health's evaluation of the present complaints procedure and its consultation paper on possible changes, and analyse what changes you consider would be essential.

3. To what extent do you consider that complaints relating to community services need to be handled differently from those relating to hospital services?

4. Obtain a copy of Chapter 10 of the NHS Plan. How would you ensure that your clients were encouraged to be positively involved in the provision of services and the quality assurance mechanisms?

5. Consider the proposals for patient involvement set out in the NHS Plan, and how they could apply to midwifery services.

Obtain a copy of the Inquiry into the Bristol children's heart surgery, study the recommendations under the heading Respect and Honesty and consider the extent to which your department complies with its proposals.

References

1 Department of Health. 1994. *Being Heard. The report of a review committee on NHS Complaints procedures.* London: HMSO

2 Department of Health. 2001. *The NHS Complaints Procedure: National Evaluation.* London: HMSO

3 Department of Health. 2001. *Reforming the NHS Complaints Procedure: a listening document.* London: HMSO

4 Department of Health. 2000. *NHS Plan: A plan for investment, a plan for reform.* London: HMSO

5 Department of Health. 2001. *Involving Patients and the Public in Healthcare.* London: HMSO

6 Department of Health. 2001. Press release: New Voice for Patients to shape local services

7 Chief Medical Officer of the DoH. 2000. *Supporting Doctors, Protecting Patients.* London: HMSO

8 Bristol Royal Infirmary. 2001. *Learning from Bristol: the report of the public inquiry into children's heart surgery at the Bristol Royal Infirmary 1984-1995 (The Kennedy Report). Command paper CM 5207.* www.bristol-inquiry.org.uk

9 Dimond B. 2002. After Bristol: Government Support and Rejection. *British Journal of Midwifery,* 10(3)

Chapter 12
MATERNITY BENEFITS

Midwives need to know about benefits which are available during pregnancy for two reasons:

– clients may sometimes ask the midwife for information about the benefits to which they are entitled in respect of the pregnancy and child

– the midwife herself may be pregnant and therefore would need to know what her rights are as an employee.

This is an area where there are frequent revisions both to the benefits available from the Benefits Agency and also those from the statutory scheme for maternity pay and leave. The midwife should ensure that she knows where she can obtain information and that the leaflets available in the clinic are regularly reviewed and updated as necessary. The following information is only a brief outline of the benefits currently available and further details should be obtained from the Health Authority, the Department of Social Security (or Benefits Agency, as the executive arm of the DSS is known), the Local Authority and the Department of Trade and Industry. The Maternity Alliance publishes details of the benefits which are available to the pregnant woman whether in or out of work[1] which are updated annually.

Benefits are broadly available on three different bases:

1. Benefits available as of right

2. Benefits available on a means tested basis either available through Social Security or the Local Authority

3. Benefits which are work-related, where eligibility depends upon meeting certain criteria relating to length of continuous service and other conditions laid down in the legislation. (Other statutory benefits to which employees are entitled are considered in more detail in Chapter 22.)

BENEFITS PAYABLE BY THE BENEFITS AGENCY: NON-MEANS TESTED

MATERNITY ALLOWANCE

Maternity allowance is payable to pregnant women who cannot get SMP, and to the self-employed. It is only available if the woman has been employed or self-employed. It is paid for up to 18 weeks. The claimant must have been employed or self-employed for at least 26 weeks in the 66 weeks test period (i.e. the period of 66 weeks immediately preceding the week in which the baby is due) and must have earned on average at least £30 per week.

FREE MILK FOR DISABLED CHILDREN

Free milk is available for a child between 5 and 16 who is unable to attend school because of a physical or mental disability. It is not means tested.

BENEFITS PAYABLE BY THE BENEFITS AGENCY: MEANS TESTED

SURE START MATERNITY GRANTS

This is payable to assist with the costs of items for the new baby. It is a one-off payment and does not have to be paid back. It is payable if the woman or her partner is receiving income support, income-based jobseeker's allowance, working families' tax credit or disabled person's tax credit.

The claim can be made from 11 weeks before the baby is due until 3 months after the baby is born.

INCOME SUPPORT

This is available to people on a low income, who are over 16 years of age and not working (or working less than 16 hours a week).

FREE MILK AND VITAMINS

These are available to pregnant women and children under 5 years.

THE SOCIAL FUND

Help is available with exceptional expenses which are hard to pay for out of regular income. A Community Care Grant, Budgeting Loan or Crisis Loan are available for specific purposes. The loans have to be paid back but are interest free.

BENEFITS FROM THE EMPLOYER

STATUTORY MATERNITY PAY (SMP)

This scheme which commenced in April 1987 has recently been changed to comply with the European Directive on the protection of the pregnant woman at work.

To be eligible, the employee must satisfy two sets of conditions: the continuous employment rule and the earnings rule.

The continuous employment rule
The employee must

    i.   have been continuously employed by the same employer for at least 26 weeks continuing into the 15th week before the baby is due. (This is known as the qualifying week.)

    ii. give the employer notice at least 21 days before the maternity absence is due to start, and

    iii. give the employer medical evidence of the expected date of confinement. (This certificate is not available until the 27th week of the pregnancy.)

Whether or not a woman intends to return to work does not affect the entitlement to statutory maternity pay.

The earnings rule
The employee's average weekly earnings must be at least equal to the lower earnings limit for National Insurance purposes.

For how long is it paid?
Statutory maternity pay is payable for up to 18 weeks if the employee does not intend to return to work after the baby is born. This is known as the 'maternity pay period'.

The maternity pay period can start at any time from the start of the 11th week before the expected week of the confinement and can continue up to 18 weeks.

If the baby is born late this does not affect the maternity pay period.

If the baby is born early, before the maternity pay period is due to start, the maternity pay period is the 18 weeks beginning with the Sunday following the birth of the baby.

If the baby is stillborn, before the 25th week of the pregnancy, statutory maternity pay is not payable. However, statutory sick pay may be payable. If the baby is stillborn after the start of the 25th week of the pregnancy, statutory maternity pay is payable as if the baby had been born alive. (See the Still Birth Act discussed in Chapter 25.)

How much is payable?

The first 6 weeks of SMP are earnings related; the remaining weeks are paid at a standard rate. The earnings-related rate is calculated as 90% of the average weekly earnings. If this calculation results in a figure which is less than the standard rate of SMP then the standard rate is payable.

Sickness and statutory maternity pay

An employee cannot obtain both statutory sick pay and statutory maternity pay. Statutory sick pay is not payable if someone is receiving SMP.

MATERNITY LEAVE

Ordinary maternity leave

All employees are entitled to 18 weeks' ordinary maternity leave, whether or not they qualify for statutory maternity pay or maternity allowance.

Additional maternity leave

In addition, employees who have worked for the same employer for at least one year before the 11th week before their baby is due, are entitled to additional maternity leave which lasts for 29 weeks from the start of the week in which the baby is born. The employer can request her, (not earlier than 21 days before the end of her ordinary leave period), to notify him in writing of the date of the birth and whether she intends to return to work. A press announcement issued in May 2001[2] stated that a new framework of rules governing maternity leave had been drawn up, and unpaid maternity leave was being extended by three months, allowing mothers to take up to a year as maternity leave from work.

Compulsory maternity leave

It is illegal for an employer to permit a woman to work within two weeks of childbirth.

PAID TIME OFF FOR ANTENATAL CARE

All pregnant employees are entitled to reasonable paid time off for antenatal care. For the first appointment they do not need to produce their appointment card or the certificate of pregnancy but thereafter they do. There is no requirement that the employee should have worked for a minimum period.

THE RIGHT TO RETURN TO WORK

The woman is entitled to return to work after maternity leave. She must have given her employer, if so requested (not earlier than 21 days before the end of the maternity leave period) notice of her intention to return to work, in writing. The woman must give at least 21 days notice of the date on which she intends to return.

If the employer refuses to allow her to return to work, this would count as an unfair dismissal.

THE RIGHT NOT TO BE DISMISSED ON GROUNDS OF PREGNANCY

All female employees have the following rights regardless of their length of service or hours of work:

  i. protection against dismissal or selection for redundancy on grounds of pregnancy, a reason connected with the pregnancy or childbirth. This would include breastfeeding.

  ii. an automatic right to receive written reasons for dismissal if dismissed whilst pregnant or during the statutory maternity leave period, without having to request it and regardless of length of service or hours of work.

These provisions protect the woman even when she has not formally notified her employer of the pregnancy.

They do not protect her against dismissal on other grounds, eg. conduct etc. (See Chapter 22.)

PROTECTION FROM DETRIMENT

A pregnant employee is entitled not to be subjected to any detriment because she is pregnant, gave birth to a child, was suspended from work on maternity grounds, took ordinary or additional maternity leave, parental leave or time off from work to care for dependants. This protection does not apply if she failed to notify her employer (after his request) that she intended to return to work at the end of her additional maternity leave period.

RIGHTS ON SUSPENSION ON GROUNDS OF PREGNANCY, RECENTLY GIVEN BIRTH OR BREASTFEEDING

The Management of Health and Safety at Work Regulations 1999 (see Chapter 19) require employers to carry out a risk assessment designed to ensure the health and safety at work of new mothers (who have recently given birth or who are breastfeeding) or pregnant women. If the assessment shows that there are risks to the health and safety of the woman or the fetus/baby which cannot be reasonably avoided, and if there is no alternative suitable work, then the employee must be suspended for as long as is necessary to avoid the risk.

If the woman is suspended she has the following rights:

i. The right to receive normal remuneration for as long as the suspension lasts. This does not apply where suitable alternative employment has been offered and has been unreasonably refused.

ii. The right to be offered suitable alternative employment, where available.

PARENTAL LEAVE

Employees who have worked for the same employer for at least one year are entitled to 13 weeks' parental leave to care for a child. Income support may be available during this time if the claimant is sick or disabled, a lone parent, or on a low income and when the employee was working she was entitled to working families' tax credit, disabled person's tax credit, housing benefit or council tax benefit.

TIME OFF FOR DEPENDANTS

All employees have the right to take time off to deal with an emergency involving a dependant, whatever their length of service.

Neither the parental leave right nor that of time off for dependants give a right to paid leave.

CONTRACTUAL AND STATUTORY RIGHTS

An employee may be entitled to specific contractual benefits in relation to pregnancy as part of the contract of employment. These may be more generous to the employee than the statutory rights set out above. The employee has the right to choose which benefits are the most favourable and the provision of benefits by her employer under the contract offsets any due under the employer's statutory obligations. The employer cannot provide less than the statutory obligations.

CONCLUSIONS

There are frequent changes in both the type of benefit available and also the amount payable and the conditions which apply. Our membership of the European Community has led to far greater provisions being made for pregnant women who work and further enhancements of these benefits are due in October 2002.

QUESTIONS AND EXERCISES

1. Obtain a copy of the Whitley Council regulations relating to maternity benefits. Compare these with the new statutory regulations which come into force in October 2002. Which do you consider are the most favourable?

2. A single pregnant woman who intends bringing up her child on her own asks your advice in relation to the benefits to which she will be entitled after the baby is born. What advice would you give her, and to what organisations would you refer her for further information?

3. You are informed by one of your clients that she lost her job when her boss discovered that she was pregnant. What advice would you give her and to whom would you refer her?

4. You are asked to give a lecture on the rights of the pregnant woman and mother. How would you prepare for this talk and from where would you seek further information? (Refer also to Chapter 6.)

5. A colleague has told you that she is pregnant and intends to take maternity leave. What are her entitlements as a pregnant employee?

References

1 Maternity Alliance, 45 Beech Street, London EC2P 2LX. Tel 020 7588 8583; Fax 020 7588 8584; email ma@mail.pro-net.co.uk

2 Department of Trade and Industry. 2001. Press release P/2001/280 Byers announces radical overhaul of maternity rules

SECTION C

LITIGATION AND ACCOUNTABILITY

In Section C of this book, aspects of the law relating to the accountability of the midwife are considered. The midwife is accountable for her practice before the Statutory Committees of the NMC (see Chapter 4) and before her employer's disciplinary machinery if she is in breach of the terms of her contract of employment (see Chapter 22). In addition, she may face criminal proceedings if she is guilty of an offence, or civil proceedings if there is a claim brought against her or her employer in respect of her alleged negligent practice. Chapter 13 considers the general principles involved in the bringing of a civil action for compensation. Chapter 14 will consider special areas, and the final chapters in this Section of the book look at cases involving negligent sterilisation and abortion, liability in the criminal law including health and safety laws and the rights of the fetus. Finally, the law relating to the administration of medicinal products and liability in negligence will be considered.

Chapter 13
NEGLIGENCE

As patients seek compensation for alleged harm, litigation is increasing and the greatest risk area is obstetrics. In a recent report of the National Audit Office,[1] it was stated that the NHS must make provision for outstanding claims of £2.6 billion, together with an estimated liability of a further £1.3 billion where negligent episodes are likely to have occurred, but where claims have not yet been received. The report noted that the number and value of claims continues to rise, and they are taking on average about 5½ years to settle. Somewhat startlingly, it was found that nearly half the claims settled in 1999-2000 cost more in legal and other costs than the settlement itself. For settlements of up to £50,000 the costs of reaching the settlement are greater than damages awarded in over 65% of the cases.[2] In the light of this report, the Department of Health has proposed a new compensation scheme which is considered in Chapter 14. Some of the largest sums of money are awarded in birth damage cases, with examples of claims of £2 million now being awarded or agreed.

There are concerns that the fear of litigation has led to defensive medical practice and to a reluctance to enter high risk spheres of practice.[3] Even if the midwife is not personally at fault, she may well be involved and have to give evidence in a case brought because of alleged negligence by an obstetrician or other colleagues. It is therefore important for a midwife to understand the law relating to negligence, and her own position should an action in respect of her negligence be brought.

Midwives who are employed will rarely be the defendants, since the person seeking compensation, the claimant (formerly known as the plaintiff), will normally bring the action against the employer on the basis of its vicarious liability for the negligent actions of its employees whilst acting in course of employment. Independent midwives, who have no employer, would however be sued personally (see Chapter 23). Employed midwives, who act as a midwife for friends and relatives outside the course of employment could also be sued personally. This is further explained below.

NEGLIGENCE

An action for negligence is the most frequent civil action brought in order to obtain compensation. It is one of a group of civil wrongs known as 'torts'. An action would be brought in the county court where less than £50,000 was being claimed. Claims above that amount would be brought in the High Court – the Queen's Bench Division (see Chapter 1). Other torts which the midwife may come across are set out in Box 13.1.

Box 13.1 Civil actions known as 'torts'

- Action for negligence

- Action for breach of statutory duty

- Action for trespass to the person, goods or land (this is considered in Chapter 7 on consent)

- An action for nuisance

- An action for defamation (which includes libel and slander).

This chapter covers the following topics:

- The elements which the claimant must establish to prove liability in negligence

- Vicarious liability of the employer compared with personal liability of the employee

- How compensation is calculated

- Defences to an action for negligence

- The NHS Litigation Authority and the Clinical Negligence Scheme for Trusts.

In the next chapter, detailed facts from decided cases will be considered, together with some specialist areas of litigation and the procedure for litigation in the civil courts.

LIABILITY IN NEGLIGENCE

To obtain compensation in an action for negligence, the claimant must establish the elements shown in Box 13.2.

Box 13.2 Elements in an action for negligence

1. The defendant owed a duty of care to the claimant.

2. The defendant was in breach of that duty of care, and

3. As a reasonably foreseeable result of that breach,

4. Harm recognised by the courts as subject to compensation was caused.

The burden is on the claimant to establish on a balance of probabilities that each of the four elements shown in Box 13.2 are present.

DUTY OF CARE

Usually it is fairly clear if the law would recognise a duty of care as being owed to an individual in the context of healthcare. The midwife clearly has a duty of care towards all her clients. This may include others for whom she is not directly responsible but is asked to care for. It may also, depending upon her contract of employment, require her to return from off duty in a crisis. The duty will certainly involve the need to communicate with the mother, and relatives and colleagues. The duty to inform the mother about significant risks is as much part of the duty of care as treatment and midwifery procedures. The duty to inform is considered in Chapter 8.

The definition of the duty of care was raised in a House of Lords case in 1932.[4] It was concerned with the question of whether a manufacturer owed a duty of care to the ultimate consumer, regardless of who had paid for the product.

The facts in this case were that the claimant alleged that she had drunk ginger beer which contained the decomposed remains of a snail, and held the manufacturers liable for the harm she suffered. The case went to the House of Lords over the issue of whether the manufacturers owed a duty of care to her. In a majority decision, the House of Lords decided in her favour. This may seem very remote from the duty of care owed by a midwife, but the statement of Lord Justice Atkins is very important in defining duty of care. He said:

'You must take reasonable care to avoid acts or omissions which you can reasonably foresee would be likely to injure your neighbour. Who then, in law, is my neighbour? The answer seems to be persons who are so closely and directly affected by my act that I ought reasonably to have them in contemplation as being so affected when I am directing my mind to the acts or omissions which are called in question.'

Usually there is no dispute that a duty of care is owed by a midwife to her clients and the babies. However, there can be situations where the existence of a legal duty of care is disputed. For example, it follows from the statement quoted above that the midwife would have a duty of care to ensure that reasonable care was taken of toddlers brought by mothers to clinics: cupboards containing dangerous substances should not be left unlocked and within their reach. However, it also follows that no person has a duty to volunteer help, if a duty of care does not already exist.

Is there a duty to volunteer?

The law does not require an individual to volunteer help unless there is a pre-existing duty. Thus, if a midwife were on holiday in Brighton, sunning herself on the beach, and she noticed that a heavily pregnant woman a few yards away had gone into labour, the law would not require her to rush to the woman saying 'I am a midwife. Let me help'. So if in such circumstances the midwife were to refuse assistance and if the pregnant woman, realising that there was a midwife on the beach who could have assisted her and prevented harm arising, were to sue the midwife for breach of a duty to care, it is probable that such an action would fail. The existence of a duty of care owed by the holidaying midwife to the pregnant woman would not be established.

However, the UKCC has made it clear in its Guidelines for Professional Practice[5] that the Code of Professional Conduct[6] places upon the registered practitioner a professional duty at all times. This means that failure to volunteer help in certain situations could be seen as evidence of professional misconduct. Of course, once a practitioner volunteers to take on a duty of care, then she is required to follow the reasonable standard of care and could be held accountable for any failures.

Of what does the duty consist?
The duty of care would include not only duties in relation to treatment and care, and in giving information, but also duties relating to the keeping of satisfactory records, duties in relation to management of the situation, of supervision and delegation to other staff, and all actions necessary to ensure that the mother and baby will be reasonably safe. A duty would also be held to exist in relation to colleagues, to ensure that they are reasonably safe. All those elements identified by the WHO and the EC and discussed in Chapter 2 as activities of the midwife would be considered to be part of the duty of care.

The Court of Appeal has recently held that an ambulance service could owe a duty of care to an individual member of the public, once an emergency phone call providing personal details of that person had been accepted by the service.[7] The London Ambulance Service was held liable when the ambulance took 38 minutes to arrive to assist a pregnant woman who was asthmatic. The time of arrival had been falsely recorded. As a result of the delay, the woman suffered respiratory arrest with catastrophic results, including substantial memory impairment, personality change and a miscarriage.

Would there be a duty in relation to the children of the client?
Certainly, if in preparing for the delivery, whether at home or in hospital, the midwife is aware that there are young children who should be supervised, she would probably have a responsibility to ensure that a person took over the care of the children, and to take any other action which would be reasonably required in the circumstances. The duty of the occupier to visitors is considered in Chapter 19.

STANDARD OF CARE

The claimant (formerly known as the plaintiff, i.e. the person suing for compensation) has to show that the defendant acted in breach of the duty of care. This is the 'fault element' which is required under the present laws to obtain compensation. In order to show that there has been a breach, it is first necessary to establish what standard should have been followed and how the defendant's actions differed, if at all, from what it was reasonable to expect.

The courts use a test known as the 'Bolam Test' to determine the standard expected from professionals. The name derives from a case heard in 1957[8] where a psychiatric patient was given electro-convulsive therapy without any relaxant drugs or restraint. He suffered several fractures and claimed compensation against Friern Hospital Management Committee. Mr Justice McNair, in deciding how to determine the standard which should have been followed, said:

'When you get a situation which involved the use of some special skill or competence, then the test as to whether there has been negligence or not is... the standard of the ordinary skilled man exercising and professing to have that special skill. A man need not possess the highest expert skill; it is well-established that it is sufficient if he exercises the ordinary skill of an ordinary competent man exercising that particular art.'

He added later:

'He is not guilty of negligence if he has acted in accordance with a practice accepted as proper by a responsible body of medical men skilled in that particular art.'

The Bolam Test has since been applied to a variety of professions including solicitors, architects, surveyors etc. It relates to the standards which were reasonably expected at the time the alleged negligent act took place. It thus enables the standards applied by the courts to change, and for professionals to be judged against the standards of the time of the alleged negligence acts, not the standards which existed at the time of the court hearing which may be many years later.

In the actual case of Bolam, the patient lost his claim. However, were the same facts to occur in the 21st century, there would probably be an offer to settle without any attempt to defend the case, since standards are much higher now.

The Bolam Test was applied by the House of Lords in a case involving a brain-damaged baby (Whitehouse v. Jordan 1981)[9]

The facts (in brief – the full facts are discussed in the next chapter) of this case were as follows:

Stuart Whitehouse was born in January 1970 with severe brain damage. His mother alleged that the brain damage was caused because the doctor pulled too hard and too long with forceps, as a consequence of which the baby was severely disabled. The doctor denied the allegations. The mother won the case in the High Court and £100,000 was awarded.

The doctor appealed, and this was allowed by the Court of Appeal, on the grounds that an error of judgement was not negligence. The mother then appealed to the House of Lords. Amongst the issues the House of Lords had to decide was the extent to which an error of judgement was or was not negligence. In applying the Bolam Test to the facts, the House of Lords made it clear that there was no absolute rule relating to errors of judgement; they may or may not constitute negligence depending on the circumstances and what would have been the standard of the ordinary skilled man exercising and professing to have that special skill.

'If a surgeon failed to measure up to that, in any respect ('clinical judgement' or otherwise) he had been negligent and should be so adjudged.'

Further discussion of this case can be found in Chapter 14.

What if there are different opinions over the standard which should be followed?

Mr Justice McNair in the Bolam case referred to the fact that there are sometimes differences of opinion and quoted from an earlier case (Hunter v. Hanley 1955[10]):

'In the realm of diagnosis and treatment there is ample scope for genuine difference of opinion, and one man clearly is not negligent merely because his conclusion differs from that of other professional men, nor because he has displayed less skill or knowledge than others would have shown. The true test for establishing negligence in diagnosis or treatment on the part of a doctor is whether he has been proved to be guilty of such failure as no doctor of ordinary skill would be guilty of, if acting with ordinary care.'

This principle was followed in the case of Maynard v. West Midlands Regional Health Authority.[11]

Box 13.1 Maynard v. West Midlands Regional Health Authority

Mrs Maynard had been advised to have a biopsy in order to establish whether she was suffering from Hodgkin's Disease. It seemed likely that her symptoms were those of TB, but because of the possibility of the prognosis of recovery from Hodgkin's Disease being improved with earlier treatment, it was important to eliminate that possibility as soon as possible. The operation of mediastinoscopy to provide a biopsy was performed and unfortunately caused damage to her left laryngeal nerve. The biopsy was found to be negative and the patient was diagnosed as suffering from TB. She was then advised that her condition was clearly one of TB and there was no need for the biopsy to have been performed. She therefore sued the Regional Health Authority and the doctor.

Mrs Maynard lost the case, the House of Lords holding the following:

'It was not sufficient to establish negligence for the plaintiff (i.e. claimant) to show that there was a body of competent professional opinion that considered the decision as wrong, if there was also a body of equally competent professional opinion that supported the decision as having been reasonable in the circumstances.'

The lessons of this are clear for midwives.

– Firstly, the midwife must ensure that she understands what are the present standards of care which would be provided by a reasonable midwife in any specific circumstances. This means that she must be aware of the protocols, guidelines and procedures which have been drawn up both nationally and locally.

– Secondly, she must also have an understanding as to the circumstances in which any reasonable midwife would depart from the agreed protocols because of the particular circumstances of the situation. This means that midwifery will never become simply a book of regulations which must be followed. There will always be a need for professional judgement and discretion to be exercised.

– Thirdly, the midwife should ensure that her records show accurately the particular circumstances which provided the justification for departing from the agreed procedure. Should harm occur to the mother and/or child and the midwife be challenged on what she had done, she would require comprehensive clear records to defend her actions.

– Fourthly, she must keep up-to-date and ensure that her knowledge, skill and experience is constantly updated, since the standards improve and she would be judged against those expected of her at the time, not those which applied several years before.

– Fifthly, in any area of development where standards are not certain, she should obtain as much information as possible to ensure that she can care for the mother and baby safely. This is a particular issue with water births which are discussed in Chapter 6.

How do local standards relate to national standards?
The courts are concerned with applying what it is reasonable for a claimant to expect from the professionals. Expert witnesses would give evidence for both claimant and defence (there are new rules for expert evidence, see below) on what standards could have been expected. If local standards are lower than what could be expected nationally, they would not suffice. Local standards may however be higher than

national standards, where a specialist service is offered. For example, it may be that a trust advertises itself as being able to provide a specific form of childbirth not generally available, and has referrals on that basis. If in carrying out this special procedure, harm occurs as a result of negligence by a member of staff, it would not be acceptable as a defence for the trust to say that no other hospital could have performed the technique better.

How do protocols relate to the Bolam Test?

Many trusts have now devised their own protocols for midwifery practice. For example, antenatal protocols may be devised for identifying risk factors at the initial antenatal booking. If these protocols conformed to what would be the reasonable practice of a midwife following the practice accepted as proper by a responsible body of midwives, then in normal circumstances it would be expected that these protocols should be followed. However, there may well be circumstances in which the midwife would be acting reasonably in not following the protocol to the letter. Her independent professional judgement can never be replaced by reliance upon a set procedure. Compliance levels in conforming to protocols may vary for a variety of reasons.[12]

A useful consideration of the legal implications of guidelines, policies, protocols and procedures is given by Brian Hurwitz.[13] He discusses the circumstances where it is negligent not to follow guidelines and also those situations where it is negligent to follow the guidelines absolutely. Professional judgement and discretion are required and clear documentation must record the full circumstances as to why the guidelines were not entirely appropriate for the specific circumstances which existed.

Standard setting, the National Institute of Clinical Excellence (NICE) and National Service Frameworks

As the work of NICE (see Chapter 21) develops it is likely that there will be more guidance on clinically effective practice and medication. Such guidance will probably be absorbed into the Bolam Test, so that a claimant may argue that there has been a failure to follow a reasonable standard of care as indicated in the published research findings and publications of NICE. For example, in June 2001 NICE published the Clinical Guidelines on the Induction of Labour.[14] A National Guideline on fetal heart surveillance was published by NICE in May 2000.[15] Neither met with unqualified acceptance.[16] Whilst it is accepted that there may be situations, where these guidelines would not be appropriate, it is likely that in the event of harm occurring, the claimant would use failure to follow the guidelines as evidence of negligence and therefore the professional would have to give evidence of the circumstances which made following the guidelines inappropriate. This is also true of the findings of such bodies as the National Evidence-Based Midwifery Network. As their work develops in promulgating good practice, so their recommendations will be absorbed into what is considered to be reasonable practice, according to the Bolam Test[17] (see also Chapter 21).

The publication of a National Service Framework for children and maternity care will lead to the establishment of minimum standards which should be made available for mothers and children. This could increase litigation if harm can be shown to result from a failure to follow such recommended standards. The Department of Health announced[18] that the NHS Clinical Governance Support Team is working in partnership with the Royal College of Obstetrics and Gynaecology, the Royal College of Midwifery and the NHS Litigation Authority to develop a targeted multi-disciplinary, task-orientated programme involving twelve maternity units. They will produce a working model for safe and high quality care. Evidence of failure to implement such standards will inevitably be used by claimants in litigation.

The Confidential Enquiry into Stillbirths and Deaths in Infancy (CESDI) also provides information from its analysis of the causes of death which can lead to higher standards of care. For example, in its seventh Annual Report[19] it reviewed deaths following breech presentation and found that the single and most avoidable factor was suboptimal care given in labour rather than the conduct of the delivery itself. It made strong recommendations to trusts on the conduct of a breech presentation.

The Clinical Negligence Scheme for Trusts (CNST) has also laid down standards to be followed by those trusts who belong to the scheme, some specifically relating to midwifery and obstetrics (see below). Other sources of guidance, for example professional associations and government departments, could also recommend procedures and policies which could eventually be incorporated within a Bolam Test of the reasonable standard of care. For example, the Chief Medical Officer commissioned a review of the use of catheters for the intravenous feeding of sick newborn babies following the death of four babies in the Greater Manchester area in 2000. The review made fourteen recommendations including the advice that the tip of the catheter should not be positioned in the heart.

Expert evidence

Unfortunately expert evidence has not always been based on a detached, objective view of the facts, and the House of Lords ruled in the Bolitho case[20] that experts should be sure that their evidence related to the facts of the case. In this case the House of Lords stated that:

'The court had to be satisfied that the exponents of the body of opinion relied on can demonstrate that such opinion has a logical basis. In particular, in cases involving, as they often do, the weighing of risks against benefits, the judge, before accepting a body of opinion as being responsible, reasonable or respectable, will need to be satisfied that, in forming their views, the experts had directed their minds to the question of comparative risks and benefits and had reached a defensible conclusion on the matter.'

'The use of the adjectives 'responsible, reasonable and respectable' (in the Bolam case) all showed that the court had to be satisfied that the exponents of the body of opinion relied upon could demonstrate that such opinion had a logical basis.'

'It would seldom be right for a judge to reach the conclusion that views held by a competent medical expert were unreasonable.'

Following the Woolf Reforms (see below) parties to personal injury litigation are expected to agree upon an expert witness. The new civil procedure rules emphasise that the principal duty of the expert witness is to the court.

It follows from the Bolitho judgement that there may be exceptional cases where a judge decides that expert opinion given by a defendant is not reasonable. This occurred in the case of Marriott v. West Midlands Health Authority 1999.[21]

Standards of care in prison

In a recent decision[22] it was argued by the defence that women in prison could not expect the same standards of maternity care as those outside.

Box 13.2 Brooks v. Home Office

A woman who was pregnant with twins was remanded in custody at Holloway prison, where the prison medical service had responsibility for her care. Her pregnancy was classified as high risk, requiring regular monitoring by ultrasound scans and clinical examination. A scan at the prison revealed that twin 1 was 20% smaller than twin 2 and had not grown sufficiently within the previous two weeks. Following the death of the baby and her suffering psychiatric injury, the mother sued, claiming that there had been a breach of the duty of care owed to her since the doctor in charge of her care had insufficient obstetric expertise, failed to seek immediate specialist obstetric advice and permitted a five day delay before she received specialist attention.

The High Court disagreed with the proposition put by the defendants that a pregnant woman in prison was not entitled to expect the same careful standard of obstetric care and observation as if she was at liberty. However, on the facts, the woman's action failed, since it was held that the baby had died before expert opinion could reasonably have been expected to have been obtained. The loss could not therefore have been caused by the breach of duty, i.e. the baby would have died anyway, even if the reasonable standard of care had been followed.

Even though the action failed, the case has established an important principle in terms of the standard of care owed by the prison service to pregnant women and mothers, and it may be that in the future a pregnant woman who suffers harm as a result of failures within the prison service may obtain compensation. It might surprise some midwives that the defendant would have put forward a contrary proposition: how could it ever be justifiable to give a pregnant woman a lower standard of maternity care just because she is imprisoned?

In March 1996 the Royal College of Midwives[23] published a paper emphasising the duty of all those providing maternity services to ensure that the dignity of every pregnant woman is preserved, regardless of her situation or the way in which care is delivered. It was concerned that maternity care which is both safe and appropriate should be available to women in prison. The role of the midwife is to attend to women during pregnancy and childbirth and it is the midwife's responsibility to ensure high standards of care throughout that time, whatever the woman's circumstances. The subject of pregnant women in prison is considered in Chapter 6.

CAUSATION

It is not enough for the claimant to show that the duty of care which was owed was broken; the claimant must also show that there was a causal link between that duty and the harm which has occurred. This is known as 'causation'. There must be factual causation as well as the link being reasonably foreseeable. Factual causation was lacking in the case shown in Box 13.2 above.

Factual causation

If the baby would have been harmed anyway, then the fact that there has been negligence by the midwife would not, in itself, be sufficient to enable the claimant to obtain compensation. For example, a mother might be able to show that a midwife failed to act appropriately when fetal distress was identified. However, if the child would have been born brain damaged as a result of a congenital defect inherited from its parents, and the midwife's negligence has not caused any additional harm, then no compensation would be payable.

In one decided case[24] three night watchmen drank tea which made them vomit. They went to the casualty department of the local hospital. The casualty officer, on being told of the complaints by a nurse, did not see the men, but told them to go home and call in their own doctors. Some hours later, one of them died from arsenical poisoning. The court held that

- The casualty department officers owed a duty of care in the circumstances.

- The casualty doctor had been negligent in not seeing them, but

- Even if he had, it was improbable that the only effective antidote could have been administered in time to save the deceased, and

- Therefore the defendants were not liable. The patient would have died anyway.

The onus is on the claimant to establish that there is this causal link between the breach of the duty of care and the harm which occurred.

In the following case, the claimants failed to establish causation and the House of Lords ordered a new hearing on the issue of causation.

Box 13.3 Wilsher v. Essex Area Health Authority[25]

A premature baby was being treated with oxygen therapy. A junior doctor mistakenly inserted the catheter to monitor the oxygen intake into a vein rather than an artery. A senior registrar, when asked to check what had been done, failed to notice the error. The baby was given excess oxygen. The parents claimed compensation for the retrolentalfibroplasia that the baby suffered, but failed to prove that it was the excess oxygen which had caused the harm. They therefore failed in their claim. It was agreed that there were several different factors which could have caused the child to become blind, and the negligence was only one of them. It could not been presumed that it was the defendant's negligence which had caused the harm. The House of Lords ordered the case to be reheard on the issue of causation. In the event, the parties settled.

It has also been difficult for claimants to establish causation when suing for compensation for harm which it is claimed has resulted from vaccine damage.[26] This is further discussed in Chapter 28.

In a case where a boy suffering from meningitis was given an overdose of penicillin, the parents claimed compensation for loss of hearing. The House of Lords, however, held that it had not been established that the deafness was caused by the overdose of penicillin, and the parents therefore lost their claim.[27] Factual causation between a brain-damaged baby and negligent care at birth may be difficult to establish, and of crucial importance will be the evidence of early fetal distress.

An intervening cause, which breaks the chain of causation, may also prevent causation being established and therefore cause the claimant to fail in her claim.

HARM

To obtain compensation for negligence it must be established that harm has resulted from the negligent act. Harm includes personal injury and death, loss and damage of property. What types of harm do the courts recognise as being subject to compensation? Some of the forms of harm are shown in Box 13.4.

Box 13.4 Harm recognised as subject to compensation in the civil courts

- Personal injury, pain and suffering

- Death

- Loss of the ability to have children

- Loss of the opportunity to have an abortion

▶   – Having a child after being sterilised

    – Post traumatic stress syndrome or nervous shock

    – Loss or damage of property.

Post traumatic stress syndrome

Where psychiatric harm has occurred as well as physical injury then that is compensatable if a breach of the duty of care and causation can be established. However, where nervous shock (or post traumatic stress syndrome as it is now known) has occurred on its own, compensation will only be paid if a duty of care can be established. The principles of liability for nervous shock were outlined by the House of Lords in the case of McLoughlin v. O'Brian 1982.[28] More recently, the House of Lords has set out the principles in a series of cases some involving post traumatic stress syndrome suffered by those who witnessed or assisted at the Hillsborough football stadium disaster. In Alcock v. Chief Constable of South Yorkshire Police[29] the House of Lords held that a person who suffers reasonably foreseeable psychiatric illness as a result of another person's death cannot recover damages unless he can satisfy three requirements:

– that he had a close tie of love and affection with the person killed, injured or imperilled

– that he was close to the incident in time and space, and

– that he directly perceived the incident rather than, for example, hearing about it from a third person.

In Page v. Smith[30] the House of Lords made a distinction between primary and secondary victims: a claimant who was within the range of foreseeable injury was a primary victim, all other victims must satisfy the requirements set out above.

This was applied by the House of Lords in the case of White v. Chief Constable of South Yorkshire Police and Others[31] where it decided by a majority that police officers who had assisted in the aftermath of the Hillsborough disaster could not obtain compensation because they were not primary victims since they were not in the zone of danger, nor did they satisfy the requirements set out above of being secondary victims. In contrast, a girl who witnessed her mentally-ill brother stab their mother to death was given £500,000 compensation by the NHS trust who admitted liability for her severe mental breakdown.[32] An independent inquiry had found that he had been allowed to leave the ward, even though medical staff realised that he posed a danger to himself and others.

The way in which compensation for nervous shock was calculated in a case involving brain damage at birth is discussed below.

The rights of the child to bring an action are considered in Chapter 32. It should be noted here however that the law does not recognise a child's right of action for being born (eg. where a sterilisation or abortion has failed) as opposed to a right of action for being born disabled.[33]

Harm may also include financial losses such as loss of earnings. The way in which the compensation is calculated is shown below.

Establishing the facts: The thing speaks for itself

The claimant (formerly known as the plaintiff), i.e. the person bringing the action, normally has the burden of proving that there was negligence by the defendant which caused harm to her. The standard of proof in the civil courts where an action for compensation would take place is 'on a balance of probabilities'. This contrasts with the standard of proof in a criminal case, which is 'beyond reasonable doubt'.

However, where certain circumstances arise it is possible for the claimant to argue that 'the thing speaks for itself' and the defendant has the task of showing that he was not negligent. This is known as a 'res ipsa loquitur' situation. The circumstances which have to be shown by the claimant are:

– the events were under the control of the defendant

– something has occurred which would not normally occur if all reasonable care were taken

– the defendant has not offered any explanation which shows he was not negligent.

A typical example of a res ipsa loquitur situation would be where a swab is left in a patient after surgery, or where the wrong limb is amputated. If these elements can be shown by the claimant then he has made out a prima facie case that there is evidence of negligence by the defendants. The burden of proof, however, remains with the claimant to satisfy on a balance of probabilities.[34]

An example of the application of the doctrine of res ipsa loquitur from obstetrics is given below.

Box 13.5 Brown v. Merton, Sutton and Wandsworth Area Health Authority (Teaching)[35]

In the course of preparation for giving birth, the claimant underwent epidural anaesthesia in a hospital. She developed severe pain when receiving the second dose of epidural and, as a result, developed quadriplegia. She brought an action against the defendants, a Hospital Authority, who admitted that they were responsible for the management of the hospital, that the claimant was, at all material times, a patient at that hospital and that the anaesthetic was ▶

administered by their servants or agents, for whose acts they were, in law, vicariously responsible. They denied that they had been negligent and specifically denied that the claimant was able to rely upon the doctrine of res ipsa loquitur. At a preliminary hearing, it was ordered that the number of expert medical witnesses who might be called at the trial should not be limited. On appeal by the claimant, the judge ordered that the number should be limited to five for each party. The claimant appealed to the Court of Appeal.

The Court of Appeal held that the pleadings (the documents which pass between the parties in the run-up to the hearing) showed that the defendants now admitted that the treatment was wholly under the management of the defendants and that this type of accident does not happen in the ordinary course of epidural anaesthesia when proper care is used. That is an admission of liability on the pleadings, and it is not in any way protected by the optimistic proposition that inquiries are still being made in an endeavour to find out whether the defendants can hereafter dispute liability. There was therefore no issue as to liability, only as to damages. The Court of Appeal therefore amended the order by deleting any reference to the doctors who were to give evidence on the treatment, and limited it purely to the condition and prognosis of the claimant. In total, the sum of £398,629 was awarded. (It must be remembered that this was 1982 and considerably more would be awarded today.)

VICARIOUS LIABILITY

It would be usual in the case of an employed midwife for her employer to be sued in the event of her being negligent. For obvious reasons, the employer is more likely to be able to pay the compensation due as a consequence of any harm caused by her negligence. This applies even though the employer has not been negligent in any way. In order to ensure that an innocent victim obtains compensation for injuries caused by an employee, public policy dictates that the doctrine of vicarious liability applies. Under the doctrine of vicarious liability, the employer is responsible for compensation payable for the harm.

For vicarious liability to be established the elements shown in Box 13.6 must be established.

Box 13.6 Elements in vicarious liability

- There must be negligence i.e. a duty of care which has been breached and, as a reasonably foreseeable consequence, has caused harm, or some other failure by the employee

▶

- The negligent act or omission or failure must have been by an employee

- The negligent employee must have been acting in the course of employment.

EMPLOYEE

Normally there is no difficulty in defining who is an employee for the purposes of vicarious liability. The term may well include bank or agency midwives, but much would depend upon the contractual relationship established between them and the NHS trust or hospital. Independent midwives are not employees. They may have an honorary contract to work in hospital premises. This is unlikely to make the hospital legally liable for their actions. If the hospital were prepared to pay out compensation in respect of the negligence of an independent midwife, it would probably be subject to the right of indemnity by the trust against the midwife. The situation relating to independent midwives is considered in Chapter 23.

An employer is not liable for the actions of an independent contractor unless he has authorised them or is at fault in his choice of contractor. Thus, if decorators come on site and harm is caused by the negligence of one of their employees, the occupier of the site or the person who arranged for the decorators to be contracted, will not normally be responsible for their activities (see Chapter 19). Similarly, if independent midwives have an agreement that they can come into the hospital managed by an NHS trust and deliver the mother, it is unlikely that the NHS trust will consider itself to be vicariously liable for the actions of the independent midwife, though it may be vicariously liable for its own staff, or it may be directly liable through failing to provide a safe system of work, safe premises and equipment and competent staff. Much, however, depends upon the independent midwife's contract with the NHS trust and she may agree that whilst she is working on the trust's premises, she works as an employee of the trust.

COURSE OF EMPLOYMENT

Not only must the negligent person be an employee but this person must have been acting in the course of employment. This phrase is wider than 'within the job description' or 'within the rules' or 'following procedures'. Even where the employee is deliberately disobeying the orders of the employer, that action could still be construed as being in the course of employment if it is part of the work that an employee is authorised to do. Thus a midwife who failed to follow the procedures relating to water births in a domiciliary setting would be acting in the course of employment. In contrast, a midwife who supervised the delivery of a friend or relative who was not her client would be acting outside the course of employment.

Even if the midwife were failing to obey the instructions of the employer, or working contrary to agreed protocols and procedures, the courts may still hold that the employer is vicariously liable for her actions. The House of Lords has recently held that school owners, who were the employers of a warden, could be held liable for acts of sexual abuse committed by the warden of a school boarding house against pupils.[36] The reasoning was that the acts of abuse were sufficiently connected with the work that he had been employed to do that they could be regarded as having been committed within the scope of his employment, i.e. in the course of his employment.

EMPLOYER'S RIGHT OF INDEMNITY

Whilst the doctrine of vicarious liability enables the victim of negligence to obtain compensation, it does not necessarily deprive the employer of his rights against the negligent employee. If an employee has been negligent then she is in breach of her contract of employment, which requires her to take all reasonable care and skill. This breach gives the employer a right to be indemnified against the negligent employee. The House of Lords confirmed this principle in the case of Lister v. Romford Ice and Cold Storage Co. Ltd.[37]

In the health service, hospital doctors and dentists, even though employees, accepted that they were personally liable for their negligent acts and were covered by membership of the medical defence unions. However, in 1990 Health Authorities agreed to pay the compensation resulting from the negligence of employed doctors and dentists.[38] It is therefore unlikely that NHS trusts would seek to enforce their right of indemnity against midwives and other professional staff.

CALCULATION OF COMPENSATION I.E. QUANTUM (HOW MUCH?)

In some cases of negligence, liability might be accepted by the defendant, but there might be disagreement between the parties over the amount of compensation. In other cases, there might be agreement over the amount of compensation but liability is in dispute. In others, both liability and quantum might be in dispute.

If, as a result of negligence, the child has died, then the parents can only recover a sum for bereavement under the Fatal Accidents Act 1976. This currently stands at £7,500. (This sum is not payable if the fetus dies, since the unborn child does not have legal status – see Chapter 17.)

In one case where the child died, parents were able to recover for the nervous shock which they suffered as a result of the midwife's negligence.

Box 13.7 Re W (1993)[39]

The first claimant gave birth to a child on 23rd July 1989, who suffered from cerebral palsy. The baby died on 19th November 1989. The mother sued in her own right in respect of her claim for post traumatic stress disorder and on behalf of the estate of her baby for general damages and the costs of care.

The second claimant was the baby's father, who also claimed for post traumatic stress disorder. The birth was managed by midwives who failed to highlight the potential problems of delivery in advance, given:

– the mother's short stature

– that the previous children were small at birth

– that in her second labour she had a precipitate delivery of a severely distressed child

– the failure to recognise and act upon signs of fetal distress

– the failure to carry out an episiotomy

– the failure to undertake a forceps delivery, and

– the failure to maintain or properly use resuscitation equipment.

Total damages came to £40,000 which was apportioned as follows:

Mother, general damages	£8,500
Bereavement damages*	£3,500
Cost of care	£10,925
Father, general damages	£7,500

The balance was made up of interest.

* The amount now payable for bereavement has been increased to £7,500.

An example of the payments in a case of a brain-damaged baby is given below. The details of the negligence are shown in Chapter 14. In the case of Inman v. Cambridge Health Authority[40] damages were assessed as follows:

General damages	£125,000
Interest	£12,500

Past care	£58,000
Accommodation	£50,000
Other past expenses	£139,000
Future care	£600,000
Claimant's loss of earnings	£115,000
Accommodation	£40,000
Other future expenses	£225,000
Education	£50,000
Total	£1,415,000

A structured settlement was eventually agreed between the parties. The sum of £689,000 was returned to the defendants to provide £20,000 per annum to the claimant to the age of 19 years and thereafter £35,000 pa. A contingency fund of £300,000 was set up under a trust with the parents as co-trustees. The judge approved the settlement and scheme.

DEFENCES

The main defences to an action for negligence are set out in Box 13.8.

Box 13.8 Defences

- Dispute over facts

- One of elements of negligence is not present, eg. no duty, no breach, no causation, no harm

- Limitation of time

- Contributory negligence

- Exclusion of liability

- Voluntary assumption of risk.

GENERAL POINTS ON DEFENCES

An action may be commenced by the claimant who might at any stage before or during the hearing, realise that the facts of negligence and causation cannot be established, so abandon the claim. Alternatively, the defendant might find that it is difficult to dispute the claimant's claim. In such a case the defendant might either offer the claimant an ex gratia payment in the hope that the claim can be settled speedily, or if the case commences, the defendant might make a payment into court offering to settle the claim. If the claimant accepts the payment, the case will be ended at that point and the defendant will usually be liable to pay the claimant's costs up to that stage. If the claimant refuses the offer of the payment, the case continues with the claimant at risk, i.e. if the judge either finds against the claimant or awards a sum equal to or less than the defendant's payment into court, the claimant will have to pay the defendant's costs from the time that payment was made. This is because, had the claimant accepted what was clearly a reasonable sum, there would have been no wasted time and costs in having a court hearing. Case management has been introduced under new civil procedural rules which are considered in Chapter 14.

DISPUTE OVER THE FACTS

Often a case will be determined by proof of the facts. It is therefore important to understand how facts are established before a court. For the most part, facts are proved through witnesses of fact who give evidence and may then be cross-examined by the other side. Documentary evidence will also be used, but usually such documents, with exceptions, are not taken as proof of the truth of the facts contained in them. The writer of the document would give evidence so that the judge could decide the weight which could be given to them as evidential value.

Since most cases are determined by the facts, and may take many years to come to court, the importance of the records can be understood. This is further discussed in Chapter 15.

Expert witnesses would be called to give evidence on such issues as the standard which should have been followed, and on whether the alleged fault caused the harm, and also on the amount of compensation payable.

ELEMENTS OF AN ACTION FOR NEGLIGENCE NOT PRESENT

Even where the facts are agreed, the defendant might still be able to defeat a claim by showing that one of the essential elements in an action for negligence is not present. There may, for example, be a situation where there is no duty of care, or the claimant is unable to establish that the reasonable standard of care was not followed. Even where a duty of care can be shown and a breach of duty is established, it might still be impossible for the claimant to show that there was causation.

DEFENCE OF LIMITATION OF TIME

One possible defence is for the defendant to show that claimant was out of time in bringing the action.

In cases of personal injury or death, the claim form should be issued within three years of the negligent act taking place, or within three years of the claimant's date of knowledge of the injury, whichever is the later. Under Section 14 of the Limitation Act 1980 'knowledge' means that the claimant must know the following:

– that the injury was significant

– that the injury was attributable in whole or in part to the alleged wrongful act or omission

– the identity of the defendant

– the identity of any other person who caused the act or omission, if that person was not the defendant (eg. the employee, where the employer is the defendant being sued for vicarious liability).

The fact that the claimant does not know that the act was wrong as a matter of law does not prevent knowledge, for the purposes of the limitation of time, arising. However, it is not necessary for the claimant to have actual knowledge of the facts. If it would be reasonable for the claimant to have acquired this knowledge from facts observable or ascertainable by her, or from facts ascertainable by her with help from experts which it would have been reasonable for her to have consulted, then she would be deemed to have constructive knowledge such that time will then start to run against her.

There are two main exceptions to the three year time limit from the date of the knowledge (actual or constructive) of the injury and wrong: those under a mental disability and children.

Those under a mental disability

Time does not run against such persons until the disability ends or the person dies. In most cases (eg. brain damage at birth), the disability may never end until death, when the time limit starts to run.

Children

Time does not run against a child until the child becomes an adult at 18 years. This of course has profound implications in a childbirth case. Time might run against the mother immediately (in respect of harm which she has suffered), if she has the requisite knowledge, but will not run against the child until the child becomes an adult at 18 years. Where, however, the child has suffered brain damage, there is no time limit for bringing an action until the death of that person. The implications can be seen in the case of Bull and Wakeham v. Devon Area Health Authority.[41]

Box 13.9 Bull and Wakeham v. Devon Area Health Authority

In this case Stuart, one of twins, was born on 21st March 1970. The mother alleged that he was brain damaged because of failures in the care provided. The mother commenced an action on her own behalf and also, as next friend, in the name of the child, which was heard on 9th April 1987 (17 years after the birth). The writ was issued on 23rd April 1979.

The mother's claim

The judge found that the mother knew all the facts relevant to her own claim as soon as they occurred on 21st March 1970, so that was the date from which the three year period ordained by Section 11(4) of the Limitation Act 1980 ran. The judge refused to exercise his discretion to exclude the time limits under section 33 of the 1980 Act (see below). The mother's action was therefore held to be statute barred.

The child's claim

Time did not run against the child until he was an adult, i.e. 18 years. However, as a brain damaged person, time would not run against him until his disability ceased.

Stuart's claim was therefore not out of time, and could be heard, and was upheld.

From the case of Bull and Wakeham, it would be apparent to midwives that records of childbirth must be kept for at least twenty-five years after a birth, and even longer where the child is brain damaged or mentally disordered. The implications for record keeping are discussed in Chapter 15.

Judge's discretion

Under Section 33 of the Limitation Act 1980 the judge has the right to exclude the time limit, if he considers it equitable to do so, having regard to the degree to which the ordinary limitation rules prejudice the claimant and any exercise of the power would prejudice the defendant. As has been seen in the Bull and Wakeham case, the judge refused to exercise his power to exclude the time limit in the mother's favour. He said it would not be equitable to allow her action to proceed having regard to the prejudice to the Authority.

CONTRIBUTORY NEGLIGENCE

The claimant owes a duty of care to herself. This means that if the harm which has occurred is partly her own fault as well as the fault of the defendant, then the compensation which is payable can be reduced by the extent to which the claimant was responsible for the harm. The apportionment is entirely one of fact and is required by the Law Reform (Contributory Negligence) Act 1945. Section 1(1) reads as follows:

'Where any person suffers damage as the result partly of the fault of any other person or persons, a claim in respect to that damage shall not be defeated by reasons of the fault of the person suffering the damage, but the damages recoverable in respect thereof shall be reduced to such extent as the court thinks just and equitable having regard to the claimant's share in the responsibility for the damage.'

In determining contributory negligence, the court would take into account the extent to which it would have been reasonable to expect the claimant to have taken care of herself. Less care would be looked for in a child than in an adult.

In a midwifery case, contributory negligence could be seen in a client failing to comply with suggestions for medication and treatment. There may be circumstances where the contributory negligence is so extensive that minimal compensation by the defendant is payable. At the other extreme, the contributory negligence may be so minor that no reduction in compensation is justifiable.

The contributory negligence of the mother is not attributable to any claim brought in the name of the child (thereby reducing the child's claim to compensation), unless the claim is brought under the Congenital Disabilities Act. For further discussion on this see Chapter 17.

EXCLUSION OF LIABILITY

A person may attempt to exclude his/her liability for causing loss or damage by reference to a notice or ticket, or in some other way. Is this exclusion valid? Reference must be made to the effects of the Unfair Contract Terms Act 1977.

The effect of this Act, which applies to actions for tort as well as breach of contract, is that in business situations, a person cannot by reference to a contract term or notice given to persons specifically or generally exclude his liability for death or personal injury. Business includes a profession and the activities of any government department or local or public authority.

The significance for the midwife is that if a mother wishes to have a particular form of delivery which is considered hazardous, the midwife could not say, 'well, provided I am excluded from liability, I will deliver you in the manner you wish'. It has been suggested, for example with water births, that the mother should be able to choose that form of birth, but agree that the midwife should not be liable for any harm which occurs. If the midwife is negligent, she can not exclude her liability because of the effects of the 1977 Act. This also applies to the independent midwife.

In contrast, liability for loss or damage to property may be excluded, provided that it is reasonable to do so. The requirement of reasonableness is satisfied if it would be fair and reasonable to allow reliance upon the term, having regard to all the circumstances obtaining when the liability arose or (but for the notice) would have arisen. It is for the person claiming that the term satisfies the requirement of reasonableness to show that it does.

This may be of importance in the care of patients' property. If a notice is placed in an antenatal clinic that the NHS trust is not responsible for loss or damage to property however caused, this may be effective in relieving the NHS trust of liability, even if one of their employees is at fault. It would be for the trust to prove that it was reasonable for it to rely upon the notice excluding liability.

VOLUNTARY ASSUMPTION OF RISK

Another defence on which a defendant may sometimes rely is that even though duty, breach, causation and harm can be shown, the claimant voluntarily agreed to waive the right to bring an action for negligence. This is known as 'volente non fit injuria', i.e. 'to the willing, there is no wrong'.

It has been suggested that where a mother wants to have a water birth, which might be contrary to the policy of the hospital, she could, by signing a document, state that she voluntarily took on the risks involved and would not hold the midwives in any way responsible should harm occur to her or the baby. In this way, the midwife could enable the mother to have the confinement she wanted, without the risks of being sued for compensation. If the mother voluntarily assumes the risk of being injured through negligence, and the unborn child is harmed by that negligence and is subsequently born alive, if an action were to be brought in the name of the child under the Congenital Disabilities Act this could be used as a defence (see Chapter 17).

There are, however, several dangers for the midwife in relying upon this defence to cover for her failure to provide a reasonable standard of care.

– In the first place, it is only effective as a defence against the risks of which the claimant is made aware. Were other risks to occur, the mother could argue that she had not voluntarily agreed to waive a right to sue in respect of the harm caused by negligence.

– Secondly, if there is evidence that the mother was placed in a situation where she really had no real choice, it is unlikely that the defence would succeed.

– Thirdly, even if the defence were effective in defeating a claim of negligence, the midwife might still be accountable to the NMC for misconduct (see Chapter 4) and to her employer for breach of the contract of employment (see Chapter 22).

The Road Traffic Act prevents a driver requiring a passenger to travel at his own risk. Thus if a midwife offered a pregnant woman a lift on the understanding that she travelled at her own risk this would be illegal, and would not be a valid defence for the midwife to bring were the mother to sue her.

Employers have in the past claimed that employees who worked in particularly dangerous conditions voluntarily assumed the risk of being injured. The courts are however extremely reluctant to allow such a defence to prevail against the negligence of the employer who caused harm. Thus, a midwife whose back was injured as the result of the employer's failure to take care of her health and safety and to use hoists and provide training should not be defeated in her claim for compensation on the grounds that she knew that the practice of midwifery caused back injuries. (See Chapter 19 on health and safety law.)

THE CLINICAL NEGLIGENCE SCHEME FOR TRUSTS AND NHS LITIGATION AUTHORITY

The Clinical Negligence Scheme for Trusts (CNST)[42] was established by the NHS Executive in 1994, to provide a means for trusts to fund the cost of clinical negligence litigation and to encourage and support effective management of claims and risk. The scheme covers claims arising from incidents on or after 1st April 1995. The NHS Litigation Authority (NHSLA), a Special Health Authority, administers the scheme. Membership is voluntary and open to all NHS trusts in England. Each trust can choose its own level of self-retention, and the scheme will contribute to the cost of claims in excess of this figure. Funding is on a 'pay as you go' non-profit basis. Actuaries appointed by the NHSLA analyse the available data and predict the total amount expected to be paid to the member trusts in respect of damages, costs and other expenses which will be incurred in the ensuing financial year. This amount is then apportioned between the member trusts. Individual trust contributions are based on a range of criteria, such as activities, budget, numbers of doctors by discipline, nurses and other professionals. These contributions can be reduced if a trust meets certain risk management criteria (the CNST Risk Management Standards). As the scheme matures it is possible that other criteria such as claims experience will influence individual trust contributions.

STANDARDS OF CNST

The assessment is based on nine 'core' standards. In addition, there are separate standards for maternity care, mental health and ambulance services, which are applicable only to trusts which provide such services. There are three levels of criteria: Level one criteria represent the basic elements of a clinical risk management framework; levels two and three are more demanding. Many are concerned with the implementation and integration into practice of policies and procedures, monitoring them and acting on the results.

Advice on the standards and general aspects of risk management is given in the 'NHSLA Review', and at workshops and seminars.

The nine core standards are shown in Box 13.10.

Box 13.10 Core standards of CNST

Standard 1: Clinical risk management – strategy and organisation

Standard 2: Clinical incident reporting

Standard 3: Response to major clinical incidents

Standard 4: Managing complaints

Standard 5: Advice and consent

Standard 6: Health records

Standard 7: Induction, training and competence

Standard 8: Implementation of clinical risk management

Standard 9: Clinical care

STANDARD 10: MATERNITY CARE

The standard requires that there are clearly documented systems for management and communication throughout the key stages of maternity care.

Untoward outcomes in maternity have a huge cost – both in terms of personal suffering to those involved, and economic cost to the NHS. This standard therefore addresses specific issues which are relevant to the management of risk in obstetrics. The criteria draw heavily upon advice and findings from the Royal Colleges and the Confidential Enquiries. The key references are shown in the end notes.[43]

CRITERION 10.1.1
The arrangements are clear concerning which professional is responsible for the woman's care at all times.

CRITERION 10.1.2
There are referenced, evidence-based multi-disciplinary policies for the management of all key conditions/situations on the labour ward. These are subject to review at intervals of not more than three years.

CRITERION 10.1.3
There is an agreed mechanism for direct referral to a Consultant by a midwife.

CRITERION 10.1.4
There is a personal handover of care when medical shifts change.

CRITERION 10.1.5
There is a labour ward forum or equivalent, to ensure that there is a clear documented system for management and communication throughout the key stages of maternity care.

CRITERION 10.1.6
All clinicians should attend six-monthly multi-disciplinary in-service education/training sessions, on the management of labour and CTG interpretation.

CRITERION 10.2.1
There is a lead Consultant obstetrician and clinical midwife manager for labour ward matters.

CRITERION 10.2.2
The labour ward has sufficient medical leadership and experience to provide a reasonable standard of care at all times.

CRITERION 10.3.1
Emergency Caesarean section can be undertaken rapidly and in a short enough period to eliminate unacceptable delay.

CRITERION 10.3.2
There is a personal handover to obstetric locums, either by the post-holder or senior member of the team, and vice versa.

The criteria specify the level, the source of the information, provide guidance, also identify the verification data, list any links and suggest the scoring. For example, in Criterion 10.1.2, the policies shown in Box 13.11 are to be prepared.

Box 13.11 Policies under Criterion 10.1.2

Labour ward policies. A full score is awarded only if these are referenced and dated within three years.

The assessor will expect to see the following topics covered:

Antepartum haemorrhage including placental abruption

Breech presentation including version and selection for vaginal delivery (ECV may also be found within the antenatal guidelines)

Definition and repair of perineal tear

Diabetes

Eclampsia

Failed adult intubation

Major haemoglobinopathy

Management of women who decline blood products

Multiple pregnancy

Prolapsed cord

Prophylactic antibiotics for Caesarean section

Prostaglandins use

Rupture of the uterus

Severe hypertension

Severe post-partum haemorrhage

Shoulder dystocia

Thrombo-prophylaxis in Caesarean section

Unexplained intrapartum/post-partum collapse – including amniotic fluid embolism

Water birth

Some policies may cover more than one condition. That is acceptable.

The CNST gives the definitions of level of cover for Consultants, the staff cover required for the different categories of consultant units, and the staff deployment based on workload. The latter is to be seen as the framework for local interpretation.

The Royal College of Obstetricians and Gynaecologists formally endorsed the CNST's revised Standard 10 in November 2000. Professor James Drife, vice-president of the RCOG, suggests that the 'new CNST standards will be a major factor in accelerating this process and ensuring optimal care during what is, after all, the most memorable event in a woman's life'.[44]

There are clear advantages for all midwives to have access to the CNST standards, whether or not the trust in which the midwife is employed is a participant of the CNST. The standards, criteria and verification data can be used to ensure that a strategy is in place to secure minimum levels of care. If there is clear inconsistency between the recommended standards and the situation within a specific department, then midwives can discuss means of improving services, supported by the provisions of the Public Interest Disclosure Act 1998, if there appears to be inaction or even indifference on management's part.

NHS LITIGATION AUTHORITY (NHSLA)

A litigation authority has been set up for the NHS.[45] The NHS Litigation Authority (NHSLA) exercises functions in connection with the establishment and the administration of the scheme for meeting liabilities of health service bodies to third parties for loss, damage or injury arising out of the exercise of their functions. Membership and claims issues of the CNST are dealt with by the NHSLA. Risk management matters are dealt with on behalf of the NHSLA, by the CNST assessment team at Willis Ltd, working closely with and overseen by the NHSLA.

Guidance on NHS indemnity for clinical negligence claims has been issued by the NHS Executive.[46]

In a recent report of the National Audit Office,[47] recommendations were made that the NHS Litigation Authority and the Legal Services Commission should work together to speed up the completion of cases; the Department of Health, the Lord Chancellor's Department and the Legal Services Commission to resolve the smaller and medium-sized claims with a wider range of non-financial remedies and for the Department of Health to give clear guidance to NHS trusts on what information should be given to patients who have suffered adverse incidents.

The significant changes to the process of civil litigation resulting from the Woolf Reforms are considered in the next chapter.

CONCLUSION

This chapter has set out the basic principles of liability in civil actions for negligence and considered the context of litigation. The next chapter looks at some special situations.

QUESTIONS AND EXERCISES

1. Take any incident at work which could have led to an action for compensation and consider the extent to which each of the required elements were established.

2. What evidence would you consider was relevant if you were the defendant in a negligence case?

3. To what extent do you consider that an employer should be able to determine the policies to be followed by professional staff?

4. Examine the publications of NICE and the CNST on maternity standards and consider the extent to which these are reflected in your own practice.

References

1 National Audit Office. 2001. Handling clinical negligence claims in England: Report of the Controller and Auditor General. House of Commons Session 2000-2001

2 Dimond B. 2001. Litigation in the NHS: Recommendations for change. *British Journal of Midwifery*, 9(7), 443-6

3 See for example Venkatesan Ranjan MROG. 1993. Obstetrics and the fear of litigation. *Professional Care of Mother and Child*, 3(1), who quotes research where only 146 of 1,300 senior house officers in obstetrics wished to continue in that field.

4 Donoghue v. Stevenson [1932] AC 562

5 UKCC. 1996. Guidelines for Professional Practice. London: UKCC

6 UKCC. 1992. Code of Professional Conduct. London: UKCC

7 Kent v. Griffiths (No 3) [2001] QB 36

8 Bolam v. Friern Hospital Management Committee [1957] 1 WLR 582

9 Whitehouse v. Jordan [1981] 1 All ER 267

10 Hunter v. Hanley [1955] SLT 213

11 Maynard v. West Midlands Regional Health Authority [1985] 1 All ER 871

12 See for example Young AFE, Lim J, Hudson CN et al. 1992. Audit of compliance with antenatal protocols. British Medical Journal, 305(6863), 1184-6

13 Hurwitz B. 1998. Clinical Guidelines and the Law. Abingdon: Radcliffe Medical Press

14 NICE. 2001. Induction of Labour: Inherited clinical guideline D. London: NICE; www.nice.org.uk

15 NICE. 2001. The use of Electronic Fetal Monitoring: Inherited clinical guideline C. London: NICE

16 Thornton J. 2001. Not so NICE guidelines. *British Journal of Midwifery*, 9(8), 470-2; Spiby H. 2001. NICE guidelines on electronic fetal monitoring. *British Journal of Midwifery*, 9(8), 489

17 Foundation for Nursing Studies, 32 Buckingham Palace Road, London SW1W 0RE; www.fons.org; 0207 233 5750; Hunt G and Monro J. 2001. First National Evidence-Based Midwifery Network Conference. *British Journal of Midwifery*, 9(10), 676-7

18 Department of Health. 2001. Building a Safer NHS for Patients. London: HMSO; Department of Health Press release, 17 April 2001, 2001/0190

19 Confidential Enquiry into Stillbirths and Deaths in Infancy. 2000. *7th Annual Report*. London: Maternal and Child Health Research Consortium

20 Bolitho v. City and Hackney Health Authority [1997] 3 WLR 1151

21 Marriott v. West Midlands Health Authority [1999] Lloyds Rep Med 23

22 Brooks v. Home Office. Times Law Report 17 February 1999

23 Royal College of Midwives. 1996. *Caring for pregnant prisoners.* London: RCM

24 Barnett v Chelsea HMC [1968] 1 All ER 1068

25 Wilsher v. Essex Area Health Authority HL [1988] 1 All ER 871

26 Loveday v. Renton and another. The Times 31 March 1988

27 Kay v. Ayrshire and Arran Health Board [1987] 2 All ER 417

28 McLoughlin v. O'Brian [1982] 2 All ER 298

29 Alcock v. Chief Constable of South Yorkshire Police [1992] 1 AC

30 Page v. Smith [1996] AC 155

31 White v. Chief Constable of South Yorkshire Police and others [1999] 1 All ER 1 HL

32 Frean A. 2001. Sister who saw killing wins record trauma sum. *The Times* 5 November 2001 page 5

33 McKay v. Essex AHA [1982] 2 All ER 771

34 Ratcliffe v. Plymouth and Torbay HA, Exeter and Devon HA [1998] Lloyd's Rep Med 162 CA

35 Brown v. Merton, Sutton and Wandsworth Area Health Authority (Teaching) [1982] 1 All ER 650.

36 Lister and Others v. Helsey Hall Ltd. Times Law Report 10 May 2001; [2001] UKHL 22; [2001] 2 WLR 1311

37 Lister v. Romford Ice and Cold Storage Co Ltd. [1957] 1 All ER 125

38 Health Service Circular (89)34

39 Re W [1993] *Association for the Victims of Medical Accidents Medical and Legal Journal* Summer 1993

40 Inman v. Cambridge Health Authority. Kemp & Kemp. 1998. *Quantum of Damages* Vol 2. London: Sweet and Maxwell

41 Bull and Wakeham v. Devon Health Authority [1989] CA 2 February 1989 Transcript; [1993] 4 Med LR 117 CA

42 A disc setting out standards information is available from the CNST: helpline 0845 300 12230

43 Royal College of Obstetricians and Gynaecologists and Royal College of Midwives. 1999. *Towards Safer Childbirth: Minimum Standards for the Organisation of Labour Wards*. London: RCOG and RCM
    Royal College of Obstetricians and Gynaecologists. 1999. *Maintaining Good Medical Practice in Obstetrics and Gynaecology*. London: RCOG
    Confidential Enquiry Into Stillbirth and Death in Infancy (CSEDI). Annual Reports.
    Confidential Enquiries Into Maternal Death in the UK. Reports.
    Department of Health. 1993. *Changing Childbirth: Report of the Expert Maternity Group*. London: HMSO

44 Professor Drife. 2000. Safer Childbirth and the CNST. *NHSLA Review*, 20

45 National Health Service Litigation Authority (Establishment and Constitution) Order 1995 SI No 2800

46 Health Service Circular (96)48 NHS Indemnity: Arrangements for Clinical Negligence Claims in the NHS

47 National Audit Office. 2001. Handling clinical negligence claims in England: Report of the Controller and Auditor General. House of Commons Session 2000-2001

Chapter 14

SPECIFIC SITUATIONS IN NEGLIGENCE AND CIVIL COURT PROCEDURE

In the last chapter we considered the outline of the law relating to liability for negligent actions, the elements which have to be shown and the defences available. In this chapter certain specific situations will be considered which are of particular relevance to the midwife and in addition some cases relating to midwifery and obstetric practice together with the procedure which is followed in the civil courts.

This chapter covers the following areas:

- Liability for failures in communication

- Identification of the newborn and security against intruders and bogus professionals

- Protection against dangerous professional staff (Allitt situation)

- Examples of decided cases in midwifery and child care

- Conditional fee system

- Woolf Reforms of civil procedures

LIABILITY FOR FAILURES IN COMMUNICATION

The duty of care in the law of negligence may include the duty to give information. In Chapters 7 and 8, failures in communicating to the mother important information relating to treatment and care are considered in relation to the laws relating to trespass to the person and negligence, and it is seen that even though the mother has agreed in principle to have particular treatment, she may still be able to claim compensation if she is able to show that had certain risks been explained to her, she would not have agreed to that treatment and that as a result of having that treatment, the risks have occurred and she has been harmed. In Chapter 28 the midwife's duty to give information about vaccinations is discussed.

In this chapter, we look at the wider duty possessed by the midwife in relation to the giving of information. The importance of communication cannot be overestimated, and communication between midwife and mother is at the heart of the Cumberlege proposals. It is also central to the philosophy of equal partnership between patient and professional advocated in the report which followed the Inquiry into the children's heart surgery in Bristol.[1]

The Bristol Report recommends that

'Patients should always be given the opportunity and time to ask questions about what they are told, to seek clarification and to ask for more information. It must be the responsibility of employers in the NHS to ensure that the working arrangements of healthcare professionals allow for this, not least that they have the necessary time.'

It also recommends that staff should be given the training necessary to ensure good communication skills. Recommendation 59 states:

'Communication skills include the ability to engage with patients on an emotional level, to listen, to assess how much information a patient wants to know, and to convey information with clarity and sympathy.'

In Recommendation 60, the report states:

'Communication skills must also include the ability to engage with and respect the views of fellow healthcare professionals.'

Communication between mother and midwife is only one of the many forms of communication by the midwife. She must also communicate with professionals, with the public, with the children of clients and with her colleagues.

Liability for negligence in communicating can arise when it can be shown that there exists:

– a duty of care

– failure to follow a reasonable standard, and

– as a reasonably foreseeable result of the failure to communicate,

– harm arises.

The potential litigant must show that the midwife has failed to communicate appropriately and also that it is as a reasonably foreseeable result of that failure that harm has occurred. The claimant will have the burden of proving all of the required elements on a balance of probability and sometimes it might be one person's word against another's.

It may be preferable in certain situations that the word of mouth should be supported by written instructions. For example, if specific instructions are given to the client during the antenatal stage, not only is it of value for the mother to receive this in written form for future reference, it will also support the midwife's case that the necessary information was given.

Communication, however, means listening as well as speaking and it is essential that the midwife listens carefully to what the mother says. For example, the mother may express fears which the midwife discounts as being insignificant, not realising that the mother's own perceptions and background affect the significance which she attaches to symptoms and problems. This perception may be very different to the midwife's. The midwife should make sure that she asks the mother carefully about any particular worries that the mother has and takes full note of them. Clearly, if the midwife gets to know the mother well, she will be aware of the mother who makes light of incidents which may in fact be of great significance.

Dr Sweeney reported[2] that one study found that a group of patients with diabetes who were taught to be more assertive in questioning their doctor about their disease were found to manage their condition better than those who were not. The doctors in the study were uncomfortable about the greater degree of control these patients exercised during consultations. Midwives must learn to encourage full involvement and discussion with the mothers of all aspects of the pregnancy and confinement if the Cumberlege and Bristol proposals are to be implemented in spirit as well as by the letter.

INADEQUATE INFORMATION AVAILABLE

Often the midwife's task of giving information is impeded by an absence of clear professional opinion over what is the best practice. The history of guidance over vitamin K is a good example of confusion in the early stages over what was the best advice to give to mothers. Professor Jean Golding of the Institute of Child Health, Bristol, told a conference in 1992 that she had found a link between childhood cancers and administration of intramuscular (but not oral) vitamin K to newborn babies.[3] As a consequence, midwives did not know if they should be recommending that vitamin K should be taken orally rather than intramuscularly. There was evidence that oral administration was less effective than intramuscular administration, and oral administration had not been licensed. Were the risks of not recommending it greater than the risks involved in taking it? What was the legal position of the midwife if she continued to recommend it but the patient suffered harm as a result? Could the midwife be held personally liable for the resulting harm? Such were the uncertainties until the British Paediatric Association issued definitive guidelines in the report of an expert committee.[4] (We may not however have heard the end of the vitamin K controversy, as Sara Wickham shows in her article[5] which raises the issue as to whether babies are born with less vitamin K than they need, and whether babies of women receiving medical management in hospitals should be treated in the same way as those born to women in home births.) The Department of Health has issued information for parents-to-be on vitamin K.[6]

In such circumstances the midwife can only obtain the best possible advice at the time and advise the women of the controversy. Similar problems currently arise over recommending the triple vaccine; this is discussed in Chapter 28. Clearly it is important for the midwife to document the advice which was available and which she gave, and to ensure that as new guidance is published from respected organisations, this is also passed on to the women.

IDENTIFICATION OF THE NEWBORN AND SECURITY AGAINST INTRUDERS AND BOGUS PROFESSIONALS

In the early 1990s there were several cases where there were mistakes in giving the wrong baby to the mother, and where intruders entered midwifery units and stole babies. Each maternity unit has, as part of its duty of care, to ensure the implementation of a system to prevent any mix-up of babies occurring, and to prevent the admission of intruders and bogus professionals. The system must be constantly monitored and reinforced.

The system would include:

– tagging of baby and mother

– checking to ensure that tags are put in place correctly.

If a baby were to be given to the wrong mother, could that mother be forced to hand over the baby when the mistake was realised? The answer is probably yes, but it may depend upon the age of the children when the error was discovered and the welfare of the child would be the fundamental consideration.

In 1994 Abbie Humphries, a four-hour-old baby, was handed to a person pretending to be a nurse and claiming that she wished to take the baby for a hearing test.[7] Such an event would raise a prima facie case of negligence by the trust and its employees. In its defence, the trust would have to show that all reasonable care was taken to prevent such an occurrence. In determining whether there had been a breach of duty the following facts would be considered:

– What is the risk of harm?

– How serious would the harm be if it were to occur?

– What is the cost of avoiding harm?

– What were the circumstances of the defendant's business?

Such precautions as the use of electronic tags, locks on all entrances, and identity tagging for all staff working in the unit would be seen as reasonable measures to be taken to prevent the harm arising. What was reasonable for a specific trust would depend upon the hospital layout and geography.

Precautions against bogus professionals operating in the community might include:

- identity cards

- identification of personnel for mothers to check

- code names

- check by phone calls

- better confidentiality over visit times and names and addresses of patients.

PROTECTION AGAINST DANGEROUS PROFESSIONAL STAFF – THE ALLITT CASE

Major lessons can be learnt from the events at Grantham and Kesteven General Hospital between February and April 1991 which resulted in Beverly Allitt, an enrolled nurse, being convicted of the deaths of four children and causing harm to nine others. The Regional Health Authority set up its own inquiry into the situation and an independent inquiry chaired by Sir Cecil Clothier was appointed by the Secretary of State. It reported in 1994[8] and a summary of its main recommendations is shown in Box 14.1. The recommendations relate to the recruitment and selection of staff, the role of the occupational health department and the procedures to be taken when an unexpected death of a child or untoward event takes place.

Box 14.1 Main recommendations of the Clothier Inquiry

1. For all those seeking entry to the nursing profession, in addition to routine references, the most recent employer or place of study should be asked to provide at least a record of time taken off on ground of sickness.

2. In every case coroners should send copies of post-mortem reports to any Consultant who has been involved in the patient's care prior to death, whether or not demanded under Rule 57 of the Coroner's Rules 1984.

3. The provision of paediatric pathology services should be reviewed with a view to ensuring that such services be engaged in every case in which the death of a child is unexpected or clinically unaccountable, whether the post-mortem examination is ordered by a coroner or in routine hospital practice.

▶

4. No candidate for nursing in whom there is evidence of major personality disorder should be employed in the profession.

5. Nurses should undergo formal health screening when they obtain their first posts after qualifying.

6. The possibility should be reviewed of making available to occupational health departments any records of absence through sickness from any institution which an applicant for a nursing post has attended or been employed by.

7. Procedures for management referrals to occupational health should make clear the criteria which should trigger such referrals.

8. Further consideration should be given to using in practice the criteria for detecting the presence of a personality disorder and monitoring for it (i.e. the suggestion of the Chairman of the Association of NHS Occupational Physicians).

9. Consideration should be given to how GPs might, with the candidate's consent, be asked to certify that there is nothing in the medical history of a candidate for employment in the National Health Service which would make them unsuitable for their chosen occupation.

10. The Department of Health should take steps to ensure that its guide, 'Welfare of children and young people in hospital', is more closely observed

11. In the event of failure of an alarm on monitoring equipment, an untoward incident report should be completed and the equipment serviced before it is used again.

12. Reports of serious untoward incidents to District and Regional Health Authorities should be made in writing and through a single channel which is known to all involved.

APPLICATION TO MIDWIFERY

Such events might be unthinkable, but they are not unforeseeable, and even though the possibility is remote such incidents could occur in a midwifery unit, nursery or special care baby unit. The Inquiry admitted that even if all the recommendations were to be implemented,

'no measures can afford complete protection against a determined miscreant. The main

lesson from our Inquiry and our principal recommendation is that the Grantham disaster should serve to heighten awareness in all those caring for children of the possibility of malevolent intervention as a cause of unexplained clinical events'.

What is clear is the need for far greater management control over staff, their sickness records and the knowledge of their present physical and mental health. Staff, too, should be encouraged as the result of the recent legislation on whistle blowing (see Chapter 22) to raise their concerns with management without the fear of reprisals or victimisation. High standards of care should be identified, linked with an unwillingness to accept changes in patients' condition as an inevitable consequence of being ill.

The recommendation that persons with major personality disorders should not be employed, and that GPs should be asked to certify that there is nothing in a candidate's medical history which would make them unsuitable for employment in the NHS, should be handled with care. There is considerable danger that the first recommendation will lead to discrimination against all those who have suffered mental illness from being employed in health services. 'Personality disorder' is a term which seems to lack an agreed meaning amongst professionals in psychiatric practice. To add 'major' to the term therefore does not clarify who is to be regarded as employable, and who as not employable.

Unfortunately, NHS trusts and others, and GPs in determining unsuitability, may in the new scenario of risk management decide that it would be safer not to employ anyone with a history of mental illness, whatever its cause, diagnosis and prognosis. This would be a retrograde step and contrary to the Disability Discrimination Act 1995 (see Chapter 22) and the Article on Human Rights (see Chapter 6 and Appendix 1).

In addition, it would not necessarily prevent a similar situation arising, since as the Inquiry recognised, there was no evidence at the time of employment that Allitt came into the category to be excluded.

Lessons for the midwife:

- Be aware of the possibility of an Allitt situation.
- Do not be complacent if there is an unexplained deterioration of the patient.
- Ensure new staff are closely monitored.
- Ensure appropriate delegation and supervision.
- Be prepared to raise issues of concern with senior management and pursue these issues if adequate action is not taken.

The report of the Bristol Inquiry recommends that there should be openness within the NHS: that a duty of candour, i.e. a duty to tell a patient if adverse events have occurred, must be recognised as owed by all those working in the NHS to patients.

When things go wrong patients are entitled to receive an acknowledgement, an explanation and an apology.[9]

SHIPMAN

At the time of writing, an independent public inquiry is investigating the actions of Dr Shipman, a GP who was convicted of murdering 15 patients and who is alleged to have murdered hundreds more. It is hoped that the report of the Inquiry will make recommendations on how such criminal practice by health professionals could be identified at a much earlier time.

EXAMPLES OF DECIDED CASES IN MIDWIFERY AND CHILD CARE

Some cases brought in the civil courts for compensation for alleged negligence will now be considered in depth, to illustrate the detail into which the courts go to establish whether or not there is liability.

WISNIEWSKI V. CENTRAL MANCHESTER HEALTH AUTHORITY[10]

On 15th January 1988 at about 02.50 Mrs W, 31, was admitted to St. Mary's Hospital for delivery of her child. The expected date of delivery was 7th January 1988. A midwife, Sister B, carried out an abdominal examination, measured the fetal heart rate (recorded as 160 and regular), recorded the fetus's position as a cephalic presentation with the head 3-4/5ths palpable and noted contractions as irregular. She carried out a vaginal examination at 03.05 and recorded that the cervix was 1-2cm dilated, the head was about 3cm above the ischial spines, in the pelvic rim and not completely free. The midwife considered that Mrs W was a normal patient in early labour.

Mrs W was taken to the pre-delivery room. A CTG trace for the period 03.10 to 03.40 showed a fetal heart baseline of between 170 and 175 beats per minute (bpm), rising to 180 bpm but not dropping below 160 pbm. The beat to beat variability was 5 bpm. Between 03.10 and 03.40 there were two decelerations in the fetal heart rate when the rate fell to 130 bpm (at 03.23) and 110 bpm (at 03.40), although it rapidly recovered on both occasions. Sister B did not feel that she needed a doctor but contacted Dr R, the SHO, to inform him of the tachycardia. The Corometric monitor was disconnected shortly after 03.40 and Mrs W allowed to walk about the ward. The monitor was reconnected at 04.20. There was no written record of any monitoring. The trace showed less beat to beat variability and decelerators at 04.25

to 120 bpm, at 04.28 to 120 bpm, at 04.35 to 150 bpm, at 04.40 to 150 bpm and at 04.50 to 150 bpm with a slow recovery. At 05.00 Sister B carried out a further abdominal examination and recorded that there were two weak to moderate contractions every 10 minutes and the head was still 3-4/5ths palpable. She also noted tachycardia of 170 from the CTG trace. Sister B said that she did not consider that Mrs W was in established labour at 05.00.

The vaginal examination was concluded at 05.23 and revealed that the dilation of the cervix was 5 cm and that it was thin and effaced. The head of the baby was noted as being 1-2cm above the ischial spines. Sister B explained that it was hospital policy to carry out an artificial rupture of the membrane when the mother was in established labour and that was the reason why at that point she artificially ruptured the membrane; she made a note on the admission record: 'thick meconium-stained liquor'. A fetal scalp electrode was then attached and the fetal heart rate recorded as 160 and regular.

At 05.27 the CTG trace showed the fetal heart rate failing rapidly and the admission record showed that the fetal heart rate dipped to 60 bpm and did not pick up. Sister B said that she decided to call Dr R when she observed the meconium-stained liquor and that the fetal heart rate had dropped.

Dr R attended at once and many others were then summoned to help. There had been a rapid increase in contractions after the rupture of the membrane. Labour progressed very rapidly and at 05.40 Philip was born. His head descended rapidly and the cord tightened, depriving him of a blood supply for 13 minutes.

At birth his APGAR scores were nil and he showed no signs of life. Only through the highly skilled efforts of the neonatal specialists was Philip revived and the damage to him minimised beyond that which had occurred during the 13 minutes prior to his birth. At the time of the hearing Philip was 10 years old and suffered from athetoid cerebral palsy.

The judge decided in favour of the claimant. The main points of his decision were that:

1. Dr R did not attend and examine Mrs W at 03.40 and therefore did not see the CTG traces as it was not removed from the monitor.

2. It was negligent of Dr R not to attend because

   (a) There was no supervening emergency that prevented Dr R or another doctor attending

   (b) Dr R should have attended Mrs W at 03.40 examined her and considered the CTG trace before deciding what to do; no responsible medical practitioner should have done otherwise and there was no responsible body of medical opinion that would support a decision not to attend.

(c) The doctor was negligent to have relied upon the midwife and not attended to make his own judgement because Sister B was overconfident in her own abilities and not in any way qualified to make the clinical judgement required at 03.40, in that her lack of ability to make the proper assessment of treatment that a patient should receive was shown

1. by her failure to take any action at 04.50, when it was accepted by the defendants' experts that action should have been taken, and

2. by her failure to ask for a doctor to attend until 05.27, particularly in the light of what she had found on the vaginal examination at 05.20.

3. (a) It could be inferred from Dr R's failure to attend at the trial that he had no answer to criticisms made and that, if he had attended at 03.40 he would, after examination of Mrs W and the CTG trace, have concluded because of the tachycardia and decelerations that it was necessary to rupture the membrane, and concluded it was safe to do so, and thereafter proceeded to a Caesarean section

    (b) A competent doctor would, after examination of Mrs W, have concluded that an artificial rupture of the membrane should be performed and that it was safe to do so, and proceeded to a Caesarean section because the only real risk that was entailed in carrying out a rupture of the membrane at or shortly after 03.40 was the possibility of a cord prolapse; there was no risk of accelerating labour at that time

    (c) Any competent assessment of that risk would have to take into account an examination to see if the cord could be felt, the position of the head, which was not free, and the risk of the head moving.

    His failure to attend was the direct cause of the baby being born with cerebral palsy as, had he attended, he would have ruptured the membrane, noted the meconium and that would have led to a decision to perform a Caesarean section.

4. Sister B was negligent in not calling the doctor and in delaying the vaginal examination, and rupturing the membranes without asking the doctor to attend was seriously negligent.

The defendants appealed to the Court of Appeal, but lost the appeal on the grounds that:

1. It was impossible for the court to hold that the views sincerely held by the defendants' experts could not logically be supported at all; accordingly, the

views expressed by those experts could be supported and held by responsible doctors.

2. The judge did not err in drawing an adverse inference from the failure of Dr R to appear at the trial because the principles were:

   (a) In certain circumstances a court may draw adverse inferences from absence of a witness who might be expected to have material evidence to give on an issue

   (b) If a court were willing to draw such inferences they might strengthen evidence adduced on that issue by the other party – or weaken evidence adduced by the party who might reasonably have been expected to call the witness

   (c) There must be a case to answer on that issue

   (d) If the reason for the witness's absence satisfied the court then no such adverse inference might be drawn.

3. The plaintiff had established a prima facie, if weak, case that a doctor who attended the mother at 03.40 would probably have adopted the course which the plaintiff's expert witness testified was his duty. The judge was entitled to treat Dr R's absence as strengthening the case against him on that issue.

4. As to causation, the judge correctly held that since the damage that occurred was caused by hypoxia, it made no difference that the precise mechanism by which the hypoxia arose was not foreseeable.

Many points arise from this case

1. Fault must be shown

As was noted in Chapter 13, we have at present a system of fault liability, so in order to obtain compensation for negligence it must be shown that there was a breach of the duty of care. In this case, this was established and so the claimant obtained compensation. In countries where a system of no-fault liability is in place, compensation is payable if a medical accident can be shown to have occurred, whether or not there was fault by anyone. The Department of Health is considering the possibility of introducing a system of no-fault liability in clinical claims.

2. The importance of record keeping (see Chapter 15)

Since the baby was born 10 years before the court hearing, there would have been almost total reliance on what was recorded during the labour.

3. The importance of defining the scope of professional practice

Sister B was criticised for failing to obtain the doctor's attendance. She was seen as over-confident. The judge considered that, had she asked the doctor to attend when she first phoned him, then the doctor would have ruptured the membranes, seen the stained meconium and arranged for a Caesarean to have taken place immediately. The case raises the issue of what the competent midwife can be expected to do without the involvement of the doctor, and when does reasonable practice require the midwife to call in the doctor.

4. The importance of ensuring that witnesses give evidence

In this case the doctor was, at the time of the hearing, in Australia and said that there was no point in his returning because he could not provide any further evidence. The judge criticised the failure to obtain his attendance or conduct a video interview.

5. Role and importance of expert witnesses

Experts are required to give evidence to the court on the standards which they would have expected to have been followed at the time. They may also (as in this case) give evidence on causation, i.e. whether the harm which occurred could be factually attributed to the breach of duty by the defendant. (See Chapter 15 on the role of experts and witnesses of fact.)

HALLATT AND HALLATT V. NORTH WEST ANGLIA HEALTH AUTHORITY[11]

Mrs H, who was 29-30 weeks into her seventh pregnancy on 8th October 1990, visited her GP who in the light of the urine test ordered a random blood sugar test which proved to be normal. On 21st November 1990 Mrs H was examined by the clinical assistant to the Consultant obstetrician at Peterborough District Hospital. He noted the urine test showed glycosuria but was reassured by a random blood sugar result of 4.6 mmol/l. Accordingly, a glucose tolerance test was not carried out. On 26th December 1990 Mrs H gave birth to a boy weighing 12 lbs 12 oz. Vaginal delivery was stopped because of shoulder dystocia. The baby was delivered by Caesarean section, but suffered brain damage caused by oxygen deprivation and damage to the left brachial plexus. Mrs H sued for negligence on her own account and that of the baby. The High Court judge dismissed her claim on the following grounds:

– On the 8th October 1990, on the balance of probabilities, she was not suffering from gestational diabetes, but she was by 21st November 1990.

– A GTT carried out on or after that date would have disclosed that fact, and good obstetric practice would have led to the baby being delivered by Caesarean section, probably with no significant injuries or disabilities.

- Reliance on a random blood test could not stand up to critical analysis, but its use could be justified on grounds of ease and convenience, provided its limitations were recognised. In this case it was relied upon in ignorance of its limitations and, to that extent, the practice at Peterborough Hospital could not be approved.

- The claimants had not shown that the decision itself was wrong and that no reasonably competent doctor would have failed to carry out a GTT in the prevailing circumstances.

Mrs H appealed against this decision. The Court of Appeal held that:

- The question which the clinical assistant had to consider was whether the single random urine sample result on 8th October converted the case from one in which no GTT was required into one where it was.

- The clinical assistant was assessing the significance of a single and isolated observation of mild gycosuria at 29 or 30 weeks. By most criteria, that did not suffice to cross the GTT. The clinical assistant was entitled to be reassured by the negative result of the random blood test which could only go to confirm the assessment that this single incident of glycosuria did not alter the risk assessment.

Mrs H lost her appeal.

Comment on the case
- A distinction is drawn between best practice and reasonable practice. It would have been excellent practice for a GTT to have been taken on 21st November 1990 but it would not have been reasonable in the light of the evidence which existed.

- The case also shows that hindsight should not be used against the defendant. Clearly in hindsight, had a GTT been carried out on 21st November, the birth would have followed a very different course, but in the light of the knowledge available on 21st November 1990 it was not reasonable to have required a GTT.

- The issue of causation did not arise: the judge accepted that had a GTT been undertaken the gestational diabetes would have been diagnosed. The issue was simply what would the reasonable standard have been. Clearly had a no-fault system of compensation been in existence Mrs H would have been able to obtain compensation.

WHITEHOUSE V. JORDAN[12]

The defendant, a senior hospital registrar, took charge of the plaintiff's delivery as a baby after the mother had been in labour for a considerable time. The notes made by the Consultant professor in charge of the hospital maternity unit identified the pregnancy as likely to be difficult and noted that a 'trial of forceps' delivery would have to be tried before proceeding to delivery by Caesarean section. Trial of forceps was a tentative procedure, requiring delicate handling of the baby with forceps and a continuous review of the baby's progress down the birth canal, with the obligation to stop traction if it appeared that the delivery could not proceed without risk. Having examined the mother and read the professor's notes, the defendant embarked on a trial of forceps delivery. He pulled on the baby six times with the forceps coincident with the mother's contractions, but when there was no movement on the fifth and sixth pulls he decided, some 25 minutes after the commencement of the trial of forceps, to abandon that procedure and to proceed to a Caesarean section. He then quickly and competently delivered the plaintiff by Caesarean section. The plaintiff was found soon after the delivery to have sustained severe brain damage due to asphyxia. Acting by his mother as next friend, he claimed damages for negligence against the defendant, alleging that he had pulled too long and too hard on the plaintiff's head in carrying out the trial of forceps and thereby caused the brain damage.

At the trial the mother gave evidence that she was 'lifted off' the bed by the application of the forceps and although that description of what happened was rejected by the judge as being clinically impossible, on the suggestion of an expert witness he interpreted it to mean that the forceps were applied with such force that she was pulled towards the bottom of the bed in a manner inconsistent with a properly carried out trial of forceps.

The defendant gave evidence that when there was no progress on the fifth pull of the forceps he pulled once more to see if he could ease the head past what might have been only a minimal obstruction, but as there was no further progress he decided to proceed to Caesarean section and he had easily pushed the head slightly upwards to effect the Caesarean section. He denied that the head was wedged or stuck prior to the Caesarean section. The judge interpreted his evidence to mean that he had pulled too long and too hard, causing the head to become wedged or stuck.

There was also in evidence a report made by the Consultant professor shortly after the delivery, from clinical notes and after discussion with the defendant, the tenor of which was that the mother had received correct and skilled treatment and that no blame attached to anyone for the plaintiff's condition. However, in the report the professor referred three times to 'disimpaction' of the head prior to the Caesarean section. At the trial the professor gave evidence that he had used that term as meaning no more than that a gentle push of the head up the birth canal was needed before proceeding to the Caesarean section. There was no unanimity of opinion among the other medical experts as to the meaning of the term 'impacted' or whether it meant that there had been excessive or unprofessional traction with the forceps. The evidence of the medical experts made it clear, however, that the amount of force to be properly used in a trial of forceps was a matter of clinical judgement, although there should be no attempt to pull the fetus past a bony obstruction, and if the head became so stuck as to cause asphyxia, excessive force had been used. The judge inferred from the professor's use of the term 'disimpacted' that the plaintiff's head had become so firmly wedged or stuck, that in so doing or in getting the head unwedged or unstuck he had caused the plaintiff's asphyxia, and that in so using the forceps he had fallen below the standard of skill expected from the ordinary competent specialist and had therefore been negligent. The judge accordingly awarded the plaintiff £100,000 damages.

The defendant appealed.

The Court of Appeal reversed the judge's decision, on the following grounds:

1. If the judge's finding that the defendant pulled too long and too hard with the forceps during the trial of forceps was accepted, that amounted only to an error of clinical judgement and as such was not negligence in law.

2. In any event, the court was entitled to, and would, reverse that finding because it was based on an unjustified interpretation of the evidence.

The plaintiff appealed to the House of Lords.

The House of Lords held that although the view of the trial judge (who had seen and heard the witnesses) as to the weight to be given to their evidence was always entitled to great respect, where his decision on an issue of fact was an inference drawn from the primary facts and depended on the evidentiary value he gave to the witnesses' evidence and not on their credibility and demeanour, an appellate court was just as well placed as the trial judge to determine the proper inference to be drawn and was entitled to form its own opinion thereon. Since the judge's conclusion of fact that the defendant had pulled too long and too hard with the forceps was primarily an inference from the primary facts, no issue as to credibility was involved. Accordingly, his conclusion was open to reassessment by the appellate court and it was entitled to find that the evidence did not justify the inference that the defendant negligently pulled too hard and too long with the forceps. It followed that the Court of Appeal was entitled to reject the judge's finding of negligence.

The appeal would therefore be dismissed.

In addition, three judges stated that

'To say that a surgeon had committed an error of clinical judgement is wholly ambiguous and does not indicate whether he has been negligent, for while some errors of clinical judgement may be completely consistent with the due exercise of professional skill, other acts or omissions in the course of exercising clinical judgement may be so glaringly below proper standards as to make a finding of negligence inevitable. The test whether a surgeon has been negligent is whether he has failed to measure up in any respect, clinical judgement

or otherwise, to the standard of the ordinary skilled surgeon exercising and professing to have the special skill of a surgeon.'

The court also emphasised that it is necessary that expert evidence presented to the court should be, and should be seen to be, the independent product of the expert, uninfluenced as to form or content by the exigencies of litigation.

Comment

This was the only one of the three cases discussed above which went before the House of Lords. The principles which were established in the judgement on the definition of the standard of care, and when, if ever, an error of judgement can be regarded as negligence are binding on all courts in the country and can only be overruled by the House of Lords itself or by Act of Parliament.

The case shows the dangers of using words loosely. One of the experts referred to the head being impacted, when there was no clear evidence that this was so. When midwives are keeping records it is essential that they should not put down information unless there is clear evidence for what they write, and that terms are not used carelessly.

CASE OF JULIEN V. EAST LONDON AND CITY HEALTH AUTHORITY[13]

The claimant was a large baby who in 1988 suffered about ten minutes of anoxia after her head had been delivered, whilst the registrar was trying to free her shoulders. The chief allegation was that a delay of 1½ hours in the latent phase of the second stage of labour (between full dilation and effective pushing) meant that shoulder dystocia was more likely to occur than in a standard delivery, and that the Health Authority should have taken steps to ensure that it did not arise, mainly by performing a Caesarean.

The judge held that the claim failed. He stated that:

– Shoulder dystocia could only be diagnosed once it had occurred

– Evidence of an oversized baby did not mean that a Caesarean was mandatory

– The mother's weight and increased risks of morbidity had to be taken into account in deciding whether or not to perform a Caesarean, and

– As long as the mother and baby were being adequately monitored and were considered to be well, it was reasonable to allow the patient every opportunity to deliver vaginally.

The claim for at least £2.5m therefore failed.

Comment

This case shows the importance of what can be reasonably foreseen. Clearly a professional can only be expected to take precautions for those risks which are reasonably foreseeable.

WOOD V. COUNTY DURHAM AND DARLINGTON HEALTH AUTHORITY[13]

In 1989 a breech presentation had been diagnosed and arrangements were made to deliver vaginally. It was claimed that failure by the delivery team to monitor the fetal heartbeat in the last 23 minutes was negligent, because it would have alerted clinicians to sudden shearing-off of the placenta leading to hypoxia and brain damage. The judge criticised the claimant's expert and accepted defence evidence that monitoring by FSE is not practical during the delivery because it may impede the process and cause unnecessary difficulties. It was not a usual or necessary practice to continue with the FSE after crowning of the buttocks. There was nothing on the trace before it ended, to indicate that the baby was in any kind of unusual distress. The judge referred to Gibb, the standard textbook, and cited with approval 'the essence of safe breech deliveries is minimal assistance from the operator'. Inappropriate intervention in the form of attempts to hasten delivery may lead to complications and damage to the fetus. The claimant lost.

Comment

This case and the one above show clearly the nature of the burden on the claimant; the fact that they have expert evidence supporting the allegation of negligent practice will not necessarily lead to a successful claim unless fault can be shown on a balance of probability. Evidence of the reasonableness of the midwives' and obstetricians' actions would defeat a claim. The tragedy for the unsuccessful claimant is clear and there are strong arguments for the justice of a no-fault liability system of compensation.

STEELE V. PILGRIM NHS TRUST[13]

In this case, the breech delivery took place in 1996. The judge held that with breech presentations, prompt delivery of the head is essential in order to prevent hypoxia owing to constriction of the cord. However, he accepted that undue haste brings its own dangers and that the head must be allowed to descend at a natural rate. Traction can cause intracranial haemorrhage or other complications. If there is delay, however, use of forceps or the MSV manoeuvre is mandatory. The judge accepted that in 1996, a maximum of ten minutes was allowed between delivery of the umbilicus and that of the head before one of the forcing steps was required. In this case the delay was of the order of ten minutes. However, the judge decided that the delay was negligent and that the head ought to have been delivered within seven to eight minutes, mainly because the CTG had not been totally reassuring. In any event, the judge was clearly unimpressed by some of the clinicians involved in the delivery, notwithstanding the fact that the senior registrar had carried out more breech deliveries than both of the expert obstetric witnesses combined. Furthermore, he held that if properly advised beforehand, the mother would have chosen a Caesarean section, in the knowledge that this would be a breech delivery, even though she very much wanted a natural birth and in fact was originally booked for a home delivery. Indeed, the RCOG recommendation at the time (although it had subsequently changed) was that vaginal delivery in breech cases was safer than Caesarean. The judge found in favour of the claimant.

Comment

In this case the claimant won in contrast to the claimant in the previous case. It shows how each case is decided on its own particular circumstances and therefore the detailed facts of what actually happened minute by minute are extremely important.

KNIGHT V. WEST KENT HEALTH AUTHORITY[14]

The claimant brought a claim in respect of a number of medical problems attributed to the birth including damage to the perineum, persistent rectal and abdominal pains, dyspareunia, a cervical tear and fistula, depression, irritable bowel syndrome and a laparoscopy for a vaginal prolapse. She claimed that the obstetrician was in breach of his duty of care to her by attempting a long difficult pull in a forceps delivery and failing to abandon it when it was apparent that vaginal delivery could only be effected by very strong traction. In the High Court the mother won compensation of £64,059.20 with costs. The Health Authority appealed against the decision and succeeded. The Court of Appeal upheld their appeal on the grounds that the trial judge was wrong to conclude that the doctor had been negligent. He used no more than moderate and therefore an appropriate amount of force and exercised his clinical judgement in deciding that this was appropriate. In addition, given the size of the baby (11lb 2oz) the mother did not suffer any more damage than she would have had if the baby was delivered naturally. The mother did however receive compensation for the additional pain and suffering that she had endured because, on the admission of the defendants, the doctor had attended two-and-a-half hours later than he should have done. The amount to be paid for this was to be agreed between the parties.

Comment

It is unusual for the Court of Appeal to go against the trial judge's findings of fact, but here they were clearly of the view that the judge was wrong to conclude that the defendant was negligent. The defendants had admitted some negligence because of the delay in the doctor arriving, but compensation in respect of the harm caused by that would be much less than if the original finding of negligence in the management of the birth had been upheld.

INMAN V. CAMBRIDGE HEALTH AUTHORITY[15]

(The details of the award of compensation of this case are shown in Chapter 13.)

The mother was admitted to the maternity hospital for induction of labour for postmaturity on 21st October 1988. Contractions started at 23.10 hours on 22nd October. A CTG scan was commenced and from 01.50 hours showed gross dips, but medical assistance was not sought by the midwife. From 01.58 these dips were confluent and the fetal heart rate dipped to 60 bpm. Still the midwife failed to call for medical assistance. At 02.00 hours there was only a thin anterior lip of the cervix. At 02.10 hours full dilation was recorded and the midwife summoned a paediatrician, but not an obstetrician. The CTG continued to record fetal distress with a fetal heart rate of 60 bpm which then swung wildly from 60 to 80 bpm until the child was delivered at 02.37. He was severely acidotic and had suffered acute intrapartum asphyxia as a result of cord entanglement which had led to an increase in hypoxia as the head descended. The child sustained bilateral cerebral cortical damage resulting in spastic quadriplegic cerebral palsy.

A writ was issued in July 1992 and a defence served in March 1993 admitting negligence on the part of the midwife for failing to summon an obstetrician at about 02.00 hours but denying causation. An order was made for a split trial, but just prior to the case being set down for hearing, the defendants admitted liability for all of the child's cerebral palsy. The child's paediatric neurologist advised that it was too early to give an opinion on prognosis and life expectancy and therefore, pending a final settlement, a series of interim payments were made to fund his therapies and equipment, and to build a specially-designed bungalow for the child, his parents and two older brothers. The assessment of damages hearing was listed for March 1998. The claimant wished to investigate a structured settlement but the NHSLA failed to approve the annuity figures. The NHSLA finally agreed a structured settlement when threatened with the possibility of the Chief Executive of the NHSLA being called to court to explain why it was attempting to charge the claimant extra for the structure.

Comment
Like the Wisniewski case (above) this is another case of failure by the midwife to summon the obstetrician at the appropriate time. However in this case the defendants accepted that the midwife was in breach of her duty of care, but denied that this fault had caused the harm suffered by the baby. Shortly afterwards, however, the defendants accepted liability and the only outstanding issue was how much compensation should be paid (see Chapter 13). The case also illustrates the problems in setting up a structured settlement.

EVIDENCE BY MIDWIVES IN OTHER CASES

Whilst midwives can anticipate having to give evidence in court if there is a claim brought by a mother on her own behalf or on behalf of her baby, the midwife might also have to give evidence in other proceedings involving colleagues such as doctors registered with the General Medical Council. For example, in January 2001 the General Medical Council heard a case of professional misconduct brought against an obstetrician and gynaecologist in Gateshead. Mothers alleged that he had used so much force in forceps deliveries that one baby was born with a black eye and another had his head swollen to twice the normal size. Midwives at the unit had to give evidence to the GMC which decided that he should be struck off.[16] The Royal College of Obstetricians and Gynaecologists said that the case highlighted the need for trusts to employ doctors who are Members of the College and had proper practical and communication skills. The spokesman stated 'Doctors must treat women with respect at all times, particularly during labour, when a woman is most in need of sympathetic care.'

WOOLF REFORMS OF CIVIL PROCEDURES

Lord Woolf was invited to examine the deficiencies and make recommendations for reform in our procedure for civil justice. In June 1995 Lord Woolf issued an interim report on access to justice.[17] This reported on recommendations to change our system of obtaining compensation for personal injuries. His specific proposals on medical negligence include:

– training of health professionals in negligence claims

– GMC and other regulatory bodies to consider the need to clarify the professional conduct responsibilities in relation to negligence actions

– improvement of record systems to trace former staff

– use of alternative dispute mechanisms

– a separate medical negligence list for the High Court and County Courts

– specially designated court centres outside London for handling medical negligence cases

– methods to reduce delays by improving arrangements for listing of cases

– investigation of improved training for judges in medical negligence

– standard tables to be used where possible to determine quantum

– practice guide on the new case management

– pilot study to consider medical negligence claims below £10,000.

The final report was published in July 1996[18] and led to the implementation of a new procedure for civil claims in April 1999.

Features of the new scheme include:

- A new system of case management with the courts rather than the parties taking the main responsibility for the progress of cases.

- Defended cases are allocated for the purposes of case management by the courts to one of three tracks:

- small claims (up to £5,000). This provides a procedure for straightforward claims which do not exceed £5,000, without the need for substantial pre-hearing preparation and the formalities of a traditional trial and where costs are kept low.

- A new fast track with limited procedures and reduced costs (up to £10,000). Factors deciding whether a case is allocated to the fast track include: the limits likely to be placed on disclosure, the extent to which expert evidence may be necessary and whether the trial will last longer than a day. However, certain exceptions to the fast track were recommended and these included medical negligence cases.

- A new multi-track (for more complex cases over £10,000).

The court allocates each case to one of these three tracks on the basis of information provided by the claimant on the statement of case. If it does not have enough information to allocate the claim then it will make an order requiring one or more parties to provide further information within 14 days.

Case management (see below) directions are given at the allocation stage or at the listing stage.

MEDIATION

One of the results of the Woolf Reforms in civil justice is that the parties are encouraged to resolve the dispute before going to court using mediation or other forms of resolution such as Alternative Dispute Resolution. Often such processes can be linked with the complaints procedure (see Chapter 11) to avoid litigation. In mediation, an independent mediator attempts to assist the parties to bring about an agreement to resolve the dispute. Unlike arbitration, the parties are under no compulsion to accept any ruling by the independent person. The Annual Report for 2000 of the NHS Litigation Authority points out the low uptake of mediation: 'Virtually everyone engaged in civil litigation pays lip service to the benefits of mediation, but in practice it is proving extremely difficult to persuade the parties to put their words into practice.'

CASE MANAGEMENT

The overriding principle enshrined in the new Civil Procedure Rules[19] (see Box 14.2) is that all cases should be dealt with justly. The court must seek to give effect to this overriding principle when it exercises any powers under the rules and when it interprets any rule. The parties also have a duty to help the court to further this overriding objective. The court in furthering this principle of dealing with cases justly must actively manage the cases. Active management includes:

- Encouraging the parties to co-operate with each other in the conduct of the proceedings

- Identifying the issues at an early stage

- Deciding promptly which issues need full investigation and trial and accordingly disposing summarily of the others

- Deciding the order in which the issues are to be resolved

- Encouraging the parties to use an Alternative Dispute Resolution procedure if the court considers that appropriate, and facilitating the use of such procedure

- Helping the parties to settle the whole or part of the case

- Fixing timetables or otherwise controlling the progress of the case

- Considering whether the likely benefits of taking a particular step justify the cost of taking it

- Dealing with as many aspects of the case as it can on the same occasion

- Dealing with the case without the parties needing to attend court

- Making use of technology, and

- Giving directions to ensure that the trial of a case proceeds quickly and efficiently.

CLINICAL NEGLIGENCE PRE-ACTION PROTOCOL

As a consequence of the Woolf Reforms and the work of the Clinical Disputes Forum (a multi-disciplinary group formed in 1997 as a result of the Woolf recommendations) a clinical negligence pre-action protocol was drawn up which is now part of the Practice Directions which are part of the Civil Procedure Rules. This protocol requires parties to follow specific steps at the beginning of an action (three months from the notification of the claim) and they are penalised if they fail. Times are set for the response to requests for records etc.

Box 14.2 Overriding objective in civil proceedings

The rules are a new procedural code with the overriding objective of enabling the court to deal with cases justly. Dealing with a case justly includes, so far as is practicable:

1. Ensuring that the parties are on an equal footing

2. Saving expense

3. Dealing with the case in ways which are proportionate:

   (a) to the amount of money involved

   (b) to the importance of the case

   (c) to the complexity of the issues, and

   (d) to the financial position of each party

4. Ensuring that it is dealt with expeditiously and fairly, and

5. Allotting to it an appropriate share of the court's resources, while taking into account the need to allot resources to other cases.

The Lord Chancellor's Department published its first review of the new Civil Procedure Rules in April 2001.[20] It concluded that there appeared to have been a drop in the number of claims issued, that the new pre-action protocols are working well, settlements are increasing, with alternative methods of resolving claims being used.

NEW SCHEME FOR OBTAINING COMPENSATION FOR CLINICAL NEGLIGENCE

In Chapter 13 the report of the National Audit Office[21] was considered. It was stated that the NHS must make provision for almost £4 billion for outstanding claims and estimated further liabilities for claims arising out of negligent episodes which have already occurred. There is no doubt that radical measures are necessary to halt the increase in the cost of litigation and the size of claims within the NHS, and the burden that this places upon NHS funds. On 10th July 2001 the Secretary of State[22] announced that the Chief Medical Officer is to chair a committee to look at possible changes to the present system for securing compensation within the NHS, with the intention of enabling a White Paper to be published in 2002 setting out the government's reforms for obtaining compensation within the NHS. Suggestions for change include:

- a no-fault liability system

- structured settlements so that patients receive periodic payments (these are already legally possible but the NHSLA (see Chapter 13) does not favour them)

- a scheme for fixed tariffs for specific injuries (comparable to the Criminal Injury Compensation scheme which is considered in Chapter 18), and

- greater use of mediation or other ways of resolving disputes.

It remains to be seen what specific proposals the White Paper will contain and whether they will reduce the costs of compensation to the NHS.

CONCLUSION

There is no doubt that the continuing increase in claims for compensation and the burden of the current levels of payment are causing considerable anxiety to the very future and survival of the NHS. On the one hand, every reasonable action must be taken to raise standards of practice and learn from the incidents which have occurred (see the National Patient Safety Agency which is considered in Chapter 19), but on the other hand, there are very real concerns about the effectiveness of our current system for compensation, with a considerable proportion of the cost being paid to the legal professionals. Both these issues are on the agenda contained within the NHS Plan. In the meantime it is the duty of every midwife to ensure that her standards of care reflect the lessons learnt from cases of negligence analysed by lawyers[23] and researchers.[24]

QUESTIONS AND EXERCISES

1. Taking any of the cases described in detail in this chapter, consider:

    (a) whether the same standards would apply today

    (b) what evidence would be required to establish either a defence or the claimant's case

    (c) the practical lessons to be learnt for the future from such a case.

2. To what extent is your own field of practice safe from bogus professionals or the entry of strangers intent on harm?

3. What action would you take if you had concerns about a colleague's actions or omissions in relation to the safety of clients?

References

1 Bristol Royal Infirmary. 2001. *Learning from Bristol: The report of the public inquiry into children's heart surgery at the Bristol Royal Infirmary 1984-1995. Command paper CM 5207*

2 *The Times*, 14 April 1994

3 *Pharmaceutical Journal*, 16 May 1992, 641

4 British Paediatric Association. 1992. Vitamin K Prophylaxis in Infancy: Report of An Expert Committee. London: British Paediatric Association

5 Wickham S. 2000. Vitamin K: A flaw in the blueprint. *Midwifery Today*, 56, 39-41. Reprinted in *MIDIRS Midwifery Digest*, 11(3), 393-6

6 Department of Health. 2000. Vitamin K: Information for parents to be. London: HMSO; www.doh.gov.uk/vitk.htm

7 News item. *The Times*, 2 July 1994

8 Department of Health. 1994. The Allitt Inquiry. Chaired by Sir Cecil Clothier. London: HMSO

9 Bristol Royal Infirmary. 2001. *Learning from Bristol: The report of the public inquiry into children's heart surgery at the Bristol Royal Infirmary 1984-1995. Command paper CM 5207*

10 Wisniewski v. Central Manchester Health Authority CA [1998] Lloyd's Rep Med 223

11 Hallatt and Hallatt v. North West Anglia Health Authority [1998] CA Lloyds Rep Med 197

12 Whitehouse v. Jordan [1981] 1 All ER 267

13 John Mead Court circular NHSLA Review Issue 21 page 20 NHSLA 2001

14 Knight v. West Kent Health Authority [1998] Lloyd's Rep Med 18

15 Inman v. Cambridge Health Authority. Kemp & Kemp. 1998. *Quantum of Damages* Vol 2. London: Sweet and Maxwell

16 Chittenden M. 2001. Gynaecologist struck off over brutal births. *Sunday Times*, 14 January 2001

17 Lord Woolf. 1995. *Interim Report on Access to Justice Inquiry*. London: Lord Chancellor's Office.

18 Lord Woolf. 1996. *Final Report: Access to Justice*. London: HMSO

19 Grainger I and Fealy M. 1999. *Introduction to the new civil procedure rules*. London: Cavendish Publications Ltd

20 Lord Chancellor's Office. 2001. *Emerging Findings: an early evaluation of the Civil Justice Reforms*. London: Lord Chancellor's Office

21 National Audit Office. 2001. *Handling clinical negligence claims in England: Report of the Controller and Auditor General*. House of Commons Session 2000-2001 3 May 2001

22 Department of Health. 2001. Press release 2001/0313 New Clinical Compensation Scheme for the NHS

23 Jordan L. 2001. Reducing obstetric risk: Why do women sue? *MIDIRS Midwifery Digest*, 11(1), 117-9

24 Symon A. 2001. *Obstetric Litigation from A to Z*. Wiltshire: Mark Allen Publishing

Chapter 15

RECORD KEEPING, STATEMENTS AND REPORT WRITING

This chapter considers the duty of keeping clear comprehensive records, the making of statements, the compiling of reports and giving evidence in court.

DUTY OF CARE AND RECORD KEEPING

The keeping of clear comprehensive records is part of the duty of care owed to the client. Midwives have a specific statutory duty under the Midwives Rules[1] in relation to records. The duty is set out in Box 15.1.

Box 15.1 Records and the midwife

Rule 42

1. A practising midwife shall keep as contemporaneously as is reasonable detailed records of observations, care given and medicine or other forms of pain relief administered by her to all mothers and babies.

2. The records referred to in Paragraph (1) of this rule shall be kept:

   (a) in the case of a midwife employed by a Health Authority or NHS trust in accordance with any directions given by her employer

   (b) in any other case, in a form approved by the Local Supervising Authority.

3. A midwife must not destroy or arrange for the destruction of official records which have been made whilst she is in professional attendance upon a case (for the purposes of this rule called official records). If she finds it impossible or inconvenient to preserve her official records safely she must transfer them to the Local Supervising Authority or to her employing authority and details of the transfer must be duly recorded by each party to the transfer.

4. Immediately before ceasing to practise as a midwife employed by a Health

---

▶ Authority or NHS trust, a midwife shall transfer her official records to the Local Supervising Authority and details of the transfer must be duly recorded by each party to the transfer.

5. Immediately before a self-employed midwife ceases to practise, she must ensure that her official records are kept in a safe place and she may transfer them to the Local Supervising Authority and details of any such transfer must be duly recorded by each party to the transfer.

As was emphasised in Chapter 4, the Rules are part of the law of the country and are therefore automatically binding upon the midwife.

The statutory duty to keep records is amplified in the Midwife's Code of Practice.[1] This provides guidance to midwives, and whilst breach of the Rules would automatically be regarded as misconduct, breach of the guidelines may not necessarily be so. Paragraphs 26 to 28 of the Code of Practice are given in Box 15.2.

Box 15.2 Paragraphs 26-28 of the Midwife's Code of Practice

26. Your records are an essential aspect of your practice and you must comply with Rule 42 of the Midwives Rules. To maintain and improve standards of practice, your Supervisor of Midwives will periodically audit your records. Rule 42 requires that the format of records kept by midwives practising outside the National Health Service should be approved by the LSA. General advice on record keeping is published in the UKCC's Guidelines for Records and Record Keeping.[3]

27. All essential maternity records (such as those recording the care of a mother and baby during puerperium, including all test results, prescription forms and records of medicines administered) must be retained for 25 years. Decisions concerning those records which are to be regarded as essential must not be made at a local level without involving senior midwifery and medical practitioners concerned with the provision of neonatal services.

28. Those involved in determining policy at a local level must ensure that the records retained are comprehensive, including hospital and community midwifery records and those held by mothers during pregnancy and puerperium. Records must be of a kind which can facilitate an investigation which may be required as a result of action brought under the Congenital Disabilities (Civil Liability) Act 1976 or as a result of any other complaint which needs to be investigated.

Whilst Paragraph 27 of the Midwife's Code of Practice suggests keeping the records of children for 25 years, if there is any sign that the child is brain damaged or suffers from a mental disability, those records should be kept until after the death of that person, since there is no time limit on bringing an action for compensation as long as the complaint who has a mental disability is alive (see Chapter 13).

GUIDELINES FOR RECORDS AND RECORD KEEPING

The UKCC has published Guidelines for Records and Record Keeping[2] which amplify the responsibilities of the practitioner in relation to record keeping. Record keeping must be seen as an intrinsic part of the duty of caring for the patient or client. The UKCC document states that:

'Record keeping is an integral part of nursing, midwifery and health visiting practice. It is a tool of professional practice and one which should help the care process. It is not separate from this process and it is not an optional extra to be fitted in if circumstances allow.'

The UKCC document sets out clearly the purpose of record keeping and its importance, and, on page 8, sets out guidance on the content and style (Box 15.3).

Box 15.3 UKCC guidance on content and style in record keeping

Records should

– be factual, consistent and accurate

– be written as soon as possible after an event has occurred, providing current information on the care and condition of the patient or client

– be written clearly and in such a manner that the text cannot be erased

– be written in such a manner that any alterations or additions are dated, timed and signed in such a way that the original entry can still be read clearly

– be accurately dated, timed and signed, with the signature printed alongside the first entry

– not include abbreviations, jargon, meaningless phrases, irrelevant speculation and offensive subjective statements

▶ – be readable on any photocopies.

Additional guidance from the UKCC suggests that the records should:

– be written, wherever possible, with the involvement of the patient or client or their carer

– be written in terms that the patient or client can understand

– be consecutive

– identify problems that have arisen and the action taken to rectify them

– provide clear evidence of the care planned, the decisions made, the care delivered and the information shared.

The Guidance also includes assistance on audit, legal matters and complaints, access and ownership, information technology and computer-held records.

Additional advice on record keeping is given in the RCM booklet on litigation[3] which at the time of writing is being updated. This points out the need to ensure that all timings should be recorded consistently, preferably from the same clock; the need to record warnings of risks given to the mother and refusal by the mother to consent to recommended treatment or procedures; a note that abnormalities on the trace have been observed; and the procedure which should be followed if an error has been made in the records.

Additional guidance on record keeping is provided by the NHS executive.[4]

CONTEMPORANEOUS RECORDS

Records should be written up as soon as possible after the events described and in any event not more than 24 hours later. Courts require records to be contemporaneous if they are to be used in evidence. One of the greatest problems in midwifery is the fact that if a midwife is under pressure during a delivery (and in hospital she may be responsible for providing care to more than one woman at the same time) it is impossible for her to record events at the same time that the delivery takes place. She therefore relies upon being able to write up the delivery at a later stage. Sometimes midwives are known to use scraps of paper or even their arms or aprons for recording information which they later transfer into the proper record, destroying or washing out the original. This is not a recommended practice. It is preferable if the information is recorded on the document which will be retained in the woman's record. Mistakes can take place on transferring the information from one document to another. Midwives should ensure that even whilst working under pressure, they keep as complete a contemporaneous account of the events as possible.

ALTERATIONS TO RECORDS

If changes are necessary because inaccurate information has been entered, eg. the wrong woman's name, then Tippex or correction fluid should not be used, but a line should be placed through the wrong entry and the correct entry made, signed and dated clearly. Midwives may be under pressure to amend their records to accord with the doctor's account of the events. They should not under any circumstances allow their records to be altered.

ABBREVIATIONS

In its advice the UKCC makes it clear that abbreviations should not be used. This is the ideal situation, but in practice the midwife makes considerable use of abbreviations and other signs and hieroglyphics to save time. It is essential that no misunderstandings should arise over the intended meaning and there are advantages in an agreed list of abbreviations being approved by the trust, and enforced through disciplinary action if anyone uses abbreviations or signs not on the list, or uses one on the list for a different meaning.[5]

STORAGE AND DESTRUCTION OF RECORDS

Advice is given in the Midwife's Code of Practice about keeping the records for at least 25 years in the case of children. In addition, records relating to brain-damaged babies should be kept until three years after his/her death. The Department of Health has given advice relating to a variety of patient and office records.[6] There will be local policies on destruction of records which will relate to storage or microfilm facilities, but there should be senior midwifery involvement in policies relating to the destruction of midwifery records.

OWNERSHIP OF RECORDS

NHS records are owned by the Secretary of State, but the actual management and responsibility for them are delegated to the individual Health Authorities and trusts. The records are not owned by those who complete them. General Practitioners are required under their terms of service to complete the records and return them to the Health Authority or NHS Primary Care Trust when a patient dies or leaves that practice. In contrast, the records of the independent midwife are owned by her, but under the Rules, on ceasing practice, she is obliged to keep them in a safe place or transfer them to the LSA.

LITIGATION

Whilst the first objective of record keeping is the protection of the mother, inevitably in the event of a complaint or claim, the records become central to the evidence available. The fact that awards of compensation in birth injuries are amongst the highest, and that there is a greater likelihood of litigation in obstetrics and midwifery than other specialties, may put the records kept by midwives under greater scrutiny by the courts than those kept by any other professional group. In the event of a complaint or litigation, the records of other groups could also be used to complement the midwife's documentation. For example, in an emergency, if an ambulance has been sent for, the ambulance service will have full details of the time the call was made; they may also have tapes of any conversations; they may check drugs with the midwife and this would also be recorded. The midwife should not, however, rely on these records for completing her own notes of the case. This would be regarded as second-hand evidence. The ambulance records should be independent of the midwife's.

USE OF RECORDS IN LITIGATION

In any legal conflict one of the biggest areas for dispute is over the facts of what occurred. Whilst records are not in themselves proof of the truth of what occurred (records can be changed, or written incorrectly) they are used in conjunction with the evidence of the writer of the records so that the court can determine the weight which can be attached to them. The more distant in the past that the events occurred, the more dependent the witnesses will be on the documentation which was kept at the time. This is so whether the court proceedings are related to a claim for compensation being heard in the civil courts, a prosecution in the criminal courts and inquest before the coroner, fitness to practice proceedings or disciplinary proceedings brought by the employer against the employee.

ANALYSIS OF COMMENTS ON RECORD KEEPING IN THE CASE OF BULL AND WAKEHAM

One of the ways of examining the value and significance of the principles set out by the UKCC is to examine court cases where the records have come under scrutiny and ascertain the lessons which can be learnt.

An example is the case of Bull and Wakeham[7] which was heard 17 years after the birth of twins. The facts of the case were as follows.

The mother, who already had one child, went into labour at 33 weeks' gestation on 21st March 1970. On admission at 4.30pm to the maternity unit in the first stage room, two fetal hearts were detected for the first time. (This was the first time it was realised that this was a twin pregnancy.) One fetus was recorded as vertex in brim and the other as a breech presentation. At 7.27pm the first twin, a boy, called Darryl, was spontaneously delivered. A blood loss was recorded as occurring at 7.55pm. Mrs Bull was given a general anaesthetic at 8.25pm and the second twin, Stuart, was delivered by breech extraction at 8.35pm. Stuart was subsequently found to have been born with severe brain damage.

The mother claimed compensation for the harm caused to the baby and the child sued in his own right through his mother as 'next friend' (this is a legal term which applies to the person who brings an action on behalf of a person who is not competent in his/her own right). The case was heard in the High Court in April 1987 and the health authority was found to be liable. The latter appealed to the Court of Appeal and the hearing took place in February 1989.

The dispute centred on several issues:

1. Did an unidentified person pull the cord and damage the placenta after Darryl was born, thereby causing oxygen deprivation to Stuart?

2. At what point did blood loss per vagina occur, and did this cause harm to the baby?

3. Was there an unreasonable delay in the delivery of the second baby, which was prima facie evidence of negligence?

4. Was there a failure to provide either the immediate presence or the immediate availability of someone with skill, experience and authority sufficient to bring about the delivery of the second twin?

Two important points followed from the fact that the case was heard so long after the birth:

– it was impossible to trace a student midwife who had been present at the time and who could have explained some of the records which it was presumed that she had made

– the records were of great significance in evidence. Witnesses would have little personal recall of the events.

The record keeping was criticised by the judge.

The records showed the following entry:

7.26pm cervix fully dilated.

7.27pm spontaneous delivery living premature male class A. (This was the actual wording in the records.)

It was stated in evidence at the hearing by both husband and wife that no midwife was present at the moment of Darryl's birth. They also stated that shortly after his birth a nurse entered the first stage room and pulled the umbilical cord, which was uncut and still attached to the baby. These assertions were denied by that nurse, Sister Jones, who stated that she arrived just in time to deliver the baby, that she did not pull the cord and that she would not have allowed anyone else to do so. (There was no record as to whether Syntometrine was given and there is no discussion of this in the court hearings.)

Since it was impossible to trace the student midwife who was present in the maternity ward at the time and made the records, she could not be called to give evidence.

The High Court judge concluded that:

– No midwife or doctor was present at the moment when Darryl was born, though Sister Jones was there immediately afterwards

– Sister Jones clamped and cut the cord

– Someone, not Sister Jones, but probably the student midwife, pulled the cord shortly after the birth in an attempt to remove the afterbirth because she had not read the notes, did not realise that this was a double birth and did it before anyone in charge could stop her

– Damage was thereby caused to the placenta

– The person who pulled the cord was negligent

– Since the twins were uniovular and shared the same placenta, the pulling of the cord endangered the supply of oxygen to the second baby

– The second baby was born at 8.35pm and the judge accepted the medical evidence which suggested that this delay in the birth of the second twin was unacceptably long.

Further errors were noted: entries in the hospital notes at 7.55pm and 8.00pm record the hearing of the fetal heart, but did not state whether it was regular or irregular.

There was no record of a fetal heart beat being listened to between 8.00 and 8.25pm, but at 8.25pm it was noted that the fetal heart was irregular. This was the first record of any irregularity in the heart beat.

The Court of Appeal stated that they considered that the judge had put undue weight upon the absence of any statement about the regularity or otherwise of the fetal heart beat at 7.55pm and 8.00pm. There was also confusion over the time the mother suffered a blood loss. Sister Jones had recorded 7.55pm as the time of the brisk loss of blood per vaginam. The judge concluded from hearing the mother's evidence and from the notes made by the student midwife that this loss took place at 7.45pm.

However, the Court of Appeal saw no reason to doubt the record made by Sister Jones in the Kardex that the loss occurred at 7.55pm. The Kardex had been written up by Sister Jones two-and-a-half hours after the delivery. One of the Court of Appeal judges (Lord Mustill) held there was no reason for the Kardex to have been falsified and it seemed a more reliable guide to the meaning of the records than a reconstruction of 17 years after the event by reference to the position on the page of entries made by a person whose identity was not even known. The judges concluded that the loss must have occurred between 7.45pm and 7.55pm.

The result of the Court of Appeal hearing was that the decision of the trial judge was upheld, though not all his findings were accepted. Of importance in deciding that there was liability by the hospital was the delay in delivering the second child, particularly after the blood loss and the apparent lack of emergency staffing cover to provide immediate assistance. Clearly in this case, the UKCC guidelines were not followed: there was no index for tracing potential witnesses, and the records were ambiguous and not always meaningful.

In the Bull and Wakeham case it was accepted that records made two-and-a-half hours after the birth were contemporaneous with the birth. However, if Sister Jones had made a note on a piece of paper at the time that blood loss occurred, it would have been preferable if that piece of paper had been attached to the Kardex or delivery record.

CARDIOTOCOGRAPH READINGS

Cardiotocograph readings were not taken in the Bull and Wakeham case, but now intrapartum fetal wellbeing can be assessed by electronic means or by intermittent auscultation with a Pinard's stethoscope. In a multiple pregnancy it would be current practice to apply continuous electronic fetal monitoring. Where such electronic monitoring is in place, the midwife finds it useful to record upon the graph itself significant events. The advantage of this is that the graph is timed and the midwife does not need to write in the time again. In addition, some of the equipment allows the machine itself to record significant events if the appropriate buttons are pressed. The Royal College of Midwives' booklet on litigation (currently being updated) recommends that the name of the woman, the date and the time of commencement should be recorded on the CTG trace.

'If the machine is one that automatically records the time, the clock on the machine must be checked. In addition, there should be a record on the trace or in the notes to show when the trace ends, otherwise it may be said that part has gone missing.'

It would also be of value for computer-held records to be signed and dated when they are printed out. Recent cases have shown the importance attached to CTG records where these are available.

The recommendation of the UKCC that initials should either not be used or that there should be a local index record of signatures kept is important. One of the most difficult tasks in midwifery litigation, as seen from Bull and Wakeham, is to identify the staff who were involved in the alleged negligent incident and to track down their current whereabouts.

Another issue in midwifery is the possibility of discrepancy between the records of the midwife and those of the obstetricians. This may sometimes reveal a conflict of evidence. For example, the midwife might have called a doctor to see the mother. Subsequently, the doctor might deny that any such request has been made. In order to prevent such a dispute, the midwife might ask the doctor to sign in the record or on the CTG the fact that he has seen the mother. The midwife should not regard such a signature as relieving her of all responsibility if harm occurs. She is still accountable for her professional duty of care to the mother and child.

LEGAL STATUS OF RECORDS

The question is often asked as to when a record becomes a legal document. The answer is simple: whenever it is relevant in a court of law and is required in evidence. In this sense there is no limit to the nature of records which could be ordered to be produced in court. Even scraps of paper which a midwife might use to remind herself of significant events in the delivery could be ordered to be produced in court, if they are still available. X-rays, pathological test results, CTG graphs, fetal monitoring traces could all be produced in court.

However, as can be seen from the case of Bull and Wakeham, records are not evidence of the truth of what is written upon them. Normally the writer of contemporaneous records would be called to give evidence of the circumstances which led to the record being made, and could be cross-examined upon them so that the court could determine the weight which should be attached to their credibility.

In midwifery cases, as the case of Bull and Wakeham shows, it may be many years before a court action is commenced. A child can bring a court action at any time before the end of three years of attaining his majority (i.e. 18 years + 3 years).

AUDIT

Regular audit of record keeping standards is required to ensure that there is compliance with the Midwives Rules and Code of Practice. In addition, under Rule 43 the practising midwife is required to give her Supervisor of Midwives, the Local Supervising Authority and the NMC every reasonable facility to inspect her records as well as her methods of practice, her equipment and such part of her residence as may be used for professional purposes. Regular review and advice by the Supervisor of Midwives of record keeping standards could ensure that a high standard of record keeping is established and maintained. In addition, midwives might be able to establish small internal groups of colleagues who can at regular intervals examine a set of records and monitor their standard, identifying any improvements which should be made. External auditors of record keeping standards may also be brought into the organisation to assist in establishing and maintaining standards. The King's Fund in London provides such a service. In addition, the Clinical Negligence Scheme for Trusts monitors record keeping standards for its members (see below).

The Audit Commission, in its report on hospital records,[8] considered that patients were being put at risk because their medical records are not kept carefully and are sometimes lost. Failure to find records led to consultations being cancelled and to operations being postponed. It recommended that hospitals set up one main records library with good security.

CLINICAL NEGLIGENCE SCHEME FOR TRUSTS (CNST)

The CNST requires those trusts which belong to the scheme to maintain specified standards in relation to a range of topics (see Chapter 13), including record keeping. The CNST has identified hospital records as one of its core standards. The criteria for this standard are shown below:

Standard 6 : Health Records	Level	Weight
A comprehensive system for the completion, use, storage and retrieval of health records is in place. Record keeping standards are monitored through the clinical audit process.		
6.1.1 There is a unified health record which all specialties use.	1	H
6.1.2 Records are bound and stored so that loss of documents and traces are minimised for in-patients and out-patients.	1	M
6.1.3 The health record contains clear instructions regarding filing of documents.	1	M
6.1.4 Operation notes and other key procedures are readily identifiable.	1	M

6.1.5 CTG and other machine-produced recordings are securely stored and mounted. 1 M

6.1.6 There is a computer system, or other, for identifying and retrieving X-rays. 1 L

6.1.7 The storage arrangements allow retrieval on a 24 hour/ 7 day arrangement. 1 L

6.1.8 There is clear evidence of clinical audit of record keeping standards for all professional groups in at least 25% of specialties, including any high-risk specialties, within the 12 months prior to the assessment. 1 H

6.1.9 There is a mechanism for identifying records which must not be destroyed. 1 L

6.2.1 A&E records are contained within the main record for patients who are subsequently admitted. 2 L

6.2.2 There is a system for ensuring that the GP is sent a copy of the A&E record. 2 L

6.2.3 Nursing, medical and other records (eg. physiotherapy notes) are filed together when the patient is discharged. 2 M

6.2.4 There is a system for measuring efficiency in the recovery of records for in-patients and out-patients. 2 L

6.2.5 The health record contains a designated place for the recording of hypersensitivity reactions, and other information relevant to all healthcare professionals. 2 H

6.2.6 There is clear evidence of clinical audit of record keeping standards for all professional groups in 50% of the specialties, within the 12 months prior to the assessment. 2 H

6.3.1 An author of an entry in a health record is clearly and easily identifiable. 3 H

6.3.2 There is clear evidence of clinical audit of record keeping standards for all professional groups in all of the specialties, within the 12 months prior to the assessment. 3 H

6.3.3 There is a computer-based Patient Administration System. 3 L

These standards can be used as the basis for a regular internal audit of documentation, even by those units which are not members of the CNST pool, to ensure that a reasonable standard is being maintained.

PERSONAL CHECKLIST

Individual midwives might find the checklist prepared by Dot Walters for her midwifery students at the East Glamorgan District General Hospital of value. It is set out in Box 15.4.

Box 15.4 A checklist for record keeping in midwifery

Use this practice checklist as a way of highlighting those record keeping activities which may need critical evaluation.

It is assumed that you will have read all the relevant UKCC documents and 'Litigation, a risk management exercise guide' (RCM, 1993).

This checklist is prepared only as an outline to the principles of record keeping for midwives.

1. Do any actions or common practices prevent me from making contemporaneous records, eg. case notes not easily accessible?

2. Do I ever make rough notes for later transcription into the client's records eg. scraps of paper, on my hand or plastic apron?

3. Are clients' records always kept with the client, especially in a high-care or emergency situation, eg. when a client is receiving emergency treatment from medical staff, do they take away the notes for completion?

4. If giving advice by telephone, as the advisor, do I make a record of the time, date, and reason for any advice given? Do I check the outcome of the case and record this too?

5. Do I regularly evaluate my personal standard of record keeping and seek peer review?

6. Have I added my signature to the local index record of signatures? Did I update the index when I changed my surname?

7. When acting as a preceptor to students, do I always check and review their standard of record keeping?

8. Do I ever use abbreviations in the description of events, actions and clinical diagnoses?

9. Do I take up opportunities (or create opportunities) for regular re-education related to record keeping in midwifery practice?

10. Have I made any necessary changes to my practice?

ELECTRONIC HEALTH RECORDS

The Secretary of State for Health, Frank Dobson, announced on 24th September 1998 that there would be £1 billion investment to put all medical files on computer.[9] The initiative will take place over 7 years enabling records to be available for access on a 24 hour basis across the country and also permitting patients access in their own home. The initiative will link into an NHS website and there will be an expansion of NHS Direct offer the public a 24-hour telephone advice service on non-urgent health matters. £40 million is to be spent connecting GPs to the NHS Net.

On 4th February 2001 the Department of Health issued a press release which stated that by March 2005, every person in the country will have their own electronic patient record (EHR).[10] The electronic health record is defined by the Department of Health as holding summarised key data about patients, such as name, address, NHS number, registered GP and contact details, previous treatments, ongoing conditions, current medication, allergies and the date of any next appointments. It is intended that it will be securely protected, created with patient consent, with individual changes made only by authorised staff. The timetable for the electronic health record envisages that 5 million people will have their own lifelong EHR by 2003, rising to around 25 million by 2004 and then everyone by March 2005. To achieve this target there will have to be considerable training and development of many health professionals, including midwives. It is hoped that midwives will welcome the opportunities for developing their skills in this area.

Whilst the computer records will avoid problems of illegibility, considerable care will still have to be taken. In August 1998 it was reported[11] that a student suffering from meningitis may have died as a result of her name being wrongly spelt on a computer. The omission of the letter 'P' in her surname, Simpkin, meant that her records could not be accessed, and an inquiry found that she might have lived if vital results of blood tests, entered into the computerised records under the wrong name, had been seen by staff.

MOTHER-HELD RECORDS

In midwifery care it is increasingly the practice that women retain their own records during their antenatal care, bringing them to the clinics for their appointments. Whilst this practice is in general very successful there are certain concerns: what if the mother destroys the records and then sues the trust for compensation? Can the midwife leave out information, eg. previous pregnancy or abortion, if the woman so wishes? What if the records are lost? (See also Chapter 10.)

Destruction of records by mother
In a claim for compensation, the burden is on the claimant to show on a balance of probabilities that the defendant or its employees failed to follow a reasonable

standard of care, which caused harm to the claimant. The fact that the claimant has lost the records which were in her custody would therefore work against her case.

Omission of information from the records

It would be contrary to professional practice for a midwife to omit essential information from a woman's obstetric history. Leaving out details of an earlier pregnancy could influence clinical decisions about the care of a mother. For example, if it were thought that the mother was a primagravida, dealing with her Rhesus negative state would be different than if it were known that this was a second or later pregnancy. (In July 1998 a GP who allowed a patient to destroy part of her records was found guilty of serious professional misconduct by the GMC.[12] He had allowed the patient, who was involved in an acrimonious property dispute with her children, to remove a letter in which she was described as 'bad tempered' and another document referring to her drinking.) Where a woman wishes to have information deleted, or not kept on her record, because of fears that her partner may discover information of which he was ignorant, then she should be offered the opportunity to have her records kept in the hospital. Alternatively, there should be a note on her records that information kept at the hospital should be consulted before any decisions are taken. (This topic is further considered in Chapter 10.)

STATEMENT MAKING

Witnesses can refer to any contemporaneous records and contemporaneous statements in giving evidence and therefore, since it takes many years for some court hearings to take place, it is vital that comprehensive clear records have been kept and statements made. Before preparing a statement, a health professional should have advice from a senior colleague and if possible a lawyer. The elements shown in Box 15.5 should be contained in a statement.

Box 15.5 Elements to include in a statement

- Date and time of the incident

- Full name of statement maker, position, grade and location

- Full names of any persons involved, eg. patient, visitor, other staff

- Date and time the statement was made

- A full and detailed description of the events which occurred

- Signature

- Any supporting statement or document attached.

The statement writer should ensure that the statement is:

– accurate

– factual

– concise

– relevant

– clear

– legible (it will usually be typed), and

– signed.

The statement maker should read it through, checking its overall impact and whether all the relevant facts are included. A copy should be kept. Advice should be sought on its clarity and comprehensiveness, and it should not be signed unless the maker is completely satisfied that it records an accurate, clear account of what took place.

REPORT WRITING

Midwives may be required to prepare reports on a variety of topics, as managers, supervisors or individual midwives. In addition, senior midwives may be invited to provide reports as an expert witness.

Expert witnesses will normally be asked to prepare a report by a solicitor representing one of the parties to the case. This report is vital since, if it is unfavourable to the party seeking it, the outcome may be that the case is settled or even withdrawn.

Box 15.6 illustrates some of the principles to be followed in report writing.

> ### Box 15.6 Principles to be followed in report writing
>
> – Identify the purpose of the report, likely readership and the kind of language which can be used, and therefore the appropriate style to be used.
>
> – Identify the main areas to be included.
>
> – Decide the order to be followed: sometimes chronological order is appropriate, at other times subject order may be preferable.
>
> – Sign and date it, but only after reading it through and being 100% satisfied with it.

▶

▶
- Identify the different kinds of information used in the report and state the source of the material, eg. hearsay evidence, factual evidence observed or heard by the author of the report, evidence of opinion of another person, statements by others, similar fact evidence.

- Avoid the mistakes shown in Box 15.7.

Box 15.7 Common mistakes in report writing

- Lack of clarity

- Failure to follow a logical order

- Inconsistency

- Ambiguities

- Lack of signature and/or date

- Lack of dates within the report

- Wrong names included

- Confusing account

- Mix of evidence and sources

- Inaccuracies

- Opinion without facts

- Failure to cite facts to support statements

- Too complex a style for reader

- Use of inappropriate jargon

- Use of misleading abbreviations

- Failure to give conclusions

- Failure to base conclusions on the evidence

- Failure to ask someone else to read.

For most purposes the style likely to be of greatest use is one of simplicity, with short sentences, clear paragraphing and sub-paragraphing, and avoidance of jargon and meaningless cliches. The report should begin with a statement as to its purpose, the person(s) to whom it is addressed, and the name and status of the writer. If it is confidential this should be highlighted at the beginning. Other documents which are relevant should be carefully referenced.

GIVING EVIDENCE IN COURT

As a witness of fact, the midwife may be required to give direct evidence over a matter with which she has been involved. If she is asked to give evidence, an employed midwife would be assisted by senior midwifery management and the solicitors to the trust. In giving evidence she should ensure that she keeps to the facts and does not offer an opinion. She may need guidance and training in how to respond to cross-examination. It is vital that she does not give facts which are outside her knowledge.

The following are key points for witness of fact.

Preparation
- Ensure that the records are available, identify significant entries with post-it notes, but do not mark or staple or pin anything to the records. Read them through so that you are familiar with them.

- Try to obtain assistance from a lawyer or senior manager in preparation for the court hearing, so that you are prepared for giving evidence in chief and answering questions under cross-examination.

- Try to visit the court in advance to familiarise yourself with its location, car parking, toilets, catering facilities etc.

At the court before the hearing
- Be prepared for a long wait, and take work to do or something to occupy yourself.

- Dress appropriately and comfortably, but not too casually.

- Try to relax.

Giving evidence
- Keep calm.

- Give answers clearly and without exaggeration.

- Tell the truth.

- Do not feel that you are there to represent only one side; you must answer the questions honestly, even though it might put the side cross-examining you in a good light.

- Take time over your answers, and do not make up replies if you are unable to answer the question raised.

- Do not answer back or allow yourself to be flustered during the cross-examination.

- If you do not understand any legal jargon which is used, ask for an explanation.

- Keep to the facts and do not express an opinion.

- Ask for time to refer to the records if this is necessary.

EXPERT WITNESS

An expert witness is invited to give evidence of opinion on any issue which is subject to dispute. This could include the standards of care which would have been expected according to the Bolam Test (see Chapter 13), or the opinion may relate to what caused the harm suffered by the mother or baby. Expert opinion may also be brought in if there is a dispute over the assessment of compensation. An article by Georgina Lessing-Turner[13] discussed the training available for a midwife who wishes to become an expert witness.

At present, where an expert has prepared a report for a solicitor in anticipation or in the course of litigation, that report and any correspondence connected with it are protected by legal professional privilege (see Chapter 10) and it cannot be ordered to be disclosed in court or the expert compelled to appear by the other side. However, once the report is disclosed to the court, it loses its professional privilege (which continues to attach to any correspondence between the parties which has not been disclosed). As a result of the changes in civil procedure following the Woolf reforms (see Chapter 14) where an expert's report is used in evidence, all amendments and changes to that report must also be disclosed.

The Woolf reforms recommended that experts should be agreed between the parties prior to any hearing, in order that the time and costs of the case could be reduced. This is not always possible in some of the large compensation claims in obstetrics and midwifery, when several different witnesses may be called as experts in different areas of practice.

CONCLUSIONS

There is perhaps insufficient sharing between colleagues of the lessons learnt from litigation, even when the defendant professionals and Health Authorities/NHS trusts win the case. Regular training in record keeping is essential for all professionals, particularly in midwifery where the peaks and troughs of activity are not predictable and when, in the pressure of the delivery, record keeping may be given a low priority. In addition, midwives should have training and assistance in making statements, writing reports and in giving evidence in court.

QUESTIONS AND EXERCISES

1. Discuss a strategy for keeping records whilst under pressure of work. Your strategy could include the use of agreed abbreviations, pre-printed forms and other devices which would be safe to adopt in speeding up record keeping.

2. With a colleague, look critically at the records kept over a two-week period. In what ways could the standard be improved?

3. Imagine that, in 15 years' time, you are being cross-examined on the care which you have provided in a particular case. Consider to what extent the records would be satisfactory as evidence in such circumstances.

4. Prepare a checklist for a report to be used in a child abuse case conference.

5. You have been asked to appear in court next week. Identify your worst fears about this request and devise ways of overcoming them.

References

1 UKCC. 1998. *Midwives Rules and Code of Practice*. London: UKCC

2 UKCC. 1998. *Guidelines for records and record keeping*. London: UKCC

3 Mason D and Edwards P. 1993. *Litigation: a risk management guide for midwives*. London: Royal College of Midwives in conjunction with Capsticks solicitors

4 NHS Training Directorate. 1992. *Keeping the record straight*. London: DoH
   NHS Training Directorate. 1994. *Just for the Record: A guide to record keeping for healthcare professionals*. London: DoH
   NHS Executive. 1999. *For the record*. Health Service Circular 1999/053

5 Dimond B. 1998. Abbreviations, record keeping and the midwife. *Practising Midwife*, 1(9), 10-11

6 NHS Executive. 1999. *For the record*. Health Service Circular 1999/053

7 Bull and Wakeham v. Devon Health Authority. Court of Appeal 2 February 1989 transcript of hearing; Bull v Devon AHA [1993] 4 Med LR 117 CA

8 Audit Commission. 1995. *Setting the Records Straight: A Study of Hospital Medical Records*. London: HMSO

9 Henderson M. 1998. £1bn scheme will put all medical files on computer. *The Times* 25 September 1998

10 Department of Health. 2001. Press release 4 February 2001. Patients to gain access to new at-a-glance Electronic Health Records.

11 Johnstone H. Spelling mistake may have cost student her life. *The Times* 28 August 1998

12 Forster P. GP allowed patient to tamper with records. *The Times* 7 July 1998

13 Lessing-Turner G. 2000. Midwives as expert witnesses. *The Practising Midwife*, 3(9), 29

Chapter 16
FAMILY PLANNING AND STERILISATION

The midwife is often the health professional who will be consulted by mothers about family planning after the birth of the baby. The duty of care includes the duty of giving advice and information, and therefore the midwife should ensure that she takes care in giving advice and information and follows the reasonable standards of practice (i.e. the Bolam Test, see Chapter 13), since she could be held liable (or her employer vicariously liable) should harm result from the mother's reliance upon her negligent advice. This chapter looks at some of the issues which have arisen in the context of family planning and sterilisations. Reference should also be made to Chapter 7, relating to consent by a minor and the Gillick case. Reference should also be made to Chapter 26, on termination of pregnancy and the extent to which the post-coital pill could be regarded as an abortion, and the fact that it is doubtful if giving advice on abortions is covered by the conscientious objection clause. Reference should also be made to Chapter 20, on medication and contraindications.

FAMILY PLANNING

The midwife should ensure that she is familiar with local provision and facilities for family planning, and give information to the mothers when asked. The midwife herself may be involved in family planning clinics. Each Health Authority has a duty to provide information about the family planning services in its area. An independent Advisory Group on Teenage Pregnancy has been appointed by the government to guide and monitor the government's strategy for teenage pregnancy.

NEGLIGENCE AND CONTRACEPTIVES

In a case reported in the Medical Protection Society Report for 1984, a General Practitioner in South Africa prescribed Trisequens, a combination drug which was intended by the makers for use in post-menopausal hormone replacement therapy. He had intended to prescribe Logynon. The patient, who had made it clear to the doctor that she did not want to become pregnant since she was the bread winner whilst her husband was still a student became pregnant before the General Practitioner realised his mistake. A settlement was offered to the patient without admission of liability. The advice given to members was that they should familiarise themselves with any pharmacologically-active substance which they prescribe.

Whilst at present the midwife is unlikely herself to be prescribing contraceptives, she may be asked by patients to comment on medicines which have been prescribed by a doctor. Should this occur, and the midwife has concerns over the appropriateness of the medication, she should take this up personally with the doctor rather than commence a dialogue via the patient. If her concerns are justified the doctor might then arrange for the treatment to be changed. Different principles would of course apply were the midwife to be responsible for administering the medication (see Chapter 20).

DIAGNOSIS OF PREGNANCY BEFORE TREATMENT

Where treatment on the reproductive organs is to be undertaken on a woman, it is essential to ensure that she is given a pregnancy test first. In a case in the MPS report for 1984, a 25-year-old woman with a history of infrequent periods was referred to a Consultant. A cervical erosion was noted and the patient listed for D & C and cautery. The registrar noted 'Please do pregnancy test prior to op.' The D & C was carried out and, three weeks later, the patient aborted spontaneously a 16-week fetus. A settlement was negotiated on the basis that the doctors knew, or should have known, before carrying out the D & C that the patient was pregnant.

NEGLIGENCE CAUSING OF INFERTILITY

In the case of Briody[1] a woman was given a sub-total hysterectomy at the age of 18, which led to her being deprived of any prospect of conceiving and bearing a child naturally. The hospital was held liable, but the judge had rejected a claim for the costs of an own-egg surrogacy to be carried out in California and had also rejected an alternative surrogacy proposal using donor eggs. B sought to overthrow this decision with fresh evidence that her own eggs had been successfully fertilised with her partner's sperm and that she now had the opportunity of a surrogate birth in England. The Court of Appeal dismissed her appeal, on the grounds that the chances of a successful pregnancy using the embryos created from her eggs and her partner's sperm were extremely slight. Whilst everybody had the right under the Human Rights Act 1998 Schedule 1 Article 8 to have the chance to have a child by natural means, no one had the right to be supplied with a child.

STERILISATION

Compensation may be claimed following an operation for sterilisation in the following situations:

– Negligent advice leading to a sterilisation being performed

- A sterilisation being carried out negligently and leading to a baby being born

- A sterilisation being carried out without negligence but no warning having been given about the possibility of its being not 100% effective

- A sterilisation having been carried out with a warning.

Whilst the midwife would not herself be responsible for carrying out the surgery for sterilisation, she may be involved in the information which is given to the patient prior to the operation.

NEGLIGENT ADVICE

On 31st October 1987 Mrs Roberta Biles won £55,000 from North East Thames and Barking, Havering and Brentwood Health Authorities for a sterilisation operation which should not have been carried out. The facts were that when she was 19, she was advised by a doctor that having a baby could kill her and she was therefore sterilised. She had undergone ten operations and four times had had test-tube baby treatment without success. Seven years later when she went for a routine check-up, she discovered that the sterilisation had been unnecessary. The defendants admitted liability but contested the amount of damages. Damages were awarded for probable permanent infertility, for the physical pain and suffering of various operations and painful examinations which she had undergone, and for the scarring as a result of the sterilisation. She was also awarded damages for impairment of sexual function due to the physical and emotional pain and the regime of trying for a test-tube baby.

INADEQUATE PRE-OPERATION COUNSELLING

In the case of Wells v. Surrey Area Health Authority (The Times, 29th July 1978), a Roman Catholic woman was sterilised in the course of a Caesarean. She was given the form to sign just before she went into the operation, and was awarded £3,000 compensation on the grounds that she had been inadequately counselled about the implications of the operation.

Clearly the midwife has an important role to play, where sterilisation is being contemplated during the Caesarean operation, to ensure that the woman has been given all the relevant information.

Absence of consent

Before proceeding with an operation for sterilisation the consent of the patient must be obtained (the consent of minors and the mentally disordered is considered below). In the case of Devi v. West Midlands Regional Health Authority 1980[2] the patient underwent a gynaecological operation with consent. She was a Roman Catholic and objected to sterilisation operations. During the operation, the surgeons discovered that she would be in danger if she were to become pregnant and therefore decided to perform a sterilisation operation. She sued for trespass to the person. Since the doctor had made no attempt to revive her and obtain her consent to the procedure, she succeeded in her claim.

NEGLIGENT STERILISATION

If it can be established that the surgeon failed to follow the accepted approved standard of care of a reasonable professional in undertaking a sterilisation operation, and that as a reasonably foreseeable consequence of that failure, harm was caused, then compensation would be payable. Damages can be awarded where the sterilisation is carried out negligently whether or not the woman goes on to have the baby. In the case of Chaunt v. Hertfordshire Health Authority 1982[3] the plaintiff terminated the pregnancy which followed a negligent sterilisation but was entitled to compensation for the additional pain and suffering occasioned by the termination. There is, however, no requirement that the woman is expected to have a termination following a negligent sterilisation.

Damages for an unwanted baby?

One view has been taken that whilst compensation would be payable for the additional pain and suffering in undergoing another pregnancy and labour, damages were not payable for the costs of bringing up a normal healthy child, since that would be contrary to public policy. This was the view taken by Judge Jupp in the case of Udale v. Bloomsbury 1983.[4] A different view was taken by Judge Peter Pain in the case of Thake v. Maurice (see below).

In the case of Emeh v. Kensington and Chelsea and Westminster Health Authority 1985,[5] following a negligently performed sterilisation, the woman refused to have an abortion and the question arose as to whether she was therefore entitled to have compensation for the costs of bringing up the unplanned child. The Court of Appeal held that she was.

The facts of Emeh were as follows:

In May 1976, the plaintiff, who had three normal children, underwent a sterilisation operation at the defendant's hospital. In January 1977 she discovered that she was about 20 weeks pregnant and she refused to have an abortion. She subsequently gave birth to a child with congenital abnormalities who required constant medical and parental supervision. She claimed for the pregnancy and the birth, and for the upkeep of the child. The trial judge held that the operation had been performed negligently and that therefore she was entitled to the damages accrued before she discovered that she was pregnant, but that she was not, by reason of her failure to have an abortion, entitled to the damages accruing thereafter, apart from the cost of undergoing a second sterilisation operation. She appealed to the Court of Appeal. This held that:

- Since the avoidance of the further pregnancy and the birth was the object of the sterilisation operation it was unreasonable, after the period of pregnancy which had elapsed, to expect the plaintiff to undergo an abortion and, therefore, the plaintiff's failure to do so was not so unreasonable as to eclipse the defendant's wrongdoing;

- It was not contrary to public policy to recover damages for the birth of the child, and therefore

- The plaintiff was entitled to recover damages for her financial loss caused by the negligent performance of the sterilisation operation.

As a result of the decision in the Emeh case it was possible for the parents to claim the cost of educating the child privately if that was their standard of living, as well as the costs of caring for the child and the loss of future and past earnings. This ruling was followed in the case of Allen v. Bloomsbury Health Authority.[6] However, this has now changed, as a result of the House of Lords decision in McFarlane v. Tayside Health Board.[7]

Box 16.1 McFarlane v. Tayside Health Board: Damages for healthy unplanned child

Mr McFarlane had a vasectomy and after 6 months was told that he was sterile and could dispense with contraceptive precautions. Subsequently Mrs M gave birth to a healthy daughter and they sued for compensation including the costs of rearing the child and for the pain and suffering caused to Mrs M in carrying and giving birth to the child. The House of Lords held that the costs of rearing a healthy child were not recoverable, but that Mrs M could recover damages for her prenatal pain and suffering and consequential financial loss.

The ruling in the McFarlane case does not apply when the unplanned child is disabled. In the case of Nunnerley and another v. Warrington Health Authority and another,[8] (held before the decision of the McFarlane case was known) the mother was given negligent advice which led to the unwanted birth of a child who was born disabled. The High Court judge held that the plaintiffs' claim for damages should not be limited to the costs of the care which they themselves had a legal duty to provide, but damages were payable for the cost of care beyond 18 years. The judge held that the normal principle of compensation should apply, i.e. the claimants were entitled to be put in the position that they would have been in, but for the wrong done to them.

Failure to carry out a pregnancy test pre sterilisation. Groom v. Selby[9]
In the case of Groom v. Selby, the claimant underwent a sterilisation operation on 5th October 1994. No pregnancy test was carried out before the operation and in

fact she had conceived on about 29th September 1994. She saw her GP on 21st November, complaining of abdominal pain and a green discharge, but she was not examined for a pregnancy nor was she given a pregnancy test. A second GP diagnosed the pregnancy when she was 15 weeks pregnant. The claimant said that, had the pregnancy been diagnosed at an earlier stage, she would have had a termination but did not feel that she could undergo this at 15 weeks. The baby was born healthy but subsequently developed salmonella meningitis complicated by bilateral frontal brain abscesses and convulsions and episodes of septicaemia. The mother claimed against the first GP because of negligence in failing to diagnose the pregnancy or to recommend a pregnancy test.

The High Court judge held that the birth of a baby who subsequently suffered from disabilities was a reasonably foreseeable consequence of the defendant's actions and whilst the mother could not have successfully claimed for the costs of caring for a healthy baby, she could recover for the additional costs involved in caring for a disabled child, but not for the past and future cost of her basic maintenance.

The House of Lords decision in the McFarlane case was applied by the Court of Appeal in the case of Parkinson v. St James and Seacroft University Hospital NHS Trust.[10] In this case, a woman who underwent a laparoscopic sterilisation procedure subsequently became pregnant and had a disabled baby. It was held that she was able to recover for the damages for the costs of providing for his special needs and the care relating to his disability, but that she could not recover for the basic costs of his maintenance. The Court of Appeal has recently held[11] that a disabled mother was entitled to recover damages uniquely referable to her disability when a negligently performed sterilisation led to her giving birth to a healthy child. In this case the mother was severely visually handicapped.

In contrast, a claimant was unable to obtain compensation for giving up her job to have an unplanned baby. In this case[11] the claimant attended the surgery for a course of contraception by way of injection. The nurse failed to carry out a pregnancy test. It was accepted that this was negligent and that had the claimant been aware that she was pregnant, she would have had a termination. The claimant gave birth to a healthy daughter. She gave up employment to look after the child and sought to recover damages in respect of the loss of earnings consequent upon her decision to stay at home to look after the child. She failed in her action and her appeal to the Court of Appeal failed. The court applied the ruling in the McFarlane case and held that the claim for economic loss of future earnings was too remote.

Wrongful life: action by baby

It has been decided that the baby has no right of action to sue for the fact that had an operation to perform the sterilisation been properly performed, it would not have been born. In the following case the mother was wrongly informed that the baby was not disabled and therefore she did not have an abortion.

Case 16.2 McKay v. Essex Area Health Authority[13]

Mrs McKay was pregnant and suspected that she had contracted German measles in the early weeks of her pregnancy. Blood tests were arranged to see if she had been infected. Unfortunately, she was wrongly informed that she had not been infected. She did not therefore have an abortion. When the baby was born it was found to be disabled as a result of the effect of German measles. The Court of Appeal held that the child's claim for wrongful life (i.e. if there had been no negligence the child would have been aborted) could not be sustained. Although the child was born before the Congenital Disabilities Act 1976 was passed (see chapter 17), the Court held that the Act would not change the situation. The child did not have an entitlement against those who failed to give the correct information which would have led to a termination of the pregnancy. The child only has a right when he/she has been disabled as the result of negligence. The decision did not affect the right of the mother to claim for the reasonably foreseeable results of the negligence and her claim therefore proceeded.

Negligent termination of pregnancy

In the case of Scuriaga v. Powell[14] doctors were negligent in terminating the pregnancy of the plaintiff. When it was discovered that the plaintiff was still pregnant with one out of two fetuses, it was too late to carry out an abortion. The mother obtained compensation for pain, suffering and loss of future and past earnings.

NO WARNING ABOUT THE STERILISATION NOT BEING 100% EFFECTIVE

Even where the sterilisation operation has been carried out with all reasonable care and skill, compensation may still be payable if the patient had not been warned that the operation might not be 100% effective. However, the burden is on the claimant to prove that there has been a breach of the duty of care to provide the appropriate information.

In the case of Thake v. Maurice 1984[15] no warnings were given that an operation for a vasectomy might not be 100% successful. The claimant therefore sued for breach of contract. The facts were as follows:

Mr Thake, a railway guard, and his wife and four children lived in a three-bedroomed council house. When a fifth child was expected Mr Thake discussed with a surgeon the possibility of undergoing a vasectomy. Because of the long NHS waiting list it was agreed that the operation would be performed privately at a cost of £20. It was made clear to Mr Thake that he would become permanently sterile. Both husband and wife signed forms consenting to the operation and declaring that they had been told of its purpose and effects. Tests on Mr Thake subsequently showed him to be sterile. However, two years after the operation Mrs Thake became pregnant again, but did not realise her condition until it was too late to have an abortion. The couple claimed compensation. There was no suggestion that the operation had been performed negligently, but suitable warnings had not been given. The judge found in favour of Mr Thake, holding that on the facts the contract was not merely a contract to perform a vasectomy but was a contract to make Mr Thake irreversibly sterile and the defendants had failed to give an appropriate warning of the possibility of failure.

The defendants appealed to the Court of Appeal[16] which by a majority verdict decided that a reasonable person would have left the consulting room believing that Mr Thake would be sterilised by the operation, but not that he had been given a guarantee that he would be absolutely sterile. Mr Thake lost his case.

Case 16.3 Gold v. Haringey Health Authority[17]

Mrs Gold decided when pregnant with her third child that she would not have any more children, and a Consultant obstetrician discussed with her the possibility of her being sterilised. He did not discuss the possibility of her husband undergoing a vasectomy, which had a slightly lower failure rate, nor did he discuss the risk of the operation failing. After the birth of the third child she was sterilised. However, it was not a success and she later gave birth to a fourth child. Her claim against the Health Authority for negligence on the grounds that (a) she had not been warned of the risk of failure of the operation and (b) there had been negligent misrepresentation in giving her an assurance that the operation was irreversible, succeeded initially and she was awarded £19,000 in compensation by the trial judge. However, the defendants' appeal was upheld. The Court of Appeal held that the standard of care to be followed by the doctor in giving warnings was the standard of the reasonable professional, and applied the Bolam Test. In 1979 there was a substantial body of doctors who would have given her the same advice and not warned her of the risk of failure. Nor could the statement that the operation was irreversible be regarded as a representation that the operation was bound to achieve its objectives.

A claim also failed in the case of Eyre v. Measday[18] where the plaintiff and her husband decided that they did not wish to have any more children and in consulting a gynaecologist privately were told that the operation was intended to be irreversible. They were not advised of the very small chance of failure. The plaintiff failed in her claim for compensation following the birth of a child, the Court of Appeal deciding that it was not a contract to render her absolutely sterile but rather a contract to perform a particular operation.

Conclusions on warnings

Nowadays it would be recommended practice for the doctor discussing an operation for sterilisation to warn of the risk of failure, and to give no warranties about irreversible sterility. Consent forms for such purpose have been introduced by the NHS management executive[19] but specific forms for such treatments have not been drafted under the current guidance.[20]

Do both partners have to give consent?

It will have been noticed that in the Thake v. Maurice case both husband and wife signed the form. This is not a legal requirement: there is no necessity for one partner to give consent to a sterilisation operation proceeding on the other. Clearly counselling of both together would be good practice, but an operation should not be refused on the grounds that the partner not undergoing the procedure is refusing to give consent to the other having the operation. If there is effective counselling, then the professional should not be involved in any matrimonial proceedings between the couple.

The child or young person and sterilisation

Where it is planned to carry out a sterilisation on a child or young person, care should be taken to ensure that a valid consent is given. Whilst the parents could give consent on the minor's behalf, the minor should have independent representation to ensure that the operation is in her/his best interests. In the case Re B (1987)[21] the House of Lords agreed that a girl of 17 years could have a sterilisation with the consent of the parents. (See Chapter 7 for further discussion of this case.)

The mentally incapacitated adult and sterilisation

In the case Re F (1989)[22] the House of Lords held that where the adult lacked the mental competence to make their own decisions, then the carers could act out of necessity in the best interests of the patient and follow the reasonable standard of care (i.e. the Bolam Test). However, where a therapeutic sterilisation was being contemplated then a declaration should be sought from the court. At present there is a vacuum in the statutory law relating to decision making on behalf of mentally incapacitated adults. This should be filled when the government's proposals are incorporated into legislation.[23] (See Chapters 7 and 33.)

Sterilisation as a last resort

In the case of S (1998)[24] her mental and emotional state meant that she was unable to look after herself and she was vulnerable to sexual exploitation. Her mother applied for a declaration that it would be lawful to sterilise her. The application was refused on the grounds that the risk of pregnancy was not an identifiable risk but rather a speculative risk. Risk had to be assessed on the basis of circumstances that existed or could be reasonably foreseen to exist. The President of the Family Division (Sir Stephen Brown) held that the risk of pregnancy was not so great so as to require sterilisation, with the consequent imposition of necessary invasive procedures which carried the risk of fatality.

Lesser measures than sterilisation may be in the best interests of the patient. In the case Re S (2000),[25] the judge had to decide whether it was in the best interests of S to be fitted with an intrauterine device called Mirena which would significantly reduce her heavy periods and which was supported by the Official Solicitor, or to have a hysterectomy, which the mother wished her to have. The judge decided that the subtotal hysterectomy was in the best interests of S, because the intrauterine device would require a series of general anaesthetics every 5 to 7 years, and her mother might not be available to provide S with support in later years. However, this decision was overruled by the Court of Appeal.[26] The Court of Appeal held that the judge had failed to give proper weight to the unanimous medical evidence which supported the less invasive Mirena coil treatment and declared that this was in the patient's best interests.

In contrast to the decisions on sterilisation of a woman with learning disabilities in Re S, the Court of Appeal decided that it was not in the best interests of a man who had Down's syndrome to be sterilised.[27] The best interests of the patient encompassed medical, emotional and all other welfare issues. The best interests of the man were not the equivalent of the best interests of a woman because of the obvious biological differences.

CONCLUSIONS

Most of the legal uncertainties in this area which existed over the last 10 years, such as liability if warnings or inadequate warnings were not given, the amount of compensation for birth of an unplanned but healthy child, and sterilisation of children and those with learning disabilities have now been resolved. The midwife may well continue to be involved in discussions with clients over resource issues and the availability of family planning, fertilisation services (see Chapter 27) and facilities for termination of pregnancy (see Chapter 26).

QUESTIONS AND EXERCISES

1. Review your procedures for advising and giving information to clients who have expressed a wish to be sterilised.

2. A client expecting her fourth child has been informed that she will probably have to have a Caesarean operation. On hearing this, she decided that she would wish to be sterilised at the same time. Her husband has however made it clear that he would not agree to her being sterilised. What is the legal position?

3. To what extent do you consider that the midwife's role should include advice on family planning? What is the position if the midwife is opposed on religious grounds to family planning?

4. You are aware that a mother with a daughter of 14 years of age who suffers from severe learning disabilities wants her daughter to be sterilised. What is the legal position?

References

1 Briody v. St Helens and Knowsley AHA (Claim for damages and costs) sub nom Briody v. St Helens and Knowsley AHA [2001] EWCA Civ 1010 [2001] 2 FCR 481 CA

2 Devi v. West Midlands RHA [1980] 80 Current Law 687

3 Chaunt v. Hertfordshire Health Authority [1982] 132 NLJ 1054

4 Udale v. Bloomsbury [1983] 2 All ER 522

5 Emeh v. Kensington and Chelsea and Westminster Health Authority [1985] 2 WLR 233

6 Allen v. Bloomsbury HA [1993] 1 All ER 651

7 McFarlane v. Tayside Health Board [1999] 4 All ER 961 HL

8 Nunnerley and another v. Warrington Health Authority and another [2000] Lloyds' Rep Med 170; Times Law Report 26 November 1999

9 Groom v. Selby [2001] Lloyds Rep Med 39

10 Parkinson v. St James and Seacroft University Hospital NHS Trust [2001] Lloyds Rep Med 309

11 Rees v. Dartington Memorial Hospital NHS Trust. Times Law Report 20 February 2002

12 Greenfield v. Flather and others [2001] Lloyd's Rep Med 143

13 McKay v. Essex AHA [1982] 2 All ER 771

14 Scuriaga v. Powell [1979] 123 Sol Journal 406

15 Thake v. Maurice [1984] 2 All ER 513

16 Thake v. Maurice [1986] 1 All ER 497

17 Gold v. Haringey Health Authority [1987] All ER 888

18 Eyre v. Measday [1986] 1 All ER 488

19 Department of Health. 1990. A Guide to Consent for Examination and Treatment (HSC (90)22) as amended by HSC (92)32

20 Department of Health. 2001. Reference Guide to Consent for Examination or Treatment; www. doh.gov.uk/consent.
Department of Health. 2001. *Good practice in consent: implementation guide.* London: HMSO

21 Re B [1987] (a minor)(wardship: sterilisation) 2 All ER 206

22 Re F v. West Berkshire HA [1989] 2 All ER 545

23 Lord Chancellor's Office. 1999. *Making Decisions.* London: Lord Chancellor's Office

24 Re S (medical treatment: adult sterilisation) [1998] 1 FLR 944

25 Re S (sterilisation: patient's best interests) [2000] 1 FLR 465

26 Re S (sterilisation: patient's best interests) [2000] 2 FLR 389 CA

27 Re A (male sterilisation) [2000] 1 FLR 549

Chapter 17

THE STATUS AND RIGHTS OF THE UNBORN

The law protects the unborn child by making it a criminal offence to harm it (subject to exceptions under the Abortion Act 1967 as amended – see Chapter 26), but has been reluctant to recognise the unborn child as having the rights of a person, i.e. having a legal personality.

CRIMINAL LAW

The unborn child is specifically protected in the criminal law by the Infant Life Preservation Act 1929. This statute makes it a criminal offence for any person who, with intent to destroy the life of a child capable of being born alive, by any wilful act causes a child to die before it has an existence independent of its mother. There is a defence if the act which caused the death of the child was done in good faith for the purposes only of preserving the life of the mother. There is also a defence if the unborn child died during a lawful abortion (see Chapter 26).

Under Section 58 of the Offences Against The Person Act 1861, it is illegal for a woman being with child unlawfully to administer to herself any poison or use any instrument unlawfully with intent to procure a miscarriage; it is also unlawful for any other person to attempt to cause a miscarriage by similar means, whether or not the woman is actually pregnant. 'Unlawfully' excludes an abortion legally carried out under the Abortion Act 1967 (see Chapter 26.)

Section 59 of the Offences Against The Person Act 1861 makes it illegal for anyone to supply a poison or any instrument knowing that it is to be used unlawfully to procure the miscarriage of any woman, whether or not she is with child.

Section 60 of the 1861 Act makes it an offence to conceal the birth of a child.

These Sections are further discussed in Chapter 26, on abortion.

LEGAL STATUS OF THE FETUS

The fetus is not regarded as having an independent legal personality. As a result of this, principle actions cannot be brought in its name before its birth. Only after it is born, can legal action be brought in its behalf.

HUMAN RIGHTS ACT 1998

Article 2 of the European Convention states that

'Everyone's right to life shall be protected by law. No one shall be deprived of his life intentionally, save in the execution of a sentence of a court following his conviction of a crime for which this penalty is provided by law.'

This right does not however apply to the unborn child, so it could not be argued successfully that termination of a pregnancy is a breach of Article 2. In contrast, in the Republic of Ireland, the Bill of Rights of the Irish Constitution recognises the right to life of the unborn child.

CRIMINAL OFFENCE IN CAUSING THE DEATH OF A FETUS

In the Scottish case of Hamilton v. Fife Health Board (1992)[1] Lord Prosser held that where a child died in consequence of injuries sustained when he was a fetus as a result of the fault of another person, he was not 'a person dying in consequence of person injuries sustained by him' because at the time when the injuries were sustained he was not a person. This was a decision in interpreting the provisions of the Damages (Scotland) Act 1976. In a case reported in 1992[2] a woman who allegedly kicked her neighbour, who was 36 weeks pregnant, in the stomach, killing her unborn baby, was cleared of manslaughter. In the trial of Claudette Morgan the judge told the jury that it could not convict the accused if the child was born dead. For a charge of murder or manslaughter to succeed, the baby would have to be born alive and then die of injuries sustained in the womb.

Box 17.1 Death of baby because of pre-birth injuries[3]

In a case in 1994, a violent assault with a knife was carried out on a pregnant woman. She gave birth to a premature child who did not survive. The Court of Appeal held that an intention to cause serious injury to the mother could be transferred to the child once born so that the assailant could be guilty of murder. The House of Lords however rejected the concept of `transferred malice' and held that the accused could not be found guilty of murder of the child once born. At the time of the attack, the fetus did not have a legal personality.

Lord Mustill stated:

'It is sufficient to say that it is established beyond doubt for the criminal law, as for the civil law (Burton v. Islington Health Authority, De Martell v. Merton and Sutton Health Authority[4])(see Box 17.3 below) that the child en ventre sa mere (in his or her mother's stomach) does not have a distinct human personality, whose extinguishment gives rise to any penalties or liabilities at common law.'

It is not possible to make an unborn child a ward of court (see Box 17.3 below).

THE MOTHER AND CRIMINAL OFFENCES AGAINST THE CHILD

If the mother smokes or eats or otherwise acts in such a way during the pregnancy that she harms the fetus, is she guilty of a criminal offence?

The answer is probably no, unless her actions can be brought within the Offences against the Persons Act 1861 or the Infant Life Preservation Act 1929. It would probably be difficult for the prosecution to establish the requisite mens rea or mental element which these charges require for a prosecution to succeed.

CIVIL LAW

CONGENITAL DISABILITIES (CIVIL LIABILITY) ACT 1976

This Act, which is shown in Appendix 2, gives a right of action to the baby who is born disabled as a result of an occurrence before its birth, which affected either parent in having a healthy baby or affected the mother or the child during the pregnancy.

The main features of the Act are shown in Box 17.2.

Box 17.2 Main features of the Congenital Disabilities Act

- An action is given to the child,

- if it is born alive,

- for harm caused by negligent actions to the father or mother,

- which resulted in the child being born disabled.

- The mother is only liable if she was negligent whilst driving a car.

- Liability to the child can be excluded to the same extent and subject to the same restrictions as liability in the parent's own case

- If the disability arises from an event pre-conception, then the defendant is not liable if both parents knew of the risk of the child being born disabled.

▶ However, if the father is the defendant, this does not apply if he knew of the risk but the mother did not.

– The defendant is not liable... if when responsible in a professional capacity for treating or advising the parent, he took reasonable care having regard to the then received professional opinion applicable to the particular case; but this does not mean that he is answerable only because he departed from received opinion.

– The mother is not liable to the child, unless she was driving a motor vehicle and is in breach of her duty of care to the unborn child and as a consequence the child is born disabled.

LIABILITY OF THE MOTHER TO THE CHILD

The mother of the child is only liable under the Act if when driving a motor vehicle and knowing (or ought reasonably to know) herself to be pregnant she is negligent and in consequence of this negligence the child is born with disabilities. The child could then sue in respect of those disabilities. In practice, of course, the child would be suing the insurance company with whom the mother was insured.

LIABILITY OF THE PROFESSIONAL

It can be seen from Box 17.1 that the professional who takes reasonable care when acting in a professional capacity for treating or advising the parent would not be liable to the child if born disabled. The statute uses the test of the 'then received professional opinion to that particular class of case' which is comparable to the Bolam Test discussed in Chapter 13. However, as in Bolam itself and Maynard's case the fact that a professional departs from the received opinion is not in itself evidence of negligence. Documentation would have to show clearly the reasons why the professional acted in the way she did and the justification for not following the usual practice.

In February 2001 a girl, then aged 8, received £2.43 million from Buckinghamshire Health Authority for injuries she sustained when she was stabbed in the head with an amniocentesis needle whilst a fetus of 16 weeks' gestation. She was born profoundly brain damaged and could barely communicate.[5]

Exclusions to liability and defences under the Act

It must be emphasised that the child's action under the Congenital Disabilities Act is derivative, i.e. it relies upon a negligent act against the mother or father which results in the child being born disabled. If there would be no liability of the defendant to the parent, then there is no liability to the child. (The exception to this is the mother's duty to the child when driving a car.) The Unfair Contract Terms Act prevents any exclusion of liability for negligence which causes personal injury or death. Voluntary assumption of risk and contributory negligence may however be effective as defences (see Chapter 13).

COMMON LAW AND CIVIL LIABILITY TO THE UNBORN CHILD

Prior to the commencement of the Congenital Disabilities (Civil Liability) Act 1976, it was possible for a child, if born alive, to bring a case at common law (i.e. judge-made law) in respect of pre-birth negligence or illegal activities. This is shown in the case below.

Box 17.3 B v. Islington Health Authority 1991[6]

The facts of this case were that an operation for dilation and curettage was carried out when the plaintiff was an embryo in her mother's womb. She was born disabled with brain damage and asphyxia after a failed forceps delivery. The birth occurred before the Congenital Disabilities (Civil Liability) Act 1976 was passed and therefore the child had to bring a claim at common law. This claim was recognised. A duty of care was therefore recognised as existing towards an unborn child and this becomes actionable at the suit of the child when born alive.

It was held that children with disabilities caused by alleged negligent medical treatment before they were born had a cause of action against the health authorities.

However, under Section 4(5) of the Congenital Disabilities (Civil Liability) Act 1976, the common law is replaced in respect of all births after the Act was brought into force on 22nd July 1976. The consequence of this is that a child can only sue the mother in respect of prebirth injuries caused by the mother's negligence, if she were negligent whilst driving a car, i.e. action can only be brought under the 1976 Act.

NO POWER TO MAKE A FETUS A WARD OF COURT

There is no power for the courts to make the baby a ward of court whilst still in utero. The Court of Appeal has held that there is no jurisdiction to make the unborn child of a mentally disturbed woman a ward of court. It rejected the local authority's application that the court should extend wardship jurisdiction where a viable child was at risk.

Box 17.4 Re F (in utero) 1988[7]

In this case, the mother was aged 36 and had suffered from severe mental disturbance since 1977. Throughout 1982 she had led a nomadic existence, wandering around Europe. She had returned in 1983 and had been settled in a flat in south London. Her only means of support was supplementary benefit. The local authority was concerned about the baby expected towards the end of January. Early in January, the mother disappeared. The local authority instituted wardship proceedings. The Court of Appeal were of the opinion that they did not have the power to institute wardship proceedings in relation to a fetus. They pointed to the difficulties of enforcing such an order against the expectant mother.

AN ACTION FOR WRONGFUL LIFE?

What, however, if the child should never have been born, for example if a sterilisation or abortion operation does not proceed correctly? Does the child have a right of action for wrongful life?

Such a case was McKay v. Essex AHA (1982)[8] which is considered in Chapter 16. It was held that a child did not have an action because he or she should not have been born. In this case, the mother was wrongly informed that the baby she was carrying was not disabled and therefore she did not have an abortion.

CONCLUSIONS

The principle that the unborn child has no legal personality has major implications for the law in this area and there are likely to be constant pressures for change in this area from such groups as the Society for the Protection of the Unborn Child.

QUESTIONS AND EXERCISES

1. Do you consider that the unborn child should have clear rights to be protected from an unacceptable lifestyle of the mother?

2. If you were concerned about an unborn baby because the mother was a drug addict, what action would you take?

3. To what extent does the Congenital Disabilities Act give protection to the midwife against litigation being brought in the name of a brain damaged baby?

References

1 Hamilton v. Fife Health Board. Times Law Report January 28 1992

2 R v. Morgan. The Times, 21 May 1992

3 A-G's Reference (No 3 of 1994) [1997] 3 All ER 936

4 Burton v. Islington Health Authority; De Martell v. Merton and Sutton Health Authority [1992] 10 BMLR 63; [1993] QB 204

5 News item. *The Times,* 27 February 2001

6 B v. Islington Health Authority [1991] 1 All ER 325

7 Re F (in utero) [1988] 2 All ER 193

8 McKay v. Essex AHA [1982] 2 All ER 771

Chapter 18
CRIMINAL LIABILITY

This chapter considers the accountability of the midwife in the criminal courts and looks at the following topics:

– Coroner's jurisdiction

– Murder

– Manslaughter

– The case of R v. Cox[1]

– Other crimes

– Criminal proceedings

– Criminal injury compensation.

In Chapter 1 it was explained that criminal offences may be statutory (eg. theft) or derived from the common law (eg. murder). In order to establish that the accused is guilty of the offence with which he or she is charged, the prosecution must prove beyond reasonable doubt that both the actual physical requirements of the offence (i.e. the actus reus) and the required mental element (mens rea) are present. When a client – mother or baby – dies in the course of being cared for by health professionals, the death could be classified as accidental death, voluntary manslaughter, involuntary manslaughter or murder.

CORONER'S JURISDICTION

The death, unless it has resulted from natural causes and can therefore be certified by the doctor caring for the patient, would be reported to the coroner, who then has the responsibility for deciding whether to request a post-mortem and whether or not an inquest should be held. The coroner will also decide whether or not a jury should be summoned to decide upon the cause of death. The purpose of the inquest is to decide:

– the identity of the deceased

– how, where and when the deceased came by his death, and

– the particulars required by the Registration Acts to be registered concerning his death.

The finding of any person guilty of murder, manslaughter or infanticide is specifically prohibited by the Coroners Act 1988 Section 11(6).

Following an unexpected death, there would probably be an inquest carried out by the coroner. If criminal offences are suspected, the coroner has the power to adjourn the hearing. The Director of Public Prosecutions may also ask the coroner to adjourn the hearing. Following the coroner's hearing, the papers in the case may be placed before the Crown Prosecution Service (CPS). The CPS has the right to decide if proceedings should be brought in the criminal courts against the defendant. If a midwife is asked to provide a statement and give evidence at an inquest she should seek assistance from senior management or the solicitor to the trust (see Chapter 15).

MURDER

In order to secure a conviction of murder, the prosecution have to prove beyond all reasonable doubt that the defendant must either have intended to cause death or intended to cause grievous bodily harm. Unless a situation comparable to that of the Beverely Allitt case exists, which is extremely rare, (see Chapter 14), it would be very unusual to be able to prove the intent necessary to convict of murder in a hospital case. Following a conviction for murder, a judge at the present time has no discretion over sentencing but must sentence the convicted person to life imprisonment, i.e. a life sentence is mandatory.

INVOLUNTARY MANSLAUGHTER

This may arise where death results from the negligence of a health professional, where there is no intention to kill or to cause grievous harm. There will not be a charge of murder. In such cases there may be a prosecution for involuntary manslaughter or there may be no prosecution at all. It depends upon the circumstances. If, for example, there is gross recklessness leading to the death, then there may be a prosecution for manslaughter. The following two cases illustrate two different situations.

Death by misadventure

In 1991 two junior doctors were each given a nine-month suspended prison sentence for the manslaughter of a 16-year-old with leukaemia. He died after being wrongly injected in the spine with a cytotoxic drug which should have been administered intravenously. The conviction for manslaughter was quashed by the Court of Appeal on the grounds that the jury should have been directed by the judge to decide whether the defendants were guilty of 'gross negligence' and not 'recklessness' and whether there were any mitigating circumstances such as the lack of supervision from more experienced staff.[2]

Manslaughter

In the second case Dr Adomako, the person charged, was, during the latter part of an operation, the anaesthetist in charge of the patient. At approximately 11.05am a disconnection occurred at the endotracheal tube connection. The supply of oxygen to the patient ceased and led to a cardiac arrest at 11.14am. During that period the defendant failed to notice or remedy the disconnection. He first became aware that something was amiss when an alarm sounded on the Dinamap machine, which monitored the patient's blood pressure. From the evidence it appeared that some four-and-a-half minutes would have elapsed between the disconnection and the sounding of the alarm. When the alarm sounded the defendant responded in various ways by checking the equipment and by administering atropine to raise the patient's pulse. But at no stage before the cardiac arrest did he check the integrity of the endotracheal tube connection. The disconnection was not discovered until after resuscitation measures had been commenced.

Dr Adomako accepted at his trial that he had been negligent. The issue was whether his conduct was criminal. He was convicted of involuntary manslaughter but appealed against his conviction. He lost his appeal in the Court of Appeal and then appealed to the House of Lords.[3]

The House of Lords clarified the legal situation.

The stages which the House of Lords suggested should be followed were:

– The ordinary principles of the law of negligence should be applied to ascertain whether or not the defendant had been in breach of a duty of care towards the victim who had died.

– If such a breach of duty was established, the next question was whether that breach of duty caused the death of the victim.

– If so, the jury had to go on to consider whether that breach of duty should be characterised as gross negligence and therefore as a crime. That would depend on the seriousness of the breach of duty committed by the defendant in all the circumstances in which the defendant was placed when it occurred.

– The jury would have to consider whether the extent to which the defendant's conduct departed from the proper standard of care incumbent upon him, involving as it must have done a risk of death to the patient, was such that it should be judged criminal.

The judge was required to give the jury a direction on the meaning of 'gross negligence' as had been given in the present case by the Court of Appeal.

'The jury might properly find gross negligence on proof of

– *indifference to an obvious risk of injury to health, or*

– *actual foresight of the risk coupled with either*

    - *a determination nevertheless to run it, or*

    - *an intention to avoid it but involving such a high degree of negligence in the attempted avoidance as the jury considered justified conviction, or*

– *inattention or failure to advert to a serious risk going beyond mere inadvertence in respect of an obvious and important matter which the defendant's duty demanded he should address.'*

The House of Lords held that the Court of Appeal had applied the correct test and his appeal was dismissed.

The judge has full discretion over the sentencing in a case of conviction for involuntary manslaughter.

THE CASE OF R V. DR NIGEL COX[4]

Dr Nigel Cox was convicted when he prescribed potassium chloride to a terminally ill patient, and was sentenced to a year's imprisonment which was suspended for a year. He also had to appear before disciplinary proceedings of the Regional Health Authority, his employers and before the General Medical Council.

VOLUNTARY MANSLAUGHTER

This term is used to cover the situation where the defendant has caused the death of a person with intent, but owing to special circumstances a charge or conviction of murder is not appropriate. The term covers:

– death as a result of the provocation of the accused

– death as a result of diminished responsibility of the accused

– killing as a result of a suicide pact.

HOW DOES THIS AFFECT THE MIDWIFE?

If a midwife has been responsible for an action of gross recklessness or gross negligence which has led to the death of the mother or baby, she may well face criminal proceedings, in addition to professional conduct proceedings by the NMC (see Chapter 4) and disciplinary proceedings by the employer (see Chapter 22). The criminal procedure which would be followed is considered below.

The midwife might also be involved in a criminal case because of the alleged criminal conduct of a colleague, in which case she may be asked to provide a statement and give evidence in court (see Chapter 15).

ASSISTING IN THE SUICIDE OF ANOTHER

Reference should be made to Chapter 9, where it is pointed out that it is a criminal offence to aid or abet another person in committing suicide. The same chapter discusses the legalities involved in letting a severely disabled child die.

OTHER CRIMES

The chances of the midwife being involved in criminal proceedings for murder or manslaughter are extremely rare. However, she does face the possibility of other criminal charges particularly in relation to property, motor offences or health and safety offences which are prosecuted in the criminal courts (see Chapter 19).

Community midwives are in particular vulnerable to the allegation that they have been guilty of theft of property in a person's house, particularly where they visit on their own. There should be a clear protocol against the receipt of any gifts to the midwife from clients, to protect the midwife against false accusations.

In addition the community midwife, in driving a car, will have to ensure that it is appropriately insured and that driving it at work has been agreed in advance with the insurers. The nature of the work would have to be specified, including whether or not she uses the car to drive clients and equipment. She would be responsible for any breach of the Road Traffic Acts on her own account.

If it is known that the defendant is a registered midwife, any conviction for a criminal offence would automatically be reported to the NMC. The midwife would not have any right to sue the police for breach of confidentiality.[5]

Other offences are discussed in the context of specific chapters, eg. abortion (Chapter 26), offences against the person (Chapter 17) and offences under the Human Fertilisation and Embryology Act (Chapter 29). Breaches of the Health and Safety at Work Act and the Regulations can result in criminal prosecutions, and these are discussed in the following chapter.

PROHIBITION OF FEMALE CIRCUMCISION ACT 1985

Under Section 1 of this Act it is a criminal offence for any person to:

– excise, infibulate or otherwise mutilate the whole or any part of the labia majora or labia minora or clitoris of another person, or

– to aid, abet, counsel or procure the performance by another person of any of those acts on that other person's own body.

This is subject to Section 2(1), which states that Section 1 shall not render unlawful the performance of a surgical operation if that operation:

– is necessary for the physical or mental health of the person on whom it is performed and is performed by a registered medical practitioner, or

– is performed on a person who is in any stage of labour or has just given birth and if so performed for any purposes connected with that labour or birth by

  - a registered medical practitioner or a registered midwife, or

  - a person undergoing a course of training with a view to becoming a registered medical practitioner or a registered midwife.

Under Section 2(1), in determining for the purpose of Section 2 whether an operation is necessary for the health of a person, no account shall be taken of the effect on that person of any belief on the part of that or any other person that the operation is required as a matter of custom or ritual.

Midwives may come across information that female circumcision is being carried out illegally in this country. Disclosure of this information to the appropriate authorities would be justified in the public interest and therefore an exception to the duty of confidentiality (see Chapter 10). The RCM has published a position paper on female genital mutilation.[6] The British Medical Association has published guidelines about female genital mutilation,[7] recommending that GPs should do all they can to deter families from the practice as soon as they register with a surgery. If a doctor suspects that a girl may be about to undergo circumcision in the UK or be sent 'on holiday', then the GP should inform social services' child protection units. Such advice would also apply to midwives. The NHS pays for at least 200 operations a year to reverse female circumcision.[8] Following a parliamentary hearing, the All-Party Parliamentary Group on population development and reproductive health published a report in 2000 recommending that there should be amendments to the Prohibition of Female Circumcision Act 1985 to enable persons who take girls abroad for circumcision to be prosecuted under UK law when they return.

CRIMINAL PROCEEDINGS

For serious crimes known as 'indictable only offences', criminal proceedings would commence with committal proceedings before the magistrates court. In their capacity as examining justices, magistrates have the task of determining whether there is a case to answer. If they agree that there is a case to answer, the case is then committed to the Crown Court for trial before a jury. For less serious crimes, known as summary offences, (which can only be heard before the magistrates) or offences which are triable either way (i.e. they can be heard by magistrates or in the Crown Court), the magistrates act as both judge and jury in hearing the case. If they consider that the accused is guilty, then the magistrates sentence the accused. There is power to refer to the Crown Court for sentencing if the magistrates consider the accused should receive a stiffer sentence than they have power to give.

In a Crown Court hearing, where the accused enters a 'not guilty' plea, the jury is sworn in and the case would begin with an opening speech by the prosecution lawyer. The witnesses for the prosecution give evidence in turn: initially evidence in chief (when they are questioned by the prosecution and leading questions cannot be asked); then they can be cross-examined by the defence and then re-examined by the prosecution. After the end of the prosecution case, the judge could order the jury to bring forward a 'not guilty' verdict if he is satisfied that there is insufficient evidence from the prosecution to justify a conviction. Otherwise, the case proceeds with the evidence of the defence. At present the accused does not give have to give evidence, but the prosecution can comment on that fact. After the witnesses for the defence have given evidence, there are closing speeches from the prosecution and defence and the judge then sums up for the jury, directing the jury on the law which applies, the evidence which they have heard and the responsibility upon them. If the jury brings forward a 'guilty' verdict or verdicts, the judge then sentences the accused, but may delay this stage in order to have evidence of the accused's social and financial background.

CRIMINAL INJURY COMPENSATION

A scheme to compensate those who have suffered personal injuries as the result of criminal action has been in existence since 1964. A new scheme for compensation following injuries or death as a result of a crime was established on 1st April 1996 under the Criminal Injuries Compensation Act 1995 based on a statutory scale of awards known as the 'tariff'. Claims are processed by the Criminal Injury Compensation Authority (CICA) and claims officers and adjudicators on a panel determine whether a claim can be met. The criminal injury must have been sustained in Great Britain. The assailant does not have to have been convicted of a criminal offence, but the police should have been informed of the incident. There is a discretion to refuse to pay awards where the applicant has unduly delayed in making a claim, failed to co-operate with the police in bringing the assailant to justice, or the applicant's conduct before or after the incident makes it inappropriate that a full or any award should be made, or the applicant's character as shown by his criminal convictions make it inappropriate for an award to be made. An application must be made within two years of the date of the incident giving rise to the injury, though discretion to extend this limit can be made where it is reasonable and in the interests of justice to do so.

Payments are made according to a tariff set out in the Scheme. There are 25 levels of compensation: the minimum level 1 is set at £1,000 (eg. blurred vision of eyes lasting 6 to 13 weeks), level 25 is set at £250,000 (eg. quadriplegia/tetraplegia or permanent brain damage with no effective control of functions). The death of a viable fetus is set at level 10, £5,000. Compensation is paid for loss of earnings as a direct result of the injury after the first 28 weeks of incapacity.

Information relating to the CICA should be available to all NHS staff, who should ensure that, if they are injured at work as a result of a crime, a check is made on their eligibility to receive compensation. It is important that any assaults on staff are reported to the police since information on this would be required by the CICA.

CONCLUSIONS

The Law Commission has recommended that there should be a new law of corporate manslaughter introduced so that senior managers within an organisation can be held criminally liable when persons die as a result of gross negligence by their organisation. The government has still to introduce legislation to implement these proposals. If such legislation were to be enacted then this could have major implications for the functioning of NHS trusts and senior management within them.

QUESTIONS AND EXERCISES

1. The husband of a client attacks a midwife by grabbing her arm. She is contemplating bringing proceedings against him. What is the difference between a civil action and a criminal prosecution in this context? (See also Chapters 1 and 13.)

2. A client dies following an unsuccessful Caesarean operation. What factors would lead to a prosecution being brought against the staff involved?

3. A community midwife has not insured her car for use in transporting clients. She takes a pregnant woman to hospital in an emergency situation. What are the likely repercussions? (Consider the insurance issues as well as issues of reasonable professional practice.)

4. In what circumstances would a midwife be entitled to receive compensation from the Criminal Injury Compensation Scheme?

References

1 R v. Cox [1993] 2 All ER 19

2 R v. Prentice; R. v Adomako; R.v Holloway [1993] 4 All ER 935

3 R v. Adomako House of Lords The Times Law Report July 4 1994; [1994] 2 All ER 79

4 R v. Cox The Times 22 September 1992; [1992] 12 BMLR 38

5 Woolgar v. Chief Constable of Sussex Police and another [1999] 3 All ER 604 CA

6 Royal College of Midwives. 1998. *Position Paper 20: Female genital mutilation (Female circumcision).* London: RCM

7 British Medical Association. 2001. *Guidelines on female genital mutilation.* London: BMA

8 Charter D and Kennedy D. 2000. Doctors put on alert for girl butchery. *The Times,* 21 August 2000

Chapter 19
HEALTH AND SAFETY

This chapter on health and safety is included in the section on accountability since liability for incidents relating to health and safety can lead to hearings in the four main forums which could determine the accountability of the midwife:

– to the public through the criminal law (see Chapter 18)

– to the patient/client through the civil law (see Chapter 13)

– to her employer through the contract of employment (see Chapter 22)

– to her profession through the NMC fitness to practice proceedings (see Chapter 4).

Box 19.1 shows the areas of law which relate to health and safety.

Box 19.1 Health and safety laws

Employer's duty under the contract of employment

Employee's duty under the contract of employment

Health and Safety at Work Act 1974 and subsequent regulations

Occupier's Liability Acts 1957 and 1984

Consumer Protection Act 1987

Medical Devices Regulations 1994 SI 1994 No 3017

Control of Substances Hazardous to Health SI 1999 No 437

Reporting of Injuries, Diseases and Dangerous Occurrences Regulations 1995

Not all of the areas of law shown in Box 19.1 can be covered in detail here, and the purpose of this chapter is to give the midwife a general understanding of the broad principles which apply so that she can build upon this knowledge with her own research and reading.

The obligations placed by the Acts of Parliament and the common law create similar fields of accountability to those discussed in Chapter 13. This is shown in Box 19.2.

Box 19.2 Accountability in relation to health and safety

1. Criminal laws

    – Health and Safety at Work Act 1974 and Regulations

    – Offices Shops and Railway Premises Act 1963

    – Factories Act 1961

    – Food Safety Act 1990 and other legislation

    – Environmental Protection Act 1990

    – Medical Devices Regulations 1994 SI 1994 No 3017

    – Control of Substances Hazardous to Health SI 1999 No 437

2. Civil action

    – Breach of statutory duty

    – Action for negligence

    – Occupier's Liability Act 1957

    – Occupier's Liability Act 1984

    – Consumer Protection Act 1987

3. Employer and contract of employment

    – Laws of contract

    – Statutory Protection provided by the Employment Protection Legislation

    – Rules relating to Employment Tribunals

4. Professional Registration and Codes

    – Midwives Rules

▶

- Midwife's Code of Practice

- Code of Professional Conduct

- Guidelines for Professional Practice.

CRIMINAL LAWS

The Health and Safety at Work Act 1974 is enforced through the criminal courts by the Health and Safety Inspectorate who have the power to prosecute for offences under the Act and the Regulations and who have also powers of inspection and can issue enforcement or prohibition notices. Since the abolition of the Crown's immunity (by the National Health Service Amendment Act 1986) in relation to the health and safety laws, prosecutions and notices can be brought against the Health Authorities. Trusts do not enjoy any immunity from health and safety legislation.

The basic duty on the employer is set out in Box 19.3.

Box 19.3 Duty under the Health and Safety at Work Act 1974

Section 2(1) It shall be the duty of every employer to ensure, so far as is reasonably practicable, the health, safety and welfare at work of all his employees.

Section 2(2) of the 1974 Act gives examples of the various duties which must be carried out but these do not detract from the width and comprehensiveness of the general duty.

The Act also places a specific responsibility upon the employee. This is shown in Box 19.4.

Box 19.4 Statutory duty of the employee under Section 7 of the Health and Safety at Work Act 1974

1. To take reasonable care for the health and safety of himself and of others who may be affected by his acts or omissions at work

2. As regards any duty imposed on his employer or any other person, to co-operate with him so far as is reasonable to enable that duty to be performed or complied with.

It is also a criminal offence for an employee to interfere with health and safety measures. See Box 19.5.

Box 19.5 Section 8 Health and Safety at Work Act 1974

No person shall intentionally or recklessly interfere with or misuse anything provided in the interest of health, safety or welfare in pursuance of any relevant statutory provisions.

New regulations came into force on 1st January 1993 as a result of European Directives. These are shown in Box 19.6.

Box 19.6 Health and Safety Regulations which came into force on 1st January 1993

1. Management of Health And Safety at Work Regulations 1992 (SI (1992) 2051) (revised 1999 SI 1999 No 3242)

2. Provision and Use of Work Equipment Regulations 1992 (SI (1992) 2932) (revised 1998)

3. Manual Handling Operations Regulations 1992 (SI 1992 2793)

4. Workplace (Health, Safety and Welfare) Regulations 1992 (SI (1992) 3004) (amended by SI 1999/2024)

5. Personal Protective Equipment at Work Regulations 1992 (SI (1992) 2966) (amended by SI 1999/3232)

6. Health and Safety (Display Screen Equipment) Regulations 1992 (SI (1992) 2792)

Some of these have since been updated, as shown in Box 19.6.

Box 19.7 shows the areas covered by the Regulations relating to the Management of Health and Safety at Work Act 1999.

Box 19.7 Management of Health and Safety at Work Act 1992

Regulations cover the following topics:

1. Commencement and interpretation

2. Areas exempt from the rules

3. Risk assessment

4. Principles of prevention to be applied

5. Health and safety arrangements

6. Health surveillance

7. Health and safety assistance

8. Procedures for serious and imminent danger and for danger areas

9. Contacts with external services

10. Information for employees

11. Co-operation and co-ordination

12. Persons working in host employers' or self-employed persons' undertakings

13. Capabilities and training

14. Employees duties

15. Temporary workers and other specialist categories

16. Risk assessment in respect of new and expectant mothers

17. Certificate from a registered medical practitioner in respect of new or expectant mothers

18. Notification by new or expectant mothers

19. Protection of young persons

20. Exemption certificates

▶
21. Provisions as to liability

22. Exclusion of liability

23. Extension outside Great Britain

24-27. Amendments of earlier regulations

28. Regulations to have effect as health and safety regulations

Schedule 1 General principles of prevention

The Health and Safety Commission has provided an approved Code of Practice and Guidance along with these Regulations.[1] The legal status of this Code is explained in the introduction:

'This Code has been approved by the Health and Safety Commission, with the consent of the Secretary of State... If you are prosecuted for breach of health and safety law, and it is proved that you did not follow the relevant provisions of the Code, you will need to show that you have complied with the law in some other way or a court will find you at fault. This document also includes other, more general guidance not having this special status...'

NEW AND EXPECTANT MOTHERS

The new Regulations introduce provisions for the protection of new and expectant mothers and young persons. A 'new and expectant mother' is defined as an employee who is pregnant; who has given birth within the previous six months; or who is breastfeeding. Under Regulation 16, employers have a specific duty to carry out an assessment of risk which arises by reason of their condition and if the risk cannot be avoided, then to alter her working conditions or hours of work and if this would not remove the risk, then the employer should suspend the employee as long as is necessary to avoid such a risk.

Regulation 17 states that where a new or expectant mother works at night, and there is a certificate from a registered medical practitioner or registered midwife that she should not work for any period identified in the certificate, then the employer shall suspend her from work as long as it is necessary for her health or safety. The onus is on the woman to notify the employer in writing that she is pregnant (and to provide a certificate of that fact), has given birth within the previous six months or is breastfeeding. The suspension would be on full pay.

YOUNG PERSONS

Under Regulation 19 an employer must ensure that any young person employed by him is protected at work from any risks to their health or safety which are a consequence of their lack of experience, or absence of awareness of existing or potential risks, or the fact that young persons have not yet fully matured. In addition employers are prohibited from employing a young person for work which is beyond his physical or psychological capacity, involves harmful exposure to agents which are toxic, carcinogenic, cause heritable genetic damage or harm the unborn child, or in any other way chronically affect human health; involve harmful exposure to radiation; or where there is a risk to health from extreme cold or heat, noise or vibration.

RISK ASSESSMENT: THE LAW

Not all these regulations can be covered in detail in a book like this, but Regulation 3 on risk assessment will be selected to be looked at in detail.

Regulation 3 requires:

'Every employer shall make a suitable and sufficient assessment of

(a) the risks to the health and safety of his employee to which they are exposed whilst they are at work; and

(b) the risks to the health and safety of persons not in his employment arising out of or in connection with the conduct by him of his undertaking,

for the purpose of identifying the measures he needs to take to comply with the requirements and prohibitions imposed upon him by or under the relevant statutory provisions.'

The duty also applies to independent midwives: Regulation 3 Paragraph (2) requires every self-employed person to make a suitable and sufficient assessment of

(a) the risks to his own health and safety to which he is exposed whilst he is at work; and

(b) the risks to the health and safety of persons not in his employment arising out of or in connection with the conduct by him of his undertaking,

for the purposes of identifying the measures he needs to take to comply with the requirements and prohibitions imposed upon him by or under the relevant statutory provisions.

There is a duty under Regulation 3(3) to review the assessment when there is reason to suspect that it is no longer valid or there has been significant change in the matters to which it relates.

Regulation 3(4) requires an employer to make an assessment before employing a young person (a person below 18 years).

RISK ASSESSMENT: THE APPROVED CODE OF PRACTICE (ACOP) AND GUIDANCE

The Approved Code of Practice emphasises that risk assessment must be a systematic general examination of the effect of their undertaking, their work activities and the condition of the premises. There should be a record of the significant findings of that risk assessment.

The definition of risk includes both the likelihood that harm will occur and its severity. The aim of risk assessment is to help the employer or self-employed person to determine what measures should be taken to comply with their statutory obligations laid down under the Health and Safety at Work Act 1974 and its regulations.

Suitable and sufficient is defined in the ACOP as

(a) identifying the risks arising out of work

(b) enabling the employer or the self-employed person to take reasonable steps to help themselves identify risks

(c) being appropriate to the nature of the work and having an identified period for which it is likely to be valid.

HOW IS THE RISK ASSESSMENT TO BE CARRIED OUT?

The ACOP states that there are no fixed rules about how a risk assessment should be carried out, and it will depend upon the nature of the work and the types of hazards and risks. The ACOP sets out some general principles that should be followed and these are summarised in Box 19.8.

Box 19.8 Requirements of valid risk assessment

– Ensure that all relevant risks or hazards are addressed

– Ensure all aspects of the work activity are reviewed

– Take account of non-routine operations

– Take account of the management of incidents

– Be systematic

– Take account of the way in which work is organised

– Take account of risks to the public

– Take account of the need to cover fire risks.

RECORDING

The record should represent an effective statement of hazards and risks which then leads management to take the relevant actions to protect health and safety. It should be in writing unless in computerised form and should be easily retrievable. It should include:

– a record of the preventive and protective measures in place to control risks

– what further action, if any, needs to be taken to reduce risk sufficiently

– proof that a suitable and sufficient assessment has been made.

PREVENTIVE AND PROTECTIVE MEASURES

Schedule 1 of the Regulations specifies the general principles of prevention required by the EEC and in Regulation 4. These include:

– avoiding risks

– evaluating the risks which cannot be avoided

– combating the risks at source

– adapting the work to the individual

– adapting to technical progress

- replacing the dangerous by the non-dangerous or the less dangerous

- developing a coherent overall prevention policy

- giving collective protective measures priority over individual protective measures

- giving appropriate instructions to employees.

How do these regulations relate to the role of the midwife?

For the most part, the midwife would share common health and safety hazards with other hospital or community-based employees and thus models of risk assessment and management which applied to midwifery would also apply to other health professionals. Hazards relating to the safety of equipment, cross-infection risks, safe working practices or violence at work would all apply to midwives who should be involved in the assessment of risk. The midwife could also apply these same principles of risk assessment to the care of the woman and baby, identifying any particular circumstances which could cause harm and ensuring that reasonable action is taken to prevent such an occurrence. Risk management in midwifery practice is considered by Robina Aslam.[2] It is emphasised that the focus of clinical risk management should not be the reduction of litigation but should be the enhancement of client care. The setting up of a risk management programme in a small, private birth unit is described by Patricia Scott.[3] Amongst the many benefits resulting from the scheme are:

- early recognition of risk factors

- written care plans

- improved documentation and audit of case notes

- statistics are regularly analysed eg. postpartum haemorrhage rates

- study days on CTG traces.

Reference should also be made to the work in clinical risk management of the Clinical Negligence Scheme for Trusts discussed in Chapter 13. The RCM has also published guidance for members on the assessment of risk[4] which looks at the meaning and implications of risk management in relation to midwifery care of pregnant women.

The midwife and violence

Many health professionals, including community midwives, work in fear of violence from strangers in the street as well as abuse from relatives of clients and even clients themselves. If this is a real fear in a particular locality then an assessment should be carried out.

- Is it possible to remove the risk altogether?

    If the answer to this is yes, but only by stopping all home confinements and community visits by midwives, then it could be said not to be a realistic possibility.

– What preventive action or protective measures can be taken?

> The answer to this might include the provision of two-way radios, personal alarms or, in very dangerous areas or on visits to clients who present a threat, midwives going in pairs or accompanied by another person, who may be the police. Are attacks due to the view that midwives carry drugs? Could this be prevented by necessary medication being obtained by the patients on prescription and kept at the home, so that midwives do not have to carry them?

– Review the situation to ascertain if the nature of the risk has changed (eg. the district is more violent than it was formerly assessed to be), and the extent of the success of the measures taken to prevent harm to midwives. Are any further measures necessary?

> This type of analysis will not relate only to community midwives – it could be part of a wider assessment of all community health professionals into which the community midwife could have an input. Clearly the risk assessment is dependent upon having accurate feedback from employees and others about incidents and threatening situations.

Guidance is available from the Health and Safety Commission.[5] This gives practical advice for reducing the risk of violence in a variety of settings and emphasises the importance of commitment from the highest levels of management. An appendix includes a checklist for home visiting. The RCM has also provided advice on safety in maternity units[6] and for midwives working in the community.[7] Because of the growing concerns about violence to health staff, some general practitioners in Bristol[8] have decided that violent patients will only be attended to in the police station, not in the surgery. It is unlikely that such a rule could apply to midwives attending pregnant women, but in exceptional circumstances police could be brought into antenatal clinics or onto the wards. The Secretary of State announced in November 2001[9] the publication of new national guidelines[10] on withholding treatment from violent and abusive patients. (This does not apply to patients with severe mental health problems or suffering life-threatening conditions, and is seen as a last resort.)

Domestic violence against pregnant women
Concern is growing at the numbers of pregnant women who are subjected to domestic violence.[11] Midwives may be told of the violence in confidence. However, reporting such information may be a justifiable exception to the duty of confidentiality, since it would be in the public interest (see Chapter 10) to ensure that a woman with learning disabilities and children at risk received protection.

Risk assessment and midwife-managed units
Other assessments of risk could apply only to midwifery activity. For example, it may be that the NHS trust is considering setting up a midwife-managed unit. In the

planning of this unit it would be necessary to assess which mothers should not be admitted to such a unit but should be delivered with the facilities of a district general hospital. Such an assessment would require the identification of which tests were required during the antenatal stages to identify contraindications. An analysis would then be necessary of those risks in childbirth which could occur and the measures necessary either to prevent them occurring or to reduce their seriousness. Should the unit have storage facilities for blood? What additional procedures should the midwife receive training in, in case certain risks materialised (eg. resuscitation of the newborn)? Working parties could plan procedures for coping with emergencies and the necessary co-operation with paramedical ambulance staff and staff in the operation theatres of nearby general hospitals. Reference could also be made to the RCM Stewards Briefings and newsletters prepared by the Royal College of Midwives for health and safety representatives.[12]

Conclusions on risk assessment and management

The emphasis in the guidance from the Health and Safety Commission is on the assessment of significant risks. There is a realism therefore about the Regulations which may have been lacking in health and safety audits carried out in the past. The midwives are central to the assessment process, since they have first hand knowledge of the dangers which they face.

MANUAL HANDLING REGULATIONS

Back injuries have been recognised as a major reason for sickness and staff retiring early on grounds of ill health. The Royal College of Midwives has provided guidance on manual handling.[13] The Royal College of Midwives in its handbook[14] for health and safety representatives states that back injury is the commonest single hazard for nurses and midwives:

'Nurses and midwives take almost twice as much sick leave due to back pain as the rest of the working population. 16% of all NHS sickness absence is due to back pain. One out of six nurses or midwives is said to suffer back pain or injury each year, costing an estimated 1.5 million lost working days each year. Nearly half of all working age adults experience some low back pain in any 6-week period.'

The handbook also quotes a Health and Safety Executive survey in 1982 which showed that 25% of midwives had at one time been off sick from work because of back injury, and this is about the average figure for nurse, midwives and health visitors generally. The handbook points out that community midwives are more likely to have sustained a back injury.

'There is also some evidence to suggest that back injury is even more likely among part-time, bank or agency staff, maybe because they may be older... Risk also correlates with length of service, partly because back troubles can cumulate. The longer in midwifery, the greater the chances of back injury.'

Regulations have been enacted under the Health and Safety Act 1974 and are published with guidance by the Health and Safety Executive.[15] The guidelines are not themselves the law and the booklet advises that the guidelines set out in appendix 1 'should not be regarded as precise recommendations. They should be applied with caution. Where doubt remains, a more detailed assessment should be made.'

A Working Group set up by the Health and Safety Commission has produced a booklet of guidance on manual handling of loads in the health services.[16] This document is described as 'an authoritative document which will be used by health and safety inspectors in describing reliable and fully acceptable methods of achieving health and safety in the workplace'. Part of this health services specific guidance material relates to staff working in the community.

CONTENT OF THE REGULATIONS

The duty under the regulations can be summed up as follows:

- If possible avoid the hazardous manual handling
- Make a suitable and sufficient assessment of any hazardous manual handling which cannot be avoided
- Reduce the risk of injury from this handling so far as is reasonably practicable
- Provide information about the load and centre of weight
- Review the assessment.

Avoiding the risk
Regulation 4(1) Each employer shall

(a) so far as is reasonably practicable, avoid the need for his employees to undertake any manual handling operations at work which involve a risk of their being injured.

The guidance asks the question, as an example of this, 'Can a treatment be brought to a patient rather than taking the patient to the treatment?' It may be that in the case of midwifery, it would be very difficult to remove the risk of injury entirely without reducing patient choice to unacceptable levels. For example, water births or births in alternative positions may be considered to cause unacceptable risks to the health of the midwife. In such situations it is necessary to balance the risk of harm against the freedom of choice for the mother.

Carrying out the assessment
Regulation 4(1) Each employer shall

(b) where it is not reasonably practicable to avoid the need for his employees to undertake any manual handling operations at work which involve a risk of their being injured-

(i) make a suitable and sufficient assessment of all such manual handling operations to be undertaken by them, having regard to the factors which are specified in column 1 of Schedule 1 to these Regulations and considering the questions which are specified in the corresponding entry in column 2 of that Schedule.

Schedule 1 is set out as shown in Box 19.9.

Box 19.9 Schedule 1 of Manual Handling Regulations 1992

Factors to which the employer must have regard and questions he must consider when making an assessment of manual handling operations.

Questions	Factors
1. The tasks	eg. do they involve holding or manipulating loads at a distance from trunk etc.
2. The loads	eg. are they heavy, bulky or unwieldy etc?
3. The working environment	eg. are there space constraints preventing good posture, uneven, slippery or unstable floors etc?
4. Individual capability	Does the job require unusual strength, height etc?
5. Other factors	Is movement or posture hindered by personal protective equipment or by clothing?

Application of the schedule to midwifery

The Royal College of Midwives has identified the following areas as particularly relevant to midwives:

– helping clients to breastfeed

– delivery, particularly in water births and alternative positions

– clients with epidurals

– clients who have had lower segment Caesarean sections

– baby bathing

– transfer between ward or theatre

– handicapped mothers

– lifting of equipment, in hospital, home or car.

The assessment should take into account the mother's choice of place of confinement. It may be for example that following an assessment, the mother is advised that the accommodation is unsuitable to ensure the health and safety of the mother and baby and also of the midwife during the confinement.

Management checklist

Appendix 2 of the Regulations gives an example of an assessment checklist: Section A covering the preliminary stages, Section B the more detailed assessment where necessary and Section C identifying the remedial action which should be taken.

Taking appropriate steps to reduce the risk

Regulation 4(1)

Each employer shall

> (b) where it is not reasonably practicable to avoid the need for his employees to undertake any manual handling operations at work which involve a risk of their being injured
>
>> (ii) take appropriate steps to reduce the risk of injury to those employees arising out of their undertaking any such manual handling operations to the lowest level reasonably practicable.

For example, in carrying out the assessment of risk and deciding how to minimise the risk, it might be concluded that it might be preferable to install hoists. This may include the possibility of installing a hoist for a domiciliary confinement, even though temporarily.

Employer's duty to inform employees, so far as is reasonably practicable, about the weight

Regulation 4(1)(b)(iii) requires the employer to provide the employee with information about the weight of each load and the heaviest side of any load whose centre of gravity is not positioned centrally.

Review

Regulation 4(2) requires the employer to review the assessment

(a) if there is reason to suspect that it is no longer valid; or

(b) if there has been a significant change in the manual handling operations to which it relates and where as a result of any such review changes to an assessment are required, the relevant employer shall make them.

It is in the interests of all midwives in whatever capacity they are employed and whatever their hours per week to ensure that the employer is reminded when a review becomes necessary under the above provisions.

Agency and bank midwives and independent midwives

The duty which is owed by the employer is owed not only to employees but also to temporary staff such as agency or bank midwives who are called in to assist. All such employees are entitled to be included in the risk assessment process, since as has been seen, the assessment must take into account the individual characteristics of each employee.

Midwives who are unusually small in height or not so strong as the average might require special provisions in relation to manual handling. Independent midwives are not employees and as self-employed persons would be responsible for carrying out the assessments and taking the necessary precautions for themselves and any staff whom they employ. Where they work alongside employed midwives in maternity delivery units, they should ensure that the NHS trust takes into account hazards to their health and safety and that the agreement which they have with the NHS trust reflects this duty.

What action can be taken if the employer ignores these regulations?

The Regulations are part of the health and safety provisions which form part of the criminal law. Infringement of the Regulations can lead to prosecution by the Health and Safety Inspectorate. The Inspectorate has the power to issue enforcement or prohibition notices against any corporate body or individual.

A Health Authority no longer enjoys the immunity from the criminal sanctions which it once did as a Crown Authority and therefore these enforcement provisions are available against it. Similarly, an NHS trust and its employees are subject to the full force of the criminal law.

What remedies exist for compensation?

Section 47 of the Health and Safety at Work Act 1974 prevents breach of a duty under Sections 2-8 of the Act being used as the basis for a claim in the civil courts. Breach of the Regulations can however be the basis of a civil claim for compensation unless the Regulations provide to the contrary. Even where what is alleged is a breach of the basic duties, a midwife who suffered harm as a result of the failure of the employer to take reasonable steps to safeguard her health and safety, could sue in the civil courts on the basis of the employer's duty at common law. The statutory duty to ensure the Act is implemented is paralleled by a duty at common law placed upon the employer to take reasonable steps to ensure the employee's health and safety. Contracts of employment should state clearly the duty upon the employer to take reasonable care of the employee's safety and also the employee's duty to co-operate with the employer in carrying out health and safety duties under the Act and at common law. It is of course in the long term interest of the employer to prevent back injuries thereby avoiding payment of substantial compensation to his injured employees and also reducing the incidence of sickness and absenteeism. Considerable sums of compensation have been awarded by the civil courts in recent years in situations where the employer is in breach of the duty to take reasonable care of the health and safety of the employee in manual handling.

Wiles v. Bedfordshire CC[17]

The County Court held that there was a breach of the Manual Handling Regulations 1992 Reg 4.1a when W, a residential social worker, sustained an injury when taking M, a disabled girl, to the lavatory. W lifted the girl out of her wheelchair, propping her against the wall whilst she bent down to remove her underclothes but the girl, whose upper limbs were prone to occasional involuntary spasms, threw out her hands and fell backwards onto W, who suffered a back injury. W claimed that two persons should have carried out that activity. Following the incident, staff were instructed to use a hoist and two staff when taking M to the lavatory. The judge held that even though at the precise time, W was not actually carrying out a manual handling operation, the whole task of taking M to the lavatory should be considered a manual handling operation. The employers were in breach of the Regulations by failing to avoid the need for manual handling and for failing to carry out a proper assessment or taking steps to reduce the risk of injury.

Training

This is essential to ensure that staff have the understanding to carry out the assessments and to advise on lifting and the appropriate equipment. Regular monitoring should take place to ensure that the training is effective and the policies for ensuring the safety of midwives are being implemented.

Record keeping

The guidance emphasises the importance of recording significant findings of the assessment and that the record should be kept, readily accessible, as long as it remains relevant. In addition, the Royal College of Midwives has emphasised the importance of the HA (or NHS trust) keeping adequate statistics. It recommends that the following are kept:

– numbers and incident rate of injuries

– type of injuries

– handling methods involved

– numbers of staff involved

– age and training of the injured parties

– location and time of the accident

– the cause of the accident

– the related costs, eg. time lost.

There is a statutory duty under Health and Safety Regulations for certain accidents to be notified to the appropriate authority, usually the Health and Safety Inspectorate.

In keeping records of accidents at work, the principles set out in the guidance by the UKCC[18] should be followed.

It is in the interest of every practising midwife to ensure that the regulations on manual handling are implemented comprehensively. It should be the aim of every midwife to ensure that the level of injuries is reduced. She, her employer, her colleagues and her clients stand to gain.

MEDICAL DEVICES REGULATIONS 1994

The Medical Devices Agency (MDA) was established in September 1994 to promote the safe and effective use of devices. In particular its role is to ensure that whenever a medical device is used, it is:

– suitable for its intended purpose

– properly understood by the professional user, and

– maintained in a safe and reliable condition.

What is a medical device?
The definition used by the MDA is based upon the European Directive definition:[19]

Any instrument, apparatus, material or other article, whether used alone or in combination, including the software necessary for its proper application, intended by the manufacturer to be used for human beings for the purpose of:

– diagnosis, prevention, monitoring, treatment or alleviation of disease

– diagnosis, monitoring, treatment, alleviation of or compensation for an injury or handicap

– investigation, replacement or modification of the anatomy or of a physiological process

– control of contraception

and which does not achieve its principal intended action in or on the human body by pharmacological, immunological or metabolic means, but which may be assisted in its function by such means.

Annex B to Safety Notice 9801 from the MDA gives examples of medical devices.[20]

It covers the following:

- equipment used in the diagnosis or treatment of disease, monitoring of patients, eg. syringes and needles, dressings, catheters, beds, mattresses and covers, and other equipment

- equipment used in life support eg. ventilators, defribilators

- in vitro diagnostic medical devices and their accessories eg. blood gas analysers

- equipment used in the care of disabled people eg. orthotic and prosthetic appliances, wheelchairs and special support seating, patient hoists, walking aids, pressure care prevention equipment

- aids to daily living eg. commodes, hearing aids, urine drainage systems, domiciliary oxygen therapy systems, incontinence pads, prescribable footwear

- equipment used by ambulance services (but not the vehicles themselves) eg. stretchers and trolleys, resuscitators.

Other examples of medical devices include condoms, contact lenses and care products, intra-uterine devices.

From these examples it can be seen that almost all the equipment which a midwife would use during the care of a pregnant woman would come under the definition of a medical device.

Regulations[21] require that from 14th June 1998 all medical devices placed on the market (made available for use or distribution even if no charge is made) must conform to 'the essential requirements' including safety required by law, and bear a CE marking as a sign of that conformity. Although most of the obligations contained in the Regulations fall on manufacturers, purchasers who are positioned further down the supply chain may also be liable – for example, for supplying equipment which does not bear a CE marking or which carries a marking liable to mislead people.'[22] This is the requirement of the EC Directive on medical devices.[23] The manufacturer who can demonstrate conformity with the Regulations is entitled to apply the CE marking to a medical device.

The essential requirements include the general principle that 'A device must not harm patients or users, and any risks must be outweighed by benefits.' Design and construction must be inherently safe, and if there are residual risks, users must be informed about them. Devices must perform as claimed, and not fail due to the stresses of normal use. Transport and storage must not have adverse effects. Essential requirements also include prerequisites in relation to the design and construction, infection and microbial contamination, mechanical construction, measuring devices, exposure to radiation, built-in computer systems, electrical and electronic design, mechanical design, devices which deliver fluids to a patient, and the function of controls and indicators.

In January 1998 the MDA issued a device bulletin[22] giving guidance to organisations on implementing the regulations. The MDA has powers under the Consumer Protection Act 1987 to issue warnings or remove devices from the market.

Devices are divided into three classes according to possible hazards, class 2 being further subdivided. Thus class 1 with a low risk eg. a bandage; class 2a medium risk eg. a simple breast pump; class 2b medium risk eg. a ventilator; class 3 high risk eg. an intraortic balloon.

Any warning about equipment issued by the Medical Devices Agency should be acted upon immediately. Notices from the Agency are sent to Regional General Managers, Chief Executives of HAs and NHS trusts, directors of social services, managers of independent healthcare units and rehabilitation service managers. Failure to ensure that these notices are obtained and acted upon could be used as evidence of failure to provide a reasonable standard of care.

Adverse incident reporting procedures
In 1998 the MDA issued a safety notice[24] requiring healthcare managers, healthcare and social care professionals and other users of medical devices to establish a system to encourage the prompt reporting of adverse incidents relating to medical devices to the MDA. The procedures should be regularly reviewed, updated as necessary, and should ensure that adverse incident reports are submitted to MDA in accordance with the notice.

REPORTING OF INJURIES, DISEASES AND DANGEROUS OCCURRENCES REGULATIONS 1995 (RIDDOR 95)

Regulations were introduced in 1985 to govern the reporting of injuries, diseases and dangerous occurrences. They were replaced by new Regulations which came into force on 1st April 1996. There is now one set of regulations in place of the four sets under the 1985 Regulations. The list of reportable diseases has been updated, as has the list of dangerous occurrences. It will be legally possible for reports to be made by telephone. A pilot scheme was tested out in Scotland.

Following the successful HSE pilot scheme in Scotland, in February 2000 it was announced that funding was to be made available to the HSE to set up a centralised national workplace accident and incident reporting system instead of the 500 different addresses which have to be used at present.

National Patient Safety Agency
In April 2001 the Department of Health published its proposals for establishing a National Patient Safety Agency (NPSA) which will run the mandatory reporting system for logging all failures, mistakes, errors and near misses across the health services. The Department of Health's publication, Building a Safer NHS for Patients,

sets out details of the scheme together with recommendations for an improved system for handling investigations and inquiries across the NHS. The National Patient Safety Agency will be an independent body which will have the following statutory functions:

– Collecting and analysing information on adverse events from local NHS organisations, NHS staff and patients and carers

– Assimilating other safety-related information from a variety of existing reporting systems and other sources in this country and abroad

– Learning lessons and ensuring that they are fed back into practice, service organisation and delivery

– Producing solutions to prevent harm where risks are identified, and setting out national goals and establishing ways of tracking progress towards these goals.

The aim of this new national reporting system is to ensure that adverse events, including specified near misses will be identified, recorded, analysed, reported and lessons learnt will be shared to effect change at local and national levels.

The National Patient Safety Agency will co-ordinate its work with other reporting systems (eg. RIDDOR, MDA, and adverse reactions to medicines), but these will stay in place at the present time. Professor Rory Shaw, Medical Director of Hammersmith Hospital was appointed as chairman of the NPSA in August 2001.

CONTROL OF SUBSTANCES HAZARDOUS TO HEALTH (COSHH)

All health workers have responsibilities under the Regulations Relating to the Control of Substances Hazardous to Health. The Regulations were first introduced in 1988 but have subsequently been updated, the current regulations dating from 1999.[25]

Where the Regulations have not been followed, there can be a prosecution in the criminal courts against the offender. In addition any person who has been injured as a result of a failure to ensure reasonable care was taken by the employer would have a right of civil action to claim compensation. A COSHH assessment must be carried out in accordance with the guidance issued by the Health and Safety Executive[26] which recommends a five stage assessment.

1. Gather information about the substances, the work and the working practices.

2. Evaluate the risks to health.

3. Decide what needs to be done

4. Record the assessment

5. Review the assessment

CIVIL LAW

BREACH OF STATUTORY DUTY

The injured person can bring a civil claim for breach of the statutory duty in certain cases. However breach of the general duties under the Health and Safety at Work Act 1974 does not give rise to a civil action of breach of statutory duty, but breach of the Regulations may give rise to such an action (see above).

ACTION FOR NEGLIGENCE

The person injured is more likely to bring a claim under the law of negligence (see Chapter 13) by establishing that a duty of care which is owed has been breached and that as a reasonably foreseeable consequence harm has been caused. Where an employee has been injured by alleged failures of the employer, the employee can sue for breach of contract of an implied term in the contract of employment (see below).

OCCUPIER'S LIABILITY ACTS 1957 AND 1984

These Acts are enforceable in the civil courts where harm has occurred to a visitor (1957 Act) or to a trespasser (1984 Act). Under the 1957 Act the duty of care owed by the occupier (of whom there may be several) is what is reasonable in the circumstances to ensure that the visitor will be safe for the purposes for which he is permitted to be on the premises. Extra care is required of the occupier when a child is the visitor.

CONSUMER PROTECTION ACT 1987

This enables a claim to be brought where harm has occurred as a result of a defect in a product. It is a form of strict liability in that negligence by the supplier or manufacturer does not have to be established. The claimant will however have to show that there was a defect. The supplier can rely upon a defence colloquially known as 'state of the art', i.e. that the state of scientific and technical knowledge at the time the goods were supplied was not such that the producer of products of that kind might be expected to have discovered the defect.

There have been few examples of actions being brought under the Consumer Protection Act 1987 in healthcare cases. One reported in March 1993 led to Simon Garratt being awarded £1,400 against the manufacturers of a pair of surgical scissors which broke during an operation on his knee, with the blade being left embedded. A second operation was required to remove it. Had he relied upon the law of negligence to obtain compensation he would have had to show that the manufacturers were in breach of the duty of care which they owed to him. Under the Consumer Protection Act 1987 he had to show the harm, the defect and the fact that the equipment was produced by the defendant.

The Consumer Protection Act 1987 is significant for the midwife in that she should ensure that she keeps records of the supplier of any goods (both equipment and drugs) which she provides for the client. If she is unable to cite the name and address of the supplier, she, or her employer, may become the supplier of the goods for the purposes of the Consumer Protection Act 1987 and therefore have to defend an action alleging that there was a defect in the goods which caused harm. Harm includes both personal injury and death, and loss or damage of property.

In a recent case[27] it was held that patients who had contracted hepatitis C from blood and blood products used in blood transfusions were able to bring a claim under the Consumer Protection Act 1987. This decision may well lead to greater use of the Consumer Protection Act 1987 where personal injuries are caused as a result of defective products, since negligence does not have to be established under the Consumer Protection Act 1987, only that there was a defect in the product which has caused the harm.

EMPLOYER AND CONTRACT OF EMPLOYMENT

Under the contract of employment, both employer and employee have duties in relation to health and safety. It is the employer's duty to take reasonable care for the health and safety of the employee. It is the employee's duty to obey reasonable orders (which could include instructions in relation to health and safety) and to act with reasonable care and skill. These duties are enforced on the employer's part by disciplinary procedures and ultimately dismissal and on the employee's part by an action for breach of contract or an allegation of constructive dismissal which, if the employee has the requisite length of continuous service, may result in a hearing before an employment tribunal.

Under the contract of employment the employee must obey the express terms on the contract of employment. In addition there are implied terms binding on the employee and employer.

The employee:

- must obey the reasonable instructions of the employer

- must act with all reasonable care and skill in the performance of his duties

- must respect confidential information obtained during the course of employment.

The employer must take all reasonable care for the employee's safety in:

– employing competent staff

– ensuring a safe system of work

– providing safe plant, premises and equipment.

Failure on the employer's part could lead to an action for constructive dismissal, breach of contract or an action for negligence if harm occurs.

Stress

An example of the employer's duty under the contract to take reasonable care of the employee's health and safety is the legal situation relating to stress. The following facts would have to be proved by the employee:

– The employee is under considerable pressure which is causing unacceptable stress.

– The employer is aware of that fact.

– There is reasonable action which the employer could take but has failed to take.

– As a reasonably foreseeable result of the employer's failure,

– The employee has suffered severe mental illness.

The following case illustrates these factors.

Box 19.10 Walker v. Northumberland County Council[28]

A social worker obtained compensation when his employer failed to provide the necessary support in a stressful work situation when he returned to work following an earlier absence due to stress. The employer was not liable for the initial absence, but that put the employer on notice that the employee was vulnerable and its failure to provide the assistance he needed was a breach of its duty to provide reasonable care for his health and safety as required under the contract of employment.

In a more recent case it was reported[29] that a former social worker was awarded £140,000 after stress forced her to give up her job as head of a care home. It was alleged that Worcestershire County Council had refused to accept that she was unqualified for the position and unable to cope. In contrast, in a case brought by a teacher of children with special educational needs, claiming compensation for stress and psychiatric injury, failed on the grounds that the court held that she had not provided any evidence that the head teacher was aware that she was likely to suffer any psychiatric injury as a result of her employment. Breach of the duty of care had not been established.[30]

The Court of Appeal recently overruled three decisions where awards ranging from £7,000 to £101,041 had been made on grounds of stress. The Court of Appeal stated that where an employee is bringing a claim agains the employer for breach of its contractual duty to take reasonable care of the health and safety of the employee, the employee had to show that it was reasonably foreseeable to the employer that the employee was suffering from stress which was work related, and that it was reasonable for the employer to take action, and that the employer's failure to take action had caused the harm. The employer was entitled to assume that the employee could withstand the normal pressures of the job unless he knew of some particular problem or vulnerability. Relevant factors could include the nature and extent of the work done by the employee and the signs from the employee of impending harm to health. The size and scope of the employer's operation were relevant, including the re-distribution of duties to other employees and the need to treat them fairly. The Court of Appeal also stated that an employer who offered a confidential counselling or treatment service was unlikely to be in breach of duty. The assessment of compensation would take account of any pre-existing disorder or vulnerability.

There is evidence that a high proportion of midwives consider that they are stressed in their work. In one study 78% of midwives in a labour ward reported having insufficient time to perform their duties, causing high degrees of stress.[31] The same authors concluded in another article that poor communications between doctors and midwives also caused stress.[32] Work in a neonatal unit can be particularly stressful, especially in dealing with dying babies.[33]

If a midwife considers that she is suffering from unacceptable stress, then she must ensure that she makes senior management aware of this so that reasonable action can be taken to support her. Conversely, a midwife manager should ensure that she identifies when midwives would appear to be under stress and that reasonable action is taken to support them and this is documented. (See Chapter 34 and the role of the midwife manager.) Some trusts have counselling services for staff and similar services are available from the Royal College of Midwives.[34] A useful guide for managers on stress amongst healthcare professionals is provided in a work edited by Firth-Cozens and Payne.[35]

Bullying

The duty owed by the employer to the employee to take reasonable care of the health and safety of the employee would also include the duty to protect the employee against bullying. In a recent case, £100,000 was accepted in an out-of-court settlement by a teacher who alleged that he had been bullied by the head teacher and other staff, when he was teaching in a school in Pembrokeshire.[36] The Andrea Adams Trust, a support organisation which helps health service employees has provided a fact sheet on workplace bullying.[37] Bullying may be associated with racial or other harassment (see Chapter 22). An overview of workplace bullying in midwifery departments and how it may be addressed is provided by Ruth Hadikin.[38] She provides an action checklist for targets of workplace bullying. Records are of course essential. In November 2001 it was reported that two senior midwives in

Portsmouth were dismissed following allegations of harassment and bullying.[39] Preliminary findings of research commissioned by the RCM into why midwives leave the NHS has shown evidence of bullying by senior midwives.[40]

Smoking

Health and safety duties would include the protection of the employee against working in a dangerous smoke-filled environment. Most hospitals and clinics these days follow a no-smoking policy, only allowing smoking in certain designated (and hopefully well-ventilated) areas. However a complete ban on smoking by patients can cause difficulties and potential dangers for long-term patients who are addicted, as is discussed in an article by the author.[41] The Government initiated smoking cessation services in Health Action Zones in 1999/2000 following the White Paper 'Smoking Kills' December 1998. There were three key targets: young people, adult smoking and pregnant women. The results of the first monitoring of these services were published in February 2002.[42]

Cross infection

The problems, dangers and duties which arise from cross infection are considered in Chapter 29.

RECENT ADDITIONAL STATUTORY PROTECTION

Recent changes to the law have boosted the protection of the employee in the event of disputes over health and safety matters. The law now provides a right not to suffer detriment in health and safety cases so that an employee who is concerned about a health and safety danger can, if the appropriate procedure is followed, be protected from any victimisation such as dismissal. The criteria for judging the appropriateness of the employee's actions are 'all the circumstances including, in particular, his knowledge and the facilities and advice available to him at the time'. There is also provision for the protection of health and safety representatives carrying out their duties.

A defence is available to the employer if the employee's actions were so negligent that a reasonable employer might have treated him as the employer did (Paragraph 3(3) Schedule 5 of the Trade Union Reform and Employment Rights Act 1993).

The Public Interest Disclosure Act 1998 has extended this provision to protect the whistle blower from victimisation (see Chapter 22).

PROFESSIONAL ACCOUNTABILITY BEFORE THE NMC

The Midwives Rules contain several provisions in relation to health and safety.

Rule 39 requires a midwife to be medically examined at the request of the Local Supervising Authority (see Chapter 29).

Rule 40 emphasises that she must not undertake any treatment which she has not been trained to give or which is outside her sphere of practice except in an emergency (see Chapter 5).

Rule 41 limits her role in relation to the administration of medicines and other forms of pain relief (see Chapter 20).

Rule 43 requires her to give her supervisor, the LSA and the Council every reasonable facility to inspect her methods of practice, records, equipment and premises (see Chapter 3).

In addition, the Midwife's Code of Practice gives further guidance on these rules.

The Code of Professional Conduct also has many clauses which relate to health and safety at work:

Clause 1
'act always in such a manner as to promote and safeguard the interests and wellbeing of patients and clients'

Clause 2
'ensure that no action or omission on your part, or within your sphere of responsibility, is detrimental to the interests, condition or safety of patients and clients'

Clause 3
'maintain and improve your professional knowledge and competence'

Clause 4
'acknowledge any limitations in your knowledge and competence and decline any duties or responsibilities unless able to perform them in a safe and skilled manner'

Clause 11
'report to an appropriate person or authority, having regard to the physical, psychological and social effects on patients and clients, any circumstances in the environment of care which could jeopardise standards of practice'

Clause 12
'report to an appropriate person or authority any circumstances in which safe and appropriate care for patients and clients cannot be provided'

Clause 13
'report to an appropriate person or authority where it appears that the health or safety of colleagues is at risk, as such circumstances may compromise standards of practice and care'

Clause 14
'assist professional colleagues, in the context of your own knowledge, experience and sphere of responsibility, to develop their professional competence, and assist others in the care team, including informal carers, to contribute safely and to a degree appropriate to their roles'

The Rules and the clauses contained in the Codes are enforceable through the professional conduct proceedings of the NMC (see Chapter 4).

CONCLUSION

Whilst the areas of accountability and liability have been considered separately it is of course possible that there could be criminal proceedings, civil proceedings, disciplinary proceedings and professional conduct proceedings resulting from the same health and safety incident, especially where someone has died. Most NHS organisations employ health and safety officers who provide training, guidance and information for employees and can be contacted for updates on health and safety publications. However it remains the personal and professional responsibility of the individual midwife to ensure that health and safety laws are implemented and this implementation regularly monitored.

QUESTIONS AND EXERCISES

1. Following the risk assessment regulations, identify the risks in your practice and consider the action which should be taken to prevent them or reduce them.

2. Your trust wishes to protect clients against the possibility of babies being abducted. Carry out a risk assessment on your unit and decide what action it would be reasonably practicable to take.

3. Look carefully at your working practices over a week and identify any dangers to you in relation to manual handling. What changes, if any, should be made?

4. A colleague asks you for advice because she has been injured by the relative of a client and wants to obtain compensation. What form of legal action may she have?

5. You are aware that a senior midwife has a reputation for bullying junior staff. What action would you take if you were (a) a student midwife, (b) a junior midwife.

References

1 Health and Safety Commission. 2000. *Management of health and safety at work: Approved Code of Practice and Guidance*. London: HMSO

2 Aslam R. 1999. Risk management in midwifery practice. *British Journal of Midwifery*, 7(1)

3 Scott P. 1998. Setting up a risk management programme in a small, private birth unit. *Practising Midwife*, 1(10)

4 Royal College of Midwives. 2000. *Reassessing risk: a midwifery perspective*. London: RCM

5 Health and Safety Commission. 1997. *Violence and aggression to staff in health services*. London: HSE Books

6 Royal College of Midwives. 2000. *Safety in Maternity Units*. London: RCM

7 Royal College of Midwives. 1996. *Safety for midwives working in the community*. London: RCM

8 News report. BBC1 West, 24 July 2001

9 Department of Health. 2001. Press release 2001/0509 Violent patients can now be denied NHS treatment

10 NHS Responseline 0541 555455 or www.nhs.uk/zerotolerance

11 Hunt SC and Martin AM. 2000. *Pregnant women: Violent men*. MIDIRS

12 Royal College of Midwives. Stewards Briefings, on-going

13 Royal College of Midwives. 1999. *Handle with care: a midwife's guide to preventing back injury*. 2nd edition. London: RCM

14 Royal College of Midwives. 1992. *Handbook for health and safety representatives*. London: RCM

15 Health and Safety Executive. 1992. *Manual Handling: Guidance on Regulations*. London: HMSO

16 Health and Safety Commission. 1992. *Guidance on Manual Handling of Loads in the Health Services*. London: HMSO

17 Wiles v. Bedfordshire CC CLR 365 June 2001

18 UKCC. 1998. *Guidelines for records and record keeping*. London: UKCC

19 European Union Directive 93/42/EEC

20 Medical Devices Agency. 1998. SN 9801: Reporting Adverse Incidents Relating to Medical Devices. London: MDA

21 SI 1994/3017 Medical Devices Regulations 1994 came into force 1 January 1995, mandatory from 14 June 1998. Directive 93/42/EEC.

22 Medical Devices Agency. 1998. DB 9801: Medical Device and Equipment Management for Hospital and Community Based Organisations. London: MDA

23 93/42/EEC Directive concerning medical devices

24 Medical Devices Agency. 1998. SN 9801: Reporting Adverse Incidents Relating to Medical Devices. London: MDA

25 Statutory Instrument 1999 No 437

26 Health and Safety Executive. 1993. A step by step guide to COSHH assessment. London: HMSO

27 A and others v. National Blood Authority and another. Times Law Report 4 April 2001; Lloyd's Law Rep Med [2001] 187

28 Walker v. Northumberland County Council. Times Law Report 24 November 1994 QBD

29 News item. 2001. Care Chief's £140,000 stress award. *The Times* 5 September 2001

30 Salisbury v. Kirklees MBC 21 June 2001 Current Law Digest 392 October 2001

31 Mackin P and Sinclair M. 1998. Labour ward midwives' perceptions of stress. *Journal of Advanced Nursing*, 27, 986-91

32 Mackin P and Sinclair M. Midwives' experience of stress on the labour ward. *British Journal of Midwifery*, 7(5), 323-6

33 Raeside L. 2000. Caring for dying babies: perceptions of neonatal nurses. *Journal of Neonatal Nursing*, 6(3), 93-9

34 RCM Tel 0846 605 0044. Service always available to members and their families

35 Firth-Cozens J and Payne RL (eds). 1999. *Stress in health professionals: psychological and organisational causes and interventions.* Chichester: Wiley

36 Fletcher V. 1998. Teacher 'bullied by staff' wins £100,000. *The Times*, 17 July 1998

37 Andrea Adams Trust. 2000. Factsheet on workplace bullying. Andrea Adams Trust, Maritime House, Basin Road, North Portslade, Brighton BN41 1WA. Tel/fax 01273 704 900; Email aat@btinternet.com

38 Hadikin R. 2001. *MIDIRS Midwifery Digest*, 11(3), 308-11

39 News item. 2001. *Practising Midwife*, 4(10), 6

40 Being carried out by Professor Mavis Kirkham of Sheffield University's Informed Childbearing and Health Research Group

41 Dimond B. 1996. Smoking mothers' rights and the maternity department. *Modern Midwife*, 6(6), 10-11

42 Department of Health. 2000. Press release 2002/0075.

Chapter 20
MEDICATION

The midwife has extended powers in relation to the prescribing and administration of medicines compared with the nurse/health visitor practitioner. These powers may be further expanded as midwives are one of the designated practitioners with additional powers of prescribing under recent changes to the statutory provisions for prescribing. Amendments have been made by Section 63 of the Health and Social Care Act 2001 to the Medicines Act 1968, expanding the health practitioners who will be eligible to prescribe following the recommendations of the Final Crown Report[1] (see below). This chapter looks at the specific powers of the midwife in relation to the statutory provisions dealing with medicines and the legal issues which are likely to arise.

All practising midwives should have an up-to-date copy of the British National Formulary (BNF) which is published jointly by the British Medical Association and the Royal Pharmaceutical Society of Great Britain. At the front of the BNF there is a very useful introductory section which gives guidance on prescribing for different categories of drugs and different groups of patients. In addition a directory is published annually on over-the-counter medicinal products.[2] Reference should also be made to the Appendix on Further Reading.

THE STATUTORY FRAMEWORK

The two main Acts of Parliament controlling the administration and use of medicines are the Medicines Act 1968 and the Misuse of Drugs Act 1971.

THE MEDICINES ACT 1968

This Act set up an administrative and licensing system to control the sale and supply of medicines to the public, retail pharmacies and the packing and labelling of medicinal products. It classifies medicines in the categories shown in Box 20.1.

Box 20.1 Classification of medicines under the Medicines Act 1968

1. Pharmacy only products. These can only be sold or supplied retail by someone conducting a retail pharmacy when the product must be sold for a registered pharmacy by, or under the supervision of, a registered pharmacist.

▶

▶
2. General sales list. These are medicinal products which may be sold other than from a retail pharmacy so long as the provisions relating to Section 53 of the Medicines Act are complied with. This means that the place of sale must be the premises where the business is carried out; they must be capable of excluding the public; the medicines must have been made up elsewhere and the contents must not have been opened since make-up.

3. Prescription only list. The medicines are only available on a practitioner's prescription. Schedule I of the Regulations lists the prescription only products and Part II of the Schedule lists the prescription-only products which are covered by the Misuse of Drugs Act 1971. Special provisions apply to prescriptions in hospitals.

THE MISUSE OF DRUGS ACT 1971

This Act and subsequent legislation makes provision for the classification of controlled drugs and their possession, supply and manufacture.

The Act makes it a criminal offence to carry on the manufacture, supply and possession of controlled drugs contrary to the Regulations. Controlled drugs are divided into three categories:

Class A includes, amongst others: cocaine, diamorphine, morphine, opium, pethidine and class B substances when prepared for injection.

Class B includes, amongst others: oral amphetamines, barbiturates, cannabis, codeine.

Class C includes, amongst others: most benzodiazepines, meprobamate.

The Misuse of Drugs Regulations 1985 divides controlled drugs into 5 Schedules, each specifying the requirements governing activities such as import, export, production, supply, possession, prescribing and record keeping.

Schedule 1 Cannabis, lysergic acid etc. Possession and supply are prohibited except in accordance with Home Office authority.

Schedule 2 Diamorphine, morphine, pethidine etc. Regulations control the prescriptions, safe custody and the keeping of registers.

Schedule 3 Barbiturates, subject, apart from phenobarbitone, to special prescription requirements.

Schedule 4 Benzodiazepines etc. Subject to minimum control. Not subject to safe custody and the controlled drug prescriptions requirements do not apply.

Schedule 5 Drugs containing only minute strengths of controlled drugs. Exempt from virtually all controlled drug requirements other than retention of invoice for two years.

THE MIDWIVES RULES

Rule 41 of the Midwives Rules details further legally binding regulations in relation to the administration of medicines by midwives. For convenience these are set out in Box 20.2.

> ### Box 20.2 Rule 41 Administration of medicines and other forms of pain relief
>
> 1. A practising midwife shall only administer those medicines, including analgesics, in which she has been trained as to use, dosage and methods of administration.
>
> 2. A practising midwife shall only administer medicines including inhalational analgesics by means of apparatus if she is satisfied that the apparatus has been properly maintained, and
>
>   - it has a CE marking or, if it does not have such a marking,
>
>   - it is of a type for the time being approved by the UKCC (NMC) as suitable for use by a midwife and in this paragraph, CE marking has the meaning assigned to it in the Medical Devices Regulations SI 1994 No 3017*
>
> 3. In a situation in which clinical trials involving new medicines including inhalation analgesics, or new apparatus, are taking place, a practising midwife may only participate under the direction of a registered medical practitioner.

*The Medical Devices Regulations are discussed in Chapter 19.

RECORDS

The Midwives Rules 42 requires the midwife to keep records in relation to medicines. It is set out in Box 20.3.

Box 20.3 Rule 42: Records

1. A practising midwife shall keep as contemporaneously as is reasonable detailed records of observations, care given and medicine or other forms of pain relief administered by her to all mothers and babies.

2. The records referred to in Paragraph (1) of this Rule shall be kept

    a. in the case of a midwife employed by a Health Authority or NHS trust in accordance with any directions given by her employer

    b. in any other case, in a form approved by the Local Supervising Authority.

For further details relating to the storage and transfer of records see Chapter 15.

THE MIDWIFE'S CODE OF PRACTICE

Paragraph 15 and 16 of the Midwife's Code of Practice expands upon the midwife's duty in relation to the supply, possession and use of controlled drugs. It is set out in Box 20.4.

Box 20.4 Code of Practice Paragraphs 15 and 16

Supply, possession and use of controlled drugs

15. The possession and administration of controlled drugs by midwives is covered by the Misuse of Drugs Regulations 1985 (SI 1985 No.2066); the Misuse of Drugs (Northern Ireland) Regulations 1986 (SR 1986 No.52); the Medicines Act 1968. The Misuse of Drugs Regulations provide for the supply of pethidine to midwives (and any other controlled drug listed in Schedule 5 Part III and of the Prescription Only Medicines (Human Use) Order 1997 SI 1997 No. 1830 using the supply order procedure. You can obtain supply order forms from your Supervisor of Midwives.

16. The administration of controlled drugs by midwives working in a hospital/institution should be in accordance with locally agreed policies and procedures. It may be decided locally that midwives practising in hospitals or institutions may follow the same practice as midwives working in the community.

DESTRUCTION OF CONTROLLED DRUGS

The Midwife's Code of Practice sets out in Paragraphs 17 and 18 procedures for the destruction of controlled drugs which are shown in Box 20.5.

Box 20.5 Destruction of controlled drugs

17. Regulation 26 of the Misuse of Drugs Regulations contains a procedure for witnessing the destruction of pethidine (or other controlled drugs approved in accordance with the Medicines Act 1968) which have been supplied to the midwife, but which are no longer required. The destruction is done by the midwife but only in the presence of an 'authorised person' who may be one of the following:

    – a Supervisor of Midwives in England, Wales and Northern Ireland

    – a regional pharmaceutical officer in England

    – a pharmaceutical officer of the Welsh Office

    – a chief administrative pharmaceutical officer of health boards in Scotland

    – in Northern Ireland an inspector appointed by the Department of Health and Social Services under the Misuse of Drugs Act 1971

    – medical officers in England, Scotland or Wales

    – an inspector of the Pharmaceutical Society of Great Britain

    – a police officer

    – an inspector of the Home Office drugs branch.

18. There is provision within the Misuse of Drugs Regulations for midwives to surrender stocks of unwanted controlled drugs to the pharmacist from whom they were obtained or to an Appropriate Medical Officer, but not to a Supervisor of Midwives.

CONTROLLED DRUGS AND HOME BIRTHS

Box 20.6 sets out the procedure laid down in Paragraph 19 of the Midwife's Code of Practice.

Box 20.6 Controlled drugs and home births

19. In the case of controlled drugs supplied directly to the mother on prescription from a family practitioner, the mother (to whom in law they belong) is responsible for destroying any which are unused. You should advise the mother to destroy the drugs and suggest that she does so in your presence. Alternatively, you can advise the mother to return the unused drugs to the pharmacist from whom they were obtained. You can not do this for her. You should record the advice you have given and any action taken should be recorded in the mother's notes, together with details of the nature and amounts of drugs involved.

PRESCRIPTION ONLY AND OTHER MEDICINES USED BY MIDWIVES

Guidance is given on prescription only and other medicines in Paragraphs 20 and 21 of the Midwife's Code of Practice and is shown in Box 20.7.

Box 20.7 Prescription only and other medicines used by midwives

20. Certain medicines which are normally only available on a prescription issued by a medical practitioner may be supplied to practising midwives for use in their practice only, under the Medicines Act 1968, either from a retail chemist or hospital pharmacy. These medicines are listed in Schedule 3 Parts I and III of the Prescription Only Medicines (Human Use) Order 1997, SI No. 1830.

21. If you work in the community, you may need to carry antiseptics, sedatives and analgesics, local anaesthetics, oxytocic preparations and approved agents for neonatal and maternal resuscitation. The particular medicines and controlled drugs which a community midwife can use should be determined locally in collaboration with the senior midwife and medical and pharmaceutical staff and should be listed in written local policy. You can obtain further details from your Supervisor of Midwives. You must record the return of prescription-only medicines to the supplying pharmacist and should obtain a receipt from the pharmacist. You should record the disposal of prescription only and other medicines.

ADMINISTRATION OF HOMEOPATHIC AND HERBAL SUBSTANCES

The UKCC has introduced new paragraphs relating to homeopathic or herbal substances.

Box 20.8 Administration of homeopathic and herbal substances

22. Homeopathic and herbal medicines are subject to the licensing provisions of the Medicines Act 1968, although those on the market when that Act became operative, (which applies to most of those substances now available) received product licences without any evaluation of their efficacy, safety or quality. You should ensure that you are familiar with the requirements of Rule 41(1) in relation to the administration of medicines. You must, however, respect the right of individuals to self-administer substances of their choice.

23. When a mother wishes to receive homeopathic or herbal substances and you believe that the substances might either be an inappropriate response to the presenting symptoms or could negate or enhance the effect of prescribed medicines, you must discuss this fully with the mother. Acting in the interests of the mother and with her full knowledge, you should consider contacting the relevant expert practitioner to seek advice, but must also be mindful of the need not to override the woman's rights. Please refer to Paragraph 37 for information on complementary and alternative therapies, which are not subject to the provisions of the Medicines Act 1968. (See Chapter 35 of this book.)

ADMINISTRATION OF CONTROLLED DRUGS

Further guidance on the administration of controlled drugs is given in Paragraphs 24 and 25, see Box 20.9.

Box 20.9 Administration of controlled drugs

24. When administering controlled drugs and other medicines in the NHS, you should comply with locally agreed Health Authority (or NHS trust) policies and procedures. In some Authorities, such policies may include a standing order signed by a Consultant registered medical practitioner and a senior midwife authorising the administration of controlled drugs and medicines for use by the midwife in her practice in an institution. These drugs and medicines would be similar to those carried by a midwife in her practice in the community.

25. If you are practising outside the area of your employing authority or outside the NHS, you should seek advice from your Supervisor of Midwives regarding any matters related to the supply, administration, storage, surrender and destruction of controlled drugs and other medicines. Supervisors of Midwives should periodically audit the records of controlled drugs and prescription only medicines kept by midwives. Any discrepancies must be investigated by the Supervisor.

Reference must also be made by midwives to the UKCC advisory paper, Guidelines for the Administration of Medicines.[3] This guidance, which replaces the earlier UKCC document, Standards for the Administration of Medicines[4] covers the principles in relation to the prescription, patient group directions (see below), principles for the administration of medicines, aids to support concordance (compliance aids), self-administration of medicines, complementary and alternative therapies, management of errors or incidents in the administration of medicines and the legislation.

NURSE/MIDWIFE PRESCRIBING

Following the first Crown Report,[5] the provisions of the Medicinal Products: Prescription by Nurses Act 1992 introducing nurse prescribing came into force in October 1994 when pilot schemes for prescribing by community nurses and health visitors commenced. Nurses and health visitors who have recorded their prescribing qualification on the NMC Register can prescribe against the Nurse Prescriber's Formulary. Subsequently a further Crown Report[6] recommended the recognition of patient group directions (group protocols) whereby registered nurses, midwives and other registered health practitioners could prescribe in accordance with a protocol containing the information specified in the Regulations.[7] These provide for 'Patient Group Directions' to be drawn up to make provision for the sale or supply of a prescription only medicine in hospitals in accordance with the written direction of a doctor or dentist. To be lawful, the Patient Group Direction must cover the particulars which are set out in Part 1 of Schedule 7 of the Statutory Instrument and shown in Box 20.10.

Box 20.10 Particulars for Patient Group Direction

a. the period during which the Direction shall have effect

b. the description or class of prescription only medicines to which the Direction relates

c. whether there are any restrictions on the quantity of medicine which may be supplied on any one occasion, and if so, what restrictions

d. the clinical situations which prescription only medicines of that description or class may be used to treat

e. the clinical criteria under which a person shall be eligible for treatment

▶

▶

f. whether any class of person is excluded from treatment under the Direction, and if so, what class of person

g. whether there are circumstances in which further advice should be sought from a doctor or dentist and, if so, what circumstances

h. the pharmaceutical form or forms in which prescription only medicines of that description or class are to be administered

i. the strength, or maximum strength, at which prescription only medicines of that description or class are to be administered

j. the applicable dosage or maximum dosage

k. the route of administration

l. the frequency of administration

m. any minimum or maximum period of administration applicable to prescription only medicines of that description or class

n. whether there are any relevant warnings to note, and if so, what warnings

o. whether there is any follow up action to be taken in any circumstances, and if so, what action and in what circumstances

p. arrangements for referral for medical advice

q. details of the records to be kept of the supply or the administration of medicines under the Direction.

The final report of the Crown Review was published in March 1999.[8] One of its most significant recommendations was that the legal authority in the UK to prescribe should be extended beyond currently authorised prescribers and two types of prescribers should be recognised: the independent prescriber and the dependent prescriber. In addition a UK-wide advisory body, provisionally entitled the 'New Prescribers Advisory Committee' should be established, under Section 4 of the Medicines Act, to assess submissions from professional organisations seeking powers for suitably trained members to become independent or dependent prescribers.

An 'independent prescriber' is a clinician who is responsible for the assessment of patients with undiagnosed conditions and for the decisions about the clinical management required, including prescriptions.

A 'dependent prescriber' is a clinician who takes over the continuing care of a patient which may include prescribing, after initial assessment by an independent prescriber.

A 'clinician' is a healthcare professional who is engaged in the direct examination, treatment and care of patients.

On 25th October 2000 the Department of Health issued a consultation paper to extend nurse prescribing. This was followed by legislation enacted in the Health and Social Care Act 2001 to extend prescribing powers. Section 63 amends Section 58 of the Medicines Act 1968 to enable additional persons to be eligible to prescribe, including persons registered by a board established under the Professions Supplementary to Medicine Act 1960, persons who are pharmacists and also persons who are registered in any register established, continued or maintained under an Order in Council under Section 60(1) of the Health Act 1999. The latter would include midwives registered under the Nursing and Midwifery Council. In other words, the possibility of all registered health professionals having powers to prescribe is envisaged by the amendments to the Medicines Act 1968. However, who actually in practice will be able to prescribe will depend upon the detailed regulations to be enacted by the Secretary of State. The Secretary of State has the power to draw up orders which set the conditions for prescribing and administering specified medicines. Anyone failing to obey these conditions would be guilty of a criminal offence. At the time of writing the detailed legislation is awaited. When fully implemented, these changes will have a major impact on the traditional roles played by different health professionals.

PRESCRIBING IN PREGNANCY

The BNF[9] points out that

'Drugs can have harmful effects on the fetus at any time during pregnancy. It is important to bear this in mind when prescribing for a woman of childbearing age.'

In Appendix 4 the BNF lists the drugs which are to be avoided or used with caution in pregnancy. It also makes the following recommendation:

'Drugs should be prescribed in pregnancy only if the expected benefit to the mother is thought to be greater than the risk to the fetus, and all drugs should be avoided if possible during the first trimester. Drugs which have been extensively used in pregnancy and appear to be usually safe should be prescribed in preference to new or untried drugs; and the smallest effective doses should be used. Absence of a drug from the list does not imply safety.'

Occasionally a heroic story is told of a sacrifice of a mother for the unborn baby.

One such is that of Michelle Doyle who, it is reported,[10] gave birth to a healthy boy after being told soon after she became pregnant that she was suffering from ovarian cancer. She refused cytotoxic drugs knowing that they would have harmed the baby. After the birth of the baby she had surgery for the cancer but it was too late to save her life.

Such sacrifices cannot be insisted upon and as the law stands at present, the mother can take medications which are necessary to save her life, even if they are likely to be harmful to the child. Only if she takes the drugs intending to cause a miscarriage to the baby would she be acting illegally under the criminal law. (See Chapters 17, 25 and 26.)

DRUG ADDICTS

What action does a midwife take if she discovers that one of the mothers referred to her is a drug addict? In the past, particulars of persons addicted to specific drugs had to be notified to the Chief Medical Officer or Home Office by the doctor within seven days of his considering or having reasonable grounds to believe the addiction (Misuse of Drugs (Notification of and Supply to Addicts) Regulations 1973). However this requirement was revoked by the Misuse of Drugs (Supply to Addicts) Regulations 1997. Doctors are now expected to report on a standard form a case of drug misuse to their local Drug Misuse Database (DMD). The BNF states:

'A report (notification) to the Drug Misuse Database should be made when a patient first presents with a drug problem or re-presents after a gap of six months or more. All types of problem drug misuse should be reported including opioid, benzodiazepine and CNS stimulant.'

The BNF gives contact numbers.

If a midwife suspects that one of her clients is addicted she should ensure that a medical practitioner is informed, who would send the requisite details to the DMD. Apart from the criminal offences relating to the possession and supply of illegal drugs, there are no laws in this country which enable action to be taken against a mother to prevent the fetus being harmed by drugs. Nor can the fetus be made a ward of court before it is born, as the case Re F (in utero) 1988[11] illustrates. (The case is discussed in Chapter 17.) However, the midwife would have responsibilities to ensure that appropriate care is taken of a vulnerable adult. It may be that the mother refuses all assistance offered by the midwife. If there are concerns that the mother lacks the mental capacity to make her own decisions, then action can be taken in her best interests (see Chapter 7). Close contact with social services will be essential to ensure that action is taken in the bests interests of the child once born. A report by the Audit Commission in February 2002 recommended fundamental reforms of the drug treatment services in England and Wales. At present they provided little value for the £234 million spent on helping addicts and misusers. As a consequence of this audit midwives might find that a new strategy for drug treatment services may be planned and implemented which would assist them in their work.

LIABILITY AND MEDICINAL PRODUCTS

There are unfortunately many cases where litigation arises as a result of breaches of the duty of care in relation to the prescribing or administration of medicinal products.

In examples of contested cases, £119,302 was ordered to be paid to a man who had suffered permanent brain damage because of a badly written prescription.[12] The doctor had written a prescription for Amoxil, but this was read by the pharmacist as Daonil. The doctor was held 25% liable and the employers of the pharmacist 75% liable.

In another case[13] the doctor prescribed Migril but failed to heed the manufacturer's warnings and instead of limiting the dose to not more that 12 tablets in the course of one week and not more than one every four hours, prescribed 60 tablets to be taken at two tablets every four hours. The pharmacist did not spot the error. The patient's condition deteriorated and the mistake was not noticed by another doctor in the practice who visited the patient. In the High Court compensation of £100,000 was agreed, 45% payable by the prescribing doctor, 40% by the pharmacist and the remaining 15% by the second doctor who visited. On appeal the second doctor was found not liable and his 15% contribution was accepted by the pharmacist.

In one case, bad handwriting on a prescription for a top-up epidural resulted in a junior doctor administering to a woman following a hysterectomy operation 30mg of epidural diamorphine in 10ml of saline instead of 3mg.[14] A woman of 53 had entered the Princess Grace private hospital in London for a routine hysterectomy. As a result of the drug administration error (it was also only the second time the junior doctor had added drugs to an epidural) and the fact that the junior doctor had not been trained to use the resuscitation equipment, the patient died a few days later.

Other examples of errors in medication and prescribing are described in the Journal of the Medical Defence Union[15] and reports are to be found regularly in newspapers and professional journals.

At the heart of the issue of negligence is the question of whether the accepted standard of the reasonable professional has been followed. This is known as the Bolam Test[16] and is discussed in Chapter 13. If midwives are to have extended powers of prescribing as a result of the new legislation, standards will have to be defined, protocols drawn up and procedures agreed to ensure that there are recognised standards for professional practice.[17] However the public should not expect a lower standard of care because midwives have the role of prescribing.

The Consumer Protection Act 1987 (which is discussed in Chapter 19) can be used by those who have suffered harm as a result of a defect in medication, without having to establish that there was negligence on the part of the manufacturers or suppliers.

INFLUENCE OF THE NATIONAL INSTITUTE FOR CLINICAL EXCELLENCE (NICE)

The establishment of NICE is discussed in Chapter 21. One of its main remits is to consider research relating to medicinal products and to identify effective products. Its recommendations are not binding upon the NHS, but in practice any Health Authority or NHS trust which ignored its guidelines that a specific medication was effective, would probably face an action for judicial review if it prevented the drug from being made available on the NHS within its own catchment area. In May 2000 NICE issued guidance on the use of Taxanes in the treatment of ovarian cancer. It recommended that the drug paclitaxel (Taxol) should be used to treat women who have previously received it and whose cancer has recurred or been resistant to other forms of treatment.[18] In 2000 NICE stated that it was unable to recommend Beta-interferon for patients suffering from multiple sclerosis. It subsequently confirmed this decision and the Department of Health supported pilot schemes to undertake further research into the effectiveness of the drug. .It was announced in April 2000[19] by the Department of Health that NICE is to prepare guidelines advising GPs on when to refer patients with acute lower back pain to specialists.

Whilst the guidelines of NICE are not law in the sense that patients have the right to insist that they are followed, they may well become absorbed into any definition of what is reasonable professional practice according to the Bolam Test (see Chapter 13) thus creating a presumption that they are followed. Midwives should ensure that they receive information about NICE publications and guidelines and also, if possible, have an input into the thinking behind NICE's publications.

CONCLUSION

Recent changes in prescribing powers are supporting a radical development in the traditional demarcation boundaries of health professional activities. There are now great opportunities for professional development. However, any such widening of the scope of professional practice must ensure that midwives work within their competence and they obtain the training and necessary practice under supervision (see Chapter 5). Errors and negligent practice will be followed by litigation, disciplinary and professional conduct proceedings and, in situations where there has been gross recklessness or negligence, criminal prosecution.

QUESTIONS AND EXERCISES

1. Prepare a policy in relation to the supply and administration of controlled drugs in the community.

2. In what ways would you consider that the powers of the midwife could be enhanced by the changes in prescribing legislation?

3. A client is a drug addict. What action do you take?

References

1 Department of Health. 1999. *Final report on the prescribing, supply and administration of medicines. Chaired by Dr June Crown.* London: HMSO

2 Propriety Association of Great Britain. *OTC Directory 1994/5 Treatments for common ailments. Promoting Responsible Consumer Health Care.*

3 UKCC. 2000. *Guidelines for the administration of medicines.* London: UKCC

4 UKCC. 1992. *Standards for the administration of medicines.* London: UKCC

5 Department of Health. 1989. *Report on the nurse prescribing and supply. Advisory Group chaired by Dr June Crown.* London: HMSO

6 Department of Health. 1998. *Review of prescribing, supply and administration of medicines: a Report on the supply and administration of medicines under Group Protocols.* London: HMSO

7 Prescription only Medicines (Human Use) Amendment Order 2000 SI 2000 No 1917

8 Department of Health. 1999. *Final report on the prescribing, supply and administration of medicines. Chaired by Dr June Crown.* London: HMSO

9 BMA and Royal Pharmaceutical Society of Great Britain. 2000. *British National Formulary 40.* London: HMSO

10 *The Times* 19 March 1994

11 Re F (in utero) [1988] 2 All ER 193

12 Prendergast v. Sam & Dee and others. *Independent* 17 March 1988.

13 Dwyer v. Roderick and others. *The Times* 12 November 1983

14 Kennedy D. 1996. Hospital blamed in report on overdose death. *The Times,* 3 July 1996

15 Ferner RE. 1992. Errors in prescribing and giving drugs. *Journal of the Medical Defence Union,* 1992(3)

16 Bolam v. Friern Hospital Management Committee QBD [1957] 2 ALL ER 118

17 Dimond BC. 1994. Standards setting and litigation. *British Journal of Nursing,* 3(5), 235-8

18 *Healthcare Parliamentary Monitor,* 2000, 251, 5; www.nice.org.uk/appraisals/taxguide.htm

19 *Healthcare Parliamentary Monitor,* 2000, 250

SECTION D

MANAGEMENT ISSUES

This section of the book considers the management issues in relation to the provision of maternity services. Chapter 21 will consider the statutory authorities and the regulations relating to the provision of medical maternity services by general practitioners. Subsequent chapters look at employment law, the position of the independent midwife and the laws relating to the registration of private maternity hospitals and the role of the midwifery manager.

Chapter 21

THE STRUCTURE OF THE NHS AND THE PROVISION OF HOSPITAL, COMMUNITY AND PRIMARY CARE SERVICES

In this chapter we consider the statutory framework of the National Health Service in the light of the changes which have been made under the Primary Care Act 1997, the NHS and Community Care Act, the Health Act 1999, the Health and Social Care Act 2001 and the provision of maternity medical services by General Practitioners.

Over the past ten years there have been constant changes to the NHS structure and some midwives may have found that their contracts of employment have been transferred several times between different health organisations.

The Secretary of State has the responsibility for providing NHS services within the United Kingdom and appoints the statutory bodies which have the tasks of commissioning and providing care. The Secretary of State is under a general duty[1] to

'continue the promotion in England and Wales of a comprehensive health service designed to secure improvement

(a) in the physical and mental health of the people of those countries, and

(b) in the prevention, diagnosis and treatment of illness, and for that purpose to provide or secure the effective provision of services in accordance with this Act.'

Section 3(1) of the NHS Act 1977 requires the Secretary of State to provide throughout England and Wales, to such extent as he considers necessary to meet all reasonable requirements:

(a) hospital accommodation

(b) other accommodation for the purpose of any service provided under this Act

(c) medical, dental, nursing and ambulance services

(d) such other facilities for the care of the expectant and nursing mothers and young children as he considers are appropriate as part of the health service.

The discretionary nature of this power should be recognised. The phrases 'To such extent as he considers necessary' 'to meet all reasonable requirements' qualify the duty and have meant that actions for failure to provide services brought against statutory authorities have usually failed in the context of healthcare (see Chapter 6).

The Secretary of State fulfils the task of providing a comprehensive health service by delegating the work to statutory authorities.

HEALTH AUTHORITIES

These are statutory bodies which are appointed to carry out the functions of the Secretary of State in ensuring the provision of health services. As part of their functions they undertake an assessment of needs for healthcare and services in relation to public health. Health Authorities in each district arrange for the provision of primary care services through Primary Care Groups (in Wales Local Health Groups) or Primary Care Trusts (see below). Hospital and community services are provided by NHS trusts which receive their funding from the Health Authorities. A reorganisation of the boundaries and number of Health Authorities took place following publication of the Department of Health's paper Shifting the Balance of Power within the NHS,[2] which was designed to strengthen the strategic role of Health Authorities.

The NHS and Community Care Act 1990 introduced into the law relating to healthcare, the concept of the internal market and led to the establishment of NHS trusts from whom the Health Authorities purchased services. The White Paper of 1997[3] recommended the abolition of the internal market and the GP fundholding arrangements. Following the implementation of the Health Act 1999, GP fundholders were abolished, Primary Care Groups were established and new institutions such as the Commission for Health Improvement were established. At the same time the National Institute for Clinical Excellence was set up.

NHS TRUSTS

Section 5 of the NHS and Community Care Act 1990 enabled NHS trusts to be established. These are statutory bodies appointed by the Secretary of State which are responsible for the provision of NHS services. The NHS trust can make long-term arrangements with Health Authorities and Primary Care Groups or Trusts for the provision of health services in their area.

PRIMARY CARE GROUPS AND TRUSTS

Health Authorities and GPs working with Local Authority representatives can establish Primary Care Groups to arrange for the provision of primary care services in a specific area. Under the Health Act 1999 these Primary Care Groups are able to apply for trust status. They are of diverse constitutions, sometimes taking over the administration of social services on behalf of the Local Authority for the area served by the Primary Trust. Midwifery services are sometimes included in Primary Care Groups or Trusts. There is however no uniformity: in some areas only community maternity services are transferred to the Primary Care Group or Trust; in others the hospital and community midwifery services are transferred (Ealing is an example of the latter). Under the Health and Social Care Act 2001 powers are given to enable Care Trusts to be set up which can provide both Local Authority and health services.

HOW DOES THIS AFFECT THE MIDWIFE AND MIDWIFERY SERVICES?

Many midwives may now find that they are employed by a Primary Care Group or Trust and the employment implications of this are considered in Chapter 22. Initially their contracts are likely to be as they were under Whitley Council arrangements but since trusts have the power to make local agreements for terms and conditions of service this might eventually change. Regulations relating to the transfer to a Primary Care Trust are set out in the Health Act 1999 (Schedule 1).

GENERAL PRACTITIONERS

There are about 30,000 GPs in England with on average 2,000 patients per GP. About 10% of all GPs work without partners. The majority however work in group practices which may be attached to a health centre. General Practitioners working within the NHS have an agreement with Health Authorities over the services which they provide and are obliged to follow the National Health Service (General Medical Services) Regulations 1992 No. 635 (as amended).

The NHS and Community Care Act 1990 saw the introduction of some GPs receiving approval as fundholders working in fundholding practices. However fundholding was abolished under the Health Act 1999. Under the NHS (Primary Care) Act 1977, pilot schemes were introduced to enable General Practitioners and dentists to provide personal medical and dental services outside the framework of the Health Authorities. Where Primary Care Trusts have been established they have powers to take over the administration of personal medical services. The ENB has investigated the extent to which statutory supervision of midwives enables midwives to contribute to the work of Primary Care Groups and health improvement programmes.[4] It found that only 20 Primary Care Groups in England had midwives as board members and since maternity services were not seen as a high priority for PCGs, midwives felt marginalised or overlooked by doctors or nurse members. Research also funded by the ENB has shown that GPs were the least likely health professionals to consider that midwives should undertake the lead professional role for low risk maternity care, especially in antenatal and postnatal care. However, more than 50% of the GPs questioned felt that midwives should be the lead professional in the intrapartum period.[5]

MATERNITY MEDICAL SERVICES[6]

These include:

a. the provision of personal medical services to a woman during the antenatal period

b. the provision of personal medical services to a woman during labour

c. the provision of personal medical services to a woman and to her baby, as specified in paragraph 3(b) of Schedule 5, during the postnatal period. 'Where the pregnancy has resulted in the birth of a live baby, render all necessary personal medical services to that baby during the period of 14 days following its birth, unless, during that period, another doctor has accepted the baby for inclusion in his list pursuant to an application made on the baby's behalf under Regulation 20(1).

d. the provision of a full postnatal examination.

A woman who, after a doctor has diagnosed that she is pregnant, requires the provision of maternity medical services may arrange for the provision of any or all of the services mentioned above with

– any doctor on the obstetric list (see below),

– the doctor on whose list she is included, or

– any doctor who has accepted her as a temporary resident.

Once the woman has made arrangements with a doctor for the provision of any or all of the services listed above, he shall provide such services as are specified in Part II of Schedule 5.

The arrangement for the provision of services can be terminated by:

– the woman, by informing the HA in writing or informing the doctor in writing, who must inform the HA within 7 days, or making a new arrangement with another doctor who shall notify the HA within 7 days of making the new arrangement

– the doctor making an application under Paragraph 11 of his terms of service (Termination of Responsibility for Patients Schedule 3 of 1992 Regulations), or

– where the woman is a temporary resident, by her ceasing to be resident in the doctor's area or the doctor terminating responsibility for her under Paragraph 10 of the terms of service (whichever occurs first).

The HA must notify the doctor in writing within 7 days where it has received notification from the woman or the new doctor.

'Antenatal period' is defined as being the duration of a woman's pregnancy until the onset of labour, and 'postnatal' as the period of 14 days following the conclusion of a pregnancy.

The doctor is relieved of his obligations under Paragraphs 1, 2, 3 or 4 of Part II Schedule 5

– during any period when the woman is outside the doctor's practice area and is not present at any other place where, the doctor is obliged to visit and treat her

– where it is proposed that the woman's labour should take place in a hospital, to the extent that responsibility for her care has been taken over by the hospital; and

– where the woman has been admitted to a hospital as an in-patient, to the extent that her care has been taken over by the hospital.

OBSTETRIC LIST AND MATERNITY SERVICES

A woman can ask another doctor whose list she is not on to provide obstetric or maternity services, but in this case, the doctor must be on the obstetric list held by the Health Authority. Regulations cover the establishment of an obstetric list.

QUALITY ASSURANCE MECHANISM

The White Paper on the NHS also envisaged new institutions and strategies for raising standards within the NHS. These include the concept of Clinical Governance, the Commission for Health Improvement, the National Institute for Clinical Excellence, National Service Frameworks and new arrangements for professional registration and misconduct.

THE INTRODUCTION OF CLINICAL GOVERNANCE

The White Paper on the NHS introduced the concept of Clinical Governance. It is defined as:

'A framework through which NHS organisations are accountable for continuously improving the quality of their services.' [8]

The idea of Clinical Governance is basically simple. In the past, the trust board and its Chief Executive have been responsible for the financial probity of the organisation; there has been no statutory responsibility of the trust for the overall quality of the organisation. Under the concept of Clinical Governance the board and its Chief Executive are responsible for the quality of clinical services provided by the organisation. In theory this could mean that a board is removed or a Chief Executive dismissed if a baby suffers brain damage at birth or a mother dies in childbirth as a result of negligence.

The concept of Clinical Governance is based on the statutory duty of quality under Section 18 of the Health Act 1999.

Box 21.1 Section 18 Health Act 1999

It is the duty of each Health Authority, Primary Care Trust and NHS trust to put and keep in place arrangements for the purpose of monitoring and improving the quality of healthcare which it provides to individuals.

The duty falls primarily upon the Chief Executive of each Health Authority and NHS trust to implement. In practice, each Chief Executive designates officers to be responsible for quality or Clinical Governance in specified areas of clinical practice. Government guidance was published in March 1999.[8] This follows from the original consultation document, A First Class Service: Quality in the new NHS.[9] The aim to develop quality within the NHS is to be secured in three ways:

- setting clear national quality standards

- ensuring local delivery of high quality clinical services, and

- effective systems for monitoring the quality of services.

The UKCC has published a position paper for NHS employers[10] identifying the major issues in strengthening and supporting the midwifery contribution to maternity care for women and their families which link with the concept of Clinical Governance. These major issues include clinical issues such as variations in practice and care, the management of emergencies, the absence of or failure to use the guidelines and protocols and poor quality of record keeping; issues associated with women's experience of care, such as informed choice and communication; and organisational issues such as effective use of resources, effective leadership, communication and collaboration, lack of consensus on the midwife's role and organisational constraints on providing optimum maternity care. The UKCC suggested that 'using the Clinical

Governance and supervisory frameworks together in a proactive way can lead to major benefits for the organisation overall but more particularly will improve outcomes for women...'.

THE COMMISSION FOR HEALTH IMPROVEMENT (CHI)

The Commission for Health Improvement replaces the Clinical Standards Advisory Group (CSAG) but has much wider functions and powers. Sections 19 to 24 of the Health Act 1999 establish the Commission for Health Improvement and set out its functions and powers. It is a body corporate, i.e. it can sue and be sued on its own account. The functions are listed in Box 21.2.

Section 19(2) of the Health Act 1999 gives powers to the Secretary of State to make regulations covering:

- the times at which, the cases in which, the manner in which, the persons in relation to which or matters with respect to which any functions of the Commission are to be exercised

- the matters to be considered or taken into account in connection with the exercise of any functions of the Commission

- the persons to whom any advice, information or reports are to be given or made

- the publication of reports and summaries of reports

- the recovery from prescribed persons of amounts in respect of expenditure incurred by the Commission in the exercise of any of its functions, and

- the exercise of functions of the Commission in conjunction with the exercise of statutory functions of other persons.

Box 21.2 Functions of the Commission for Health Improvement

a. Provide advice or information with respect to arrangements by Primary Care Trusts or NHS trusts for the purpose of monitoring and improving the quality of healthcare for which they have responsibility.

b. Conducting reviews of, and making reports on, arrangements by Primary Care Trusts or NHS trusts for the purpose of monitoring and improving the quality of healthcare for which they have responsibility.

c. Carrying out investigations into and making reports on, the management, provision or quality of healthcare for which Health Authorities, Primary Care Trusts or NHS trusts have responsibility.

▶

d. Conducting reviews of and making reports on, the management, provision or quality of, or access to or availability of, particular types of healthcare for which NHS bodies or service providers have responsibility, and

e. Other functions as may be prescribed relating to the management, provision or quality of, or access to or availability of, healthcare for which prescribed NHS bodies or prescribed service providers have responsibility.

ACTIVITIES OF THE CHI

One of the earliest tasks undertaken by the CHI on the day it was established was to visit Garlands Hospital in Carlisle, run by the North Lakeland Healthcare NHS Trust in Cumbria. An independent investigation[11] had found that staff had physically and mentally abused patients. The Chairman of the NHS trust was dismissed by the Secretary of State. The Secretary of State ordered CHI to visit the hospital.

A spokesman for the Commission stated that its programme for scrutinising NHS trusts could include questions about the resuscitation of older people, following complaints that some hospital doctors are ignoring guidelines.[12] CHI will have a programme of inspections so that over five years, all NHS trusts will be visited and a report published. The powers of CHI are wide: they can ask for the production of documents, require people to be interviewed by them and make strong recommendations to the Secretary of State. The NHS Reform and Healthcare Bill 2002 contains provisions for extending the powers of CHI. The existence of an NHS watchdog is a significant step in the attempt to secure high standards of patient care. There are statutory provisions for CHI to work with the Audit Commission (see below).

PERFORMANCE STANDARDS

Another initiative envisaged in the NHS Plan is the establishment of nationwide assessment of performance in the NHS. Performance ratings were established and for the first year of assessment were based on waiting times and hospital cleanliness. Hospitals were awarded stars according to their performance and the best trusts were permitted to spend their share of the £155m Performance Fund. In addition the best performing trusts were given 10 key freedoms including: less frequent monitoring from the centre, fewer and better co-ordinated inspections, development of their own investment programmes without receiving prior approval, extra cash and resources and opportunities for their Chief Executives to provide direct advice to Ministers and to join the learning set which will consider additional freedoms for their organisations. CHI will assist in the refining the criteria for assessing performance. Four failing trusts which were given a zero star rating in the CHI assessment and failed to make improvements had their management franchised to other NHS organisations. New Chief Executives were appointed. The Government announced its intention of establishing a Register of Experts who would act as 'public service entrepreneurs' (DoH Press release 2002/0069).

AUDIT COMMISSION

The Commission for Health Improvement will work alongside the Audit Commission, supporting its work by inspections and publishing advice to organisations and practitioners. An Audit Commission Report in 1997[13] made significant recommendations for all aspects of maternity services including the care of women in pregnancy, labour and birth and the care of women after childbirth and the care of newborn babies.

NATIONAL INSTITUTE FOR CLINICAL EXCELLENCE (NICE)

This statutory body was established on 1st April 1999 to promote clinical and cost effectiveness. The then Secretary of State stated that its task would be to abolish postcode variation in the country, so that there would be national standards for the provision of healthcare such as medicines. There had been a lack of uniformity in the decisions of Health Authorities over the provision of services, particularly of medicines. One of the functions of NICE is to issue clinical guidelines and clinical audit methodologies and information on good practice. The National Institute for Clinical Excellence has a major role to play in the setting of standards of practice, by disseminating the results of research of what is proved to be clinically effective, research-based practice. One of its first activities was to recommend to the Secretary of State that the expense of Relenza, a drug developed by Glaxo Wellcome for preventing 'flu, did not justify funding through the NHS, since it appeared to have little benefit for those groups most at risk: the elderly and asthma sufferers. NICE's recommendations were accepted by the Secretary of State. Subsequently, following further research, NICE recommended that the drug should be made available for the groups at risk. Its programme for 2001 included fetal monitoring and induction of labour.[14] (See Chapter 13.) NICE guidelines on Caesarean sections which are being commissioned from the National Collaborating Centre for Women's and Children's Health are to be published by the end of 2003. The difficulties faced by midwives in attempting to use evidence-based practice are illustrated by Helen Hindle in a case study concerned with group B Streptococcus in breast milk.[15]

SETTING UP OF NATIONAL SERVICE FRAMEWORKS (NSFS)

The White Paper envisaged that there would be evidence-based National Service Frameworks which set out what patients can expect to receive from the NHS in major care areas or disease groups. One of the first National Service Frameworks to be published was that for Mental Health.[16]

A National Service Framework for children and maternity services is at the time of writing awaited. Eventually NSFs will cover most of the main sphere of clinical practice. They will doubtless assist managers and clinicians in obtaining the resources to ensure a reasonable standard of care for the patients. Inevitably however they are also likely to support litigation where patients who have suffered personal injuries are able to compare local facilities unfavourably with the norm laid down in the NSF.

NHS DIRECT

The White Paper on the NHS[17] proposed the establishment of NHS Direct. The Government's aim was that by the end of the year 2000 the whole country would be covered by a 24-hour telephone advice line staffed by nurses. A director has been appointed for NHS Direct in Wales and this became operational in January 2000, with separate funding and organisation from England. The service aims to provide both clinical advice to support self-care and appropriate self-referral to NHS services as well as access to more general advice and information. In June 2001 the Department of Health announced that as part of a £5 million pilot programme, people with digital television sets will be able to get on-screen consultations with NHS Direct nurses.[18] Patients in the pilot scheme will be able to book appointments with their GPs, get general and local health information and speak to NHS Direct nurses on screen. Clearly any NHS Direct nurse responding to a call would have to question whether the caller is pregnant and ensure that she does not give advice which is outside the limits of her competence. In certain call centres it may be possible to ensure that the woman speaks to a midwife. The caller would be advised to contact her own midwife and doctor and inform them of her contact with NHS Direct.

NATIONAL PLAN FOR THE NHS

On 22nd March 2000 the Prime Minister announced to the House of Commons that there were five challenges to be faced in the NHS. These are shown in Box 21.3.

Box 21.3 Challenges for the NHS

- Partnership – making all parts of the health and social care system work better together and ensuring the right emphasis at each level of care

- Performance – improving both clinical performance and health service productivity

- Professions – increasing flexibility in training and working practices and removing demarcations, in the context of major expansion of the healthcare workforce

- Patient care – which has two components: ensuring fast and convenient access to services and empowering and informing patients so that they can be more involved in their own care

- Prevention – tackling inequalities and focussing the health system on its contribution to tackling the causes of avoidable ill health.

Following the Prime Minister's announcement, the Secretary for Health announced that he was setting up discussions with key professionals in the NHS to develop a National Plan based on these five challenges. He intended to establish six modernisation action teams with a specific remit to address variations in performance and standards across the care system.

The NHS Plan was published in July 2000[19] and set out significant proposals for the reform of the NHS, envisaging significant increase in resources and numbers of professional staff, changes in the professional registration and controls of professional standards. Significant changes in the representation of patients are considered in Chapter 6 of this book. Changes are envisaged in the relationships between the NHS and social services and the NHS and private sector. A modernisation agency has been set up to spread best practice. At the time of writing work is under way with most of the recommendations contained in the NHS Plan. Additional funding has been allocated, targeted on maternity units. The first tranch was announced in May 2001, to support maternity services and bereavement. In October 2001 it was announced[20] a further £100m would be made available for major refurbishment, new facilities for fathers and families and the modernisation of antenatal units. A list of how the money was to be allocated accompanied the press release. Two thousand extra midwives were to be recruited over the following three years and national standards would be set for maternity services. The Maternity and Neonatal Workforce Group (chaired by the Deputy Chief Medical Officer of Health, Dr Sheila Adams, and including representatives of the RCM, RCOG and Health Authorities) was established to examine the best way to provide high quality maternity services and make recommendations to Ministers.

THE BRISTOL INQUIRY

Such were the wide sweeping recommendations in the Report of the Inquiry chaired by Professor Ian Kennedy into children's heart surgery at the Bristol Royal Infirmary[21] that one commentator suggested that in future the NHS would be talked about in terms of 'Before Bristol' and 'After Bristol'. Concerns at the high death rates amongst the children receiving heart surgery in Bristol were expressed increasingly from the late 1980s onwards. Subsequently complaints were made to the General Medical Council and in 1998 two cardiac surgeons and the Chief Executive of the trust were found guilty of serious professional misconduct: one cardiac surgeon and the chief executive were struck off from the Register and the other cardiac surgeon's registration was made conditional for three years that he did not operate on children. A public inquiry was appointed in June 1998 which reported in 2001. Significant recommendations were made across several areas shown in Box 21.4.

Box 21.4 Subjects covered by recommendations of the Bristol Inquiry

1. Respect and honesty

2. A health service which is well led

3. Competent healthcare professionals

4. The safety of care

5. Care of an appropriate standard

6. Public involvement through empowerment

7. The care of children

8. Healthcare services and the treatment for children with congenital health disease.

Many of the recommendations, such as the greater respect given to the rights of the patient, the National Patient Safety Agency, and the changes to control over professional standards exercised by the Registration bodies had already been included in the NHS Plan. In its introduction to its recommendations the Inquiry makes some extremely salient points:

- There are no right answers; just, perhaps, less wrong answers
- Cultural and institutional change takes time and can be slow, requiring patience and forbearance

- Nothing can be achieved on the cheap

- There are no quick fixes, but progress is possible and can be achieved

- Change can only be brought about with the willing and active participation of those involved in healthcare; the public, patients, healthcare professionals, trusts and Health Authorities and government.

The Inquiry outlined specific principles which it wished the Report to give effect to. These are summarised in Box 21.5.

Box 21.5 Principles recognised by the Inquiry

- The patient must be at the centre of everything the NHS does.

- The commitment and dedication of staff in the NHS must be valued and acknowledged; those caring for patients must themselves be supported and cared for.

- There must be openness and transparency in everything the NHS does.

- The impact of the way in which services are organised on the quality of care which patients receive must be recognised: the quality of care depends on systems and on facilities, as well as on individual healthcare professionals.

- All those involved in healthcare... must recognise and acknowledge the contribution of the others in the service of patients.

- The safety of patients must be the foundation of the NHS's commitment to the quality of its services.

- Sentinel events, that is, errors, other adverse events, and near misses, which occur during the care of patients, must be seen as opportunities to learn, not just as reasons to blame.

- There must be clear and understood systems of responsibility and accountability: a culture of blame is no substitute for such systems.

- The quality of healthcare must be guided by agreed standards, compliance with which is regularly monitored.

- The role of central government in relation to the NHS should be:

    a. to act as its HQ in terms of management, and

    b. to create independent mechanisms for regulating the quality of healthcare and the competence of healthcare professionals.

▶

▶
> – The various independent bodies must themselves be co-ordinated so as to avoid
> the fragmentation of responsibility which arose in the past.

The next few years are likely to see the working through of the recommendations contained in the Bristol Inquiry Report.

CONCLUSION

Major changes have been taking place in the organisation and structure of the NHS in recent years. The strengthening of a primary care service with the establishment of Primary Care Trusts will have a significant impact on the delivery of maternity services and the role of the General Practitioner. In addition the new institutions of NICE, CHI, the National Service Frameworks and the strategy set out in the NHS Plan will have an important impact on the setting and the monitoring of standards within midwifery and obstetric practice. Of great significance is the Report of the Bristol Inquiry.[21] Its comprehensive and far-reaching proposals affect all aspects of patient care and professional practice (see especially Chapter 6). The NSF on maternity and children is not expected to be published in full until 2003 with implementation in 2004. An All-Party Parliamentary Group on maternity chaired by Julia Drown MP was set up in 2000 to act as a pressure discussion group on maternity issues. In July 2001 it considered midwifery-led care and in November 2001 the results of the Sentinel research on Caesarean sections (see Chapter 6). Reports of its meetings are available from the National Childbirth Trust.[22]

QUESTIONS AND EXERCISES

1. What are the advantages of the concept of Clinical Governance in the provision of maternity services?

2. Ask your HA or primary care trust for a copy of the obstetric list and analyse this in relation to the General Practitioners who you know provide medical maternity services.

3. What services does the Local Authority provide for the care of the pregnant woman, before, during and after confinement?

4. What do you consider would be the best administrative arrangement for the provision of hospital, community health and social services for the pregnant woman and her family?

5. Obtain a copy of the NSF on maternity and children's services (when published) and consider the extent to which the department within which you work meets

these standards. What action, if any, is necessary to bring the department into compliance with the NSF standards?

6. Obtain a copy of the Report of the Bristol Inquiry and discuss with colleagues the action necessary to ensure the implementation of its recommendations in your department.

References

1 Section 1 of the National Health Service Act 1977

2 Department of Health. 2001. *Shifting the Balance of Power within the NHS*. London: HMSO

3 Department of Health. 1997. *The New NHS: Modern, dependable*. London: HMSO

4 English National Board. 2000. *Midwives and Public Health: an identification of the extent to which statutory supervision of midwives enables midwives to contribute to the work of primary care groups and health improvement programmes*. London: ENB

5 Pope R and Graham L. 1999. Maternity care of low risk women: identification of continuing education needs. *Practising Midwife*, 2(7), 30-4

6 See Regulation 31 and Schedule 5 Part II of the National Health Service (General Medical Services) Regulations 1992 SI No 635

7 Department of Health. 1998. *A First Class Service: Quality in the new NHS*. London: HMSO

8 NHS Executive. 1999. Health Service Circular 1999/065 Clinical Governance: Quality in the new NHS

9 NHS Executive. 1998. Health Service Circular 1998/113 A First Class Service: Quality in the new NHS

10 UKCC. 2001. Strengthening and supporting the midwifery contribution to maternity care for women and their families. Registrar's Letter 22/2001

11 North Lakeland Healthcare NHS Trust. 2000. *Report of Independent Inquiry into Garlands Hospital*

12 *Healthcare Parliamentary Monitor*, 2000, 250, 3

13 Audit Commission. 1997. *First Class Delivery: Improving Maternity Services in England and Wales*. London: HMSO

14 NICE. 2001. Induction of Labour: Inherited clinical guideline D. London: NICE; www.nice.org.uk; NICE. 2001. The use of Electronic Fetal Monitoring: Inherited clinical guideline C. London: NICE

15 Hindle H. 2001. The clinical application of evidence-based practice. *British Journal of Midwifery*, 9(11), 672-5

16 Department of Health. 1999. *National Service Framework for mental health services*. London: HMSO

17 Department of Health. 1997. *White Paper on the NHS: Modern, dependable*. London: HMSO

18 Department of Health. 2001. Press release 2001/0289 Switch to Health Care on your TV

19 Department of Health. 2000. *The NHS Plan: A plan for investment, a plan for reform*. London: HMSO

20 Department of Health. 2001. Press release 2001/0470 Maternity Units receive £100 million to modernise and improve facilities

21 Bristol Royal Infirmary. 2001. *Learning from Bristol: the report of the public inquiry into children's heart surgery at the Bristol Royal Infirmary 1984-1995. Command Paper CM 5207*; www.bristol-inquiry.org.uk

22 Contact Catherine Eden at the National Childbirth Trust 020 8992 2616; c_eden@national-childbirth-trust.co.uk

Chapter 22
EMPLOYMENT LAW

It is important for midwives to have a good understanding of the law relating to employment, whether they are employees or independent midwives. Some may be managers who are responsible for other employees and need to know the situation from both the employer's and the employee's perspective. It is impossible in a work of this nature to go fully into the complexities of employment law. The aim is to provide an introduction and understanding of the basic principles so that when necessary the subject can be supplemented with more specialist works listed in the list of Further Reading.

Parental rights and the rights of those who look after dependants are considered in Chapter 12.

The areas to be considered are shown in Box 22.1.

Box 22.1 Topics considered in this chapter

- The contract of employment: formation and content

- Changing the contract

- Performance of the contract

- Breach of contract

- Termination of contract

- Sex, race and disability discrimination

- Male midwives

- Rights of part-time staff

- The Working Time Directive

- Whistle blowing

CONTRACT OF EMPLOYMENT

At the heart of the employment relationship is a contract. It may not always be evidenced in writing but it exists as soon as there is agreement by one person to work for another in payment of consideration. The basic principles of contract law apply and in addition there are many Acts of Parliament giving employees rights through employment and regulating the powers of employers and also the rights of workers to combine to withdraw labour. Some of the more significant Statutes are shown in Box 22.2. Recently European Directives have led to changes in employees' rights and new maternity rights are due to be implemented in October 2002 as a result of an EC directive.

Box 22.2 Acts of Parliament covering employment law

Employers Liability (Compulsory Insurance) Act 1969

Employers Liability (Defective Equipment) Act 1969

Employment Protection (Consolidation) Act 1978

Employment Acts 1980, 1982, 1988, 1989, 1990

Health and Safety At Work Act 1974

Industrial Relations Act 1971

Race Relations Act 1976

Rehabilitation of Offenders Act 1974

Sex Discrimination Acts 1975, 1986

Trade Union and Labour Relations (Consolidation) Act 1992

Trade Union Reform and Employment Rights Act 1993

Disability Discrimination Act 1995

Employment Rights Act 1996

Employment Relations Act 1999

The essential elements of a contract are:

– agreement

– consideration

– intention to be legally binding.

The law recognises that a legally enforceable contract has come into existence when an offer is accepted and the main terms are agreed. In the employment situation, the advertisement and initial applications and interviews would be regarded as preliminary negotiations, part of the invitation to treat. However, statements made then may become part of the terms of the eventual agreement. It is not until an offer is made, usually by the employer to the prospective employee, and this is accepted, that the contract comes into existence. The contract may be conditional, eg. subject to satisfactory medical examination or subject to the receipt of satisfactory references. Should the medical examination and/or the references not be satisfactory, then the relationship will end or not come into existence.

Many employers fail to put the terms of the contract into writing and thus some employees assume that they have no contract. This is not so. A contract exists in law if there has been this offer and acceptance and if there is no reason, eg. that it is contrary to public policy, for the contract to be unlawful. There is however a statutory duty for written particulars of the contract to be given to all employees within two months of commencing work. The necessary details are shown in Box 22.3.

Box 22.3 Written statement of the terms must include

– identity of the parties

– date on which the employment began

– date when the employee's period of continuous employment began

– remuneration*

– intervals at which paid*

– sick pay

– pensions

– notice or reference to the law on minimum periods of notice or any collective agreements

►

▶ – title of job or brief description of the work for which the employee is employed*

– any terms and conditions on hours of work and holidays*

– any disciplinary rules or access to a document setting them out (unless fewer than 20 employees)

– person to whom employee can apply if dissatisfied with any disciplinary decision and how such application should be made.

Additions required by the Trade Union Reform and Employment Rights Act 1993 Section 26 and Schedule 4:

– in case of non-permanent employment, the period for which it is expected to continue*

– either the place of work, or, where the employee is required or permitted to work at various places, an indication of that fact and the address of the employer*

– any collective agreement which directly affects the terms and conditions of the employment including, where the employer is not a party, the persons by whom they were made

– details if the employee is required to work outside the UK.

All the items with an asterisk must be included in a single document given to the employee. Those items without an asterisk may be contained in some other document which the employee has reasonable opportunities of reading in the course of her employment or is made reasonably accessible to her in some other way.

Changes to the particulars must be given not later than

– one month after the change, or

– where the change arises from the requirement to work outside the UK for more than a month, the time when he leaves the UK.

CONTENT OF THE CONTRACT

Not all terms are agreed at the time the offer is accepted. Box 22.4 shows the variety of terms of which the contract is made.

Box 22.4 Content of contract of employment

– Express terms agreed between the parties at the time the contract is formed.

– Express terms agreed through collective bargaining for that type of post.

– Terms implied by the law imposing duties on both employer and employee.

– Statutory rights given to employer and employee through Acts of Parliament, regulations and European Directives.

If a midwife applies for a post with an NHS trust she may be offered employment.

– She will agree with the employer the starting date, the grade and the location and her duties.

– She will be offered commencement at a specific point either on the Whitley Council grade with all the terms and conditions which have been agreed over the years, or she will be offered the terms which the trust has negotiated through local bargaining.

– As an employee she will be expected to recognise the implied duties imposed upon her by law and set out in Box 22.5. She will also have the benefit of the implied duties placed upon her employer by law and set out in Box 22.6.

– As an employee she will be entitled to specific statutory rights which are set out in Box 22.7.

IMPLIED TERMS

The common law (i.e. judge-made law) implies into a contract of employment, however long or short it is, certain duties on both employer and employee (see Box 22.5 and Box 22.6). No specific mention need be made of these during the negotiations leading up to the appointment or in the documents. Yet they are enforceable through the courts of law. If the employer is in breach of any of the implied terms, this, depending upon the circumstances, may be regarded as a fundamental breach such that the employee is entitled to see the contract as at an end (see below). If the employee is in breach of any of the implied terms disciplinary action may be taken.

Box 22.5 Duties implied by the law and imposed upon employees

– The employee is expected to obey the reasonable orders of the employer.

– The employee owes a duty of cooperation and loyalty to his employer:

▶

a. the duty to account

b. to disclose misdeeds

c. not to disclose confidential information

d. to work with care and skill.

Box 22.6 Duties implied by the law and imposed upon employers

– To cooperate with the employees (eg. not to criticise employees in front of subordinates, not to use foul language, to show proper respect for senior employees).

– To take reasonable care for the safety of his employees.

Legislation has added to the rights of the employees, and a list of some of the statutory rights is shown in Box 22.7.

Box 22.7 Statutory rights

– Written statement of particulars

– Itemised statement of pay

– Maternity benefits (see Chapter 12)

– Payment and limitations on deductions

– Time off work:

    a. to take part in Trade Union activities (unpaid)

    b. if a Trade Union official, to undertake Trade Union duties and training (paid)

    c. reasonable time off to search for work in a redundancy situation (pay for at least 2 days)

    d. to work as member of Local Authority, JP, statutory tribunal, Health Authority or school governor (unpaid)

▶

► – Holidays (Bank Holidays)

– Patents

– Guarantee payments

– Unemployment benefit

– Redundancy

– Medical suspension payment.

CHANGING THE CONTRACT

It is a rule of law that a contract cannot be changed unilaterally, i.e. if changes are to be made they must be agreed either expressly or impliedly by both parties to the contract. If, therefore, a midwife is employed as a community midwife and this is a term of her contract of employment, and she is asked to work in a hospital as a midwife or gynaecology nurse, she is entitled to refuse the change in her contract. Should the employer attempt to force this through, it would be a fundamental breach on his part. Should she agree to the change then the contract can be amended to reflect the agreement of both parties.

What about the transfer from an NHS trust to a Primary Care Trust?
An employee who is required to transfer from one NHS trust to a Primary Care Trust has protection under the Health Act 1999. In addition, protection in relation to the original terms of contract is given under the Transfer of Undertaking Regulations which ensures that the new employer is bound to accept the contractual conditions which the employees who are now transferred originally enjoyed.

Thus the same contract provisions will apply initially. The new employer is however entitled to require a change of terms if promotion is being offered. In addition, any new employee can be asked to agree terms which are different from those of the transferred employees.

What if the midwife is forced to agree changes against her will?
The midwife is legally entitled to refuse to accept any changes which were not agreed. Should the employer attempt to force them upon her, she could claim that he is in fundamental breach of the contract and claim an unfair constructive dismissal. However, she needs to look at the situation carefully: is it a redundancy situation, which means that the offer of alternative work and conditions is the

choice instead of redundancy? Is the employer's request a reasonable one and has he given reasonable notice of it? The answers to these questions would determine whether or not she would win an unfair dismissal case.

PERFORMANCE OF THE CONTRACT

Both the express and implied terms anticipate that both parties will perform their share of the contract's responsibilities. Failure to perform would be regarded as a breach unless justified by the other party's conduct.

Working to rule has been regarded by the courts as a failure to fulfil the contract even though those working to rule would regard it as technically following the contract exactly. The Court of Appeal[1] has held that withdrawal of co-operation in the form of working to rule can amount to a breach of contract. Similarly, going on strike, i.e. withdrawing labour, is a breach of contract by employees. They are however given certain protection. Should the employer dismiss some of the strikers but not all, that is an unfair dismissal for those who are dismissed. Should the employer dismiss all the strikers and then re-employ some of them, that would be an unfair dismissal of those not re-employed. The employer could sue strikers for damages but since the aim is usually to obtain a return to work this is not a preferred option and the amount of damages would be difficult to calculate. Pay would normally be withheld during a strike. Certain protection is given to trade unions which take industrial action. These are known as 'immunities'. Section 219 of the Trade Union and Labour Relations (Consolidation) Act 1992 provides as follows:

'An act done in contemplation or furtherance of a trade dispute shall not be actionable in tort on the ground only that

– it induces a breach of contract,

– that it interferes with a contract,

– that it induces any other person to interfere with its performance,

– that it constitutes a threat of breach, inducement, or interference, or

– that it constitutes a conspiracy to do any of these things.'

There is no immunity in respect of breaches of contract or crime. The words 'trade dispute' are strictly defined and secondary action where employees of firms not involved in the trade dispute are encouraged to take part is not covered by the immunity. Reference should be made to works in the Appendix on Further Reading for more information relating to the legal position of trade unions and the rights of officials and members.

BREACH OF CONTRACT

Failure to comply with the terms and conditions of contract by either party is a prima facie breach of contract.

WHERE THE EMPLOYEE IS IN BREACH

Where the employee is in breach the employer would be entitled to take disciplinary action which may include dismissal. Statutory requirements in relation to an employer with 20 or more employees include the setting out in the written statement of terms any disciplinary rules or a reasonably accessible document containing details. The employee must also be notified of a person to whom he can apply if he is dissatisfied with any disciplinary decision and how the application is to be made. Most trusts should have in place a disciplinary procedure and the midwife should ensure that she is familiar with its contents, particularly where she has a managerial function.

Counselling an employee following misconduct or unauthorised absenteeism is not usually regarded as part of the disciplinary procedure. The stages which most procedures recognise are:

– oral warning

– first written warning

– second written warning

– final warning

– suspension and/or dismissal

Not all these stages have to be followed consecutively and in cases of serious misconduct, instant dismissal or a final written warning may be justified.

Unfair dismissal

At common law (i.e. judge-made law) it would be lawful for an employer to give an employee the requisite period of notice and terminate the contract of employment without any specific reason. This would not be unlawful but could clearly be unjust. Statutory provision has therefore been made for the employee to be protected against dismissal which would be regarded as unfair.

The statute recognises that certain reasons will make the dismissal automatically fair. Other reasons may make the dismissal unfair and in certain cases the dismissal will be automatically unfair. These three categories are shown in Box 22.8.

Box 22.8 Statutory reasons for fair dismissal

    a. national security

    b. dismissal during a strike or lockout.

Statutory reasons which may make the dismissal fair:

    a. capability and qualifications

    b. misconduct

    c. redundancy

    d. illegality for the employee to continue

    e. some other substantial reason.

Automatically unfair reasons:

    a. dismissal on the ground of pregnancy or childbirth

    b. dismissal on transfer of undertaking

    c. dismissal in relation to trade union membership or activities

    d. dismissal for assertion of a statutory right.

Definition of dismissal

The definition of dismissal covers the three situations shown in Box 22.9.

Box 22.9 Definition of dismissal

1. When a contract of employment is terminated by the employer with or without notice.

2. When the contract of employment is for a fixed term and this expires without renewal of the contract.

3. When the employee terminates the contract, with or without notice, in circumstances such that he is entitled to terminate it without notice by reason of the employer's conduct. (This is known as 'constructive dismissal'.)

> In addition, leaving early when under notice, taking a new job for a trial period, lay off and short time working, and implied termination will all count as dismissal for the purposes of statutory protection of the employee against unfair dismissal.

The first situation is the usual form of dismissal. The second situation rarely results in an unfair dismissal claim, since most short-term fixed-term contracts would have a clause which removed the employee's right to make an application for unfair dismissal if the contract is not renewed.

The third situation in Box 22.9 is commonly known as 'constructive dismissal' and entitles the employee, if she has the requisite continuous service requirement, to claim unfair dismissal. This is discussed below.

Unfair dismissal: the procedures

If an employee alleges that there has been an unfair dismissal and she has worked for at least one year, she has the right to apply to an employment tribunal for unfair dismissal. If the dismissal is in the circumstances listed in the third category shown in Box 22.8 no continuous service requirement is necessary. Initially the tribunal will refer the case to the Advisory, Conciliation and Arbitration Service (ACAS) which will attempt to secure a reconciliation between the parties. In 2001 ACAS issued a guide to a new scheme to resolve unfair dismissal disputes. This new scheme is an alternative to a hearing before an employment tribunal and is set up under the Employment Rights (Dispute Resolution) Act 1998.[2]

The employer must show:

a. What was the reason for the dismissal. The onus is on the employer to establish the reason.

b. Where the reason is potentially fair (rather than automatically fair), the tribunal has to decide if the employer acted reasonably in all the circumstances in treating the reason as justifying the dismissal.

The circumstances taken into account in deciding the reasonableness of the employer's actions include:

– whether the employer followed an agreed procedure (this may include the giving of a warning)

– whether the principles of natural justice were followed, eg. the employee was allowed to speak in her own defence

– whether the employer has been consistent in his dealings with employees.

If the employee's claim for unfair dismissal is upheld, the following remedies are available:

- reinstatement

- re-engagement

- compensation.

The basic award of compensation is calculated on the number of years of continuous service of the employee.

In addition, a compensatory award provides what is just and equitable as compensation having regard to the loss suffered as a result of the dismissal.

Both the basic award and the compensatory award can be reduced owing to failure of the employee to mitigate (reduce or offset) the loss or on account of the contributory fault of the employee.

WHERE THE EMPLOYER IS IN BREACH OF CONTRACT

 Where it is the employer who is in breach of contract, the employee has the option of continuing with the contract and seeking damages for the breach or of deciding that the breach by the employer has brought the contract to an end and that therefore she is entitled to see the contract as terminated. This is the constructive dismissal situation shown in Box 22.9. If the employee has the necessary continuous service requirements, where this is required, she can pursue an action in the employment tribunal for unfair dismissal.

TERMINATION OF CONTRACT

A contract of employment can end in the ways shown in Box 22.10.

Box 22.10 Ways of ending a contract of employment
– Notice
– Performance
– Termination by agreement
– Breach of contract
– Frustration

NOTICE GIVEN BY EITHER PARTY

The employer must give:

- one week's notice to an employee who has served him for between one month and two years

- one week for each year served up to a maximum of 12 weeks for 12 years.

The employee must give:

- at least one week's notice if employed for more than one month.

(Employment Rights Act 1996 Sections 86 and 87)

It is open to the parties to agree different lengths of notice than those specified by statute. Where the parties fail to provide for notice lengths, the common law will imply a reasonable length depending upon the seniority of the post and the intervals of payment.

Sometimes, rather than provide the notice time, an employer might prefer to give the employee pay in lieu of notice.

PERFORMANCE

Where the contract is for a fixed term then the expiry of that fixed term will bring the contract to an end. However, as we have seen, failure to renew the contract counts as a dismissal.

TERMINATION BY AGREEMENT

It is possible for the parties to agree together that the contract can be ended without the set notice periods running. In this situation there would be no dismissal.

BREACH OF CONTRACT

If either party is in fundamental breach of contract this entitles the other party to see the contract as at an end. The employer might dismiss the employee (subject of course to the employee's statutory right to claim unfair dismissal); the employee might consider himself released from his contractual obligations and claim that he has been constructively dismissed.

FRUSTRATION

This is a concept in law which covers the situation where the intention of the parties when the contract was first arranged has been made impossible to perform and the contract thus comes to an end by operation of law. No notice is required nor dismissal. A lengthy prison term, which makes it impossible for the employee to perform his job, would be a frustrating event. In one case[3] an employee was suspended from medical practice and his name temporarily removed from the Register: this was considered to be a frustrating event so as to bring the contract of employment to an end by operation of law.

Where the contract is terminated through frustration the employer does not have to dismiss the employee and the employee has no claim for unfair dismissal. Because it is not always clear if the event would actually constitute frustration in law, it is wiser for an employer to assume that the contract is continuing and regard the event as potential grounds for fair dismissal and act reasonably in all the circumstances of the case. Because of the injustices of this situation, certain remedies are available under the Law Reform (Frustrated Contracts) Act 1943.

SEX, RACE AND DISABILITY DISCRIMINATION

Statutory rights to be protected against unlawful discrimination on grounds of sex or race are given by the Sex Discrimination Acts 1975 and 1986 and the Race Relations Act 1976. The Acts prevent direct discrimination, indirect discrimination and victimisation. However, there are many exceptions to unlawful discrimination. For example, discrimination is justified on grounds of sex and race where a genuine occupational qualification requires a specific sex or race. A European Council Directive[4] sets out the definition of indirect discrimination for the purposes of the principle of equal treatment and requires each Member State to take such measures as are necessary to ensure that in complaints of sex discrimination before a court or other competent authority, the burden is on the complainant initially to establish facts from which the court or competent authority may presume there has been direct or indirect discrimination. Thereafter the burden of proof shifts to the person who has allegedly discriminated against the complainant to prove that there has been no such discrimination. The Directive has been followed by statutory regulations.[5]

Midwives who care for ethnic minorities should ensure that as far as possible their specific needs should be taken into account in the provision of services for them. However there is no legal requirement that the midwife should be of a specific race. A midwife was awarded £41,720 compensation for persistent racial discrimination. Her complaints of racial discrimination were not taken seriously by her employers who failed to carry out an investigation.[6]

Reference should be made to Further Reading for further information relating to the statutory provisions on discrimination and equal pay. The RCM has published a position paper on racism and maternity services[7] and the rights of employees.[8] The Department of Health set targets for the ending of racial harassment as part of a national strategy.[9]

The Disability Discrimination Act 1995 protects disabled people from discrimination in the areas of:

– access to goods, facilities and services

– buying or renting land and property, and

– employment.

It has been brought into force in several stages and should be completely in force by 2004.

A person is disabled if they have a physical or mental impairment which has a substantial and long-term adverse effect on their ability to carry out normal day-to-day activities. Long-term means 'lasting' or likely to last at least 12 months. There must be an effect on at least one of the following aspects:

– Mobility

– Manual dexterity

– Physical co-ordination

– Continence

– Ability to lift, carry or otherwise move everyday objects

– Speech

– Hearing or eyesight

– Memory or ability to concentrate, learn or understand

– Perception of the risk of physical danger.

Discrimination occurs if a disabled person is treated less favourably than a person without a disability. A National Disability Council has been established which, following consultation, advises the Secretary of State on relevant matters as requested, and prepares Codes of Practice. In addition in April 2000 the Disability Rights Commission was established, and is funded by the Government. The Commission can sue any company that denied equal treatment to disabled people. In March 2001 the Disability Rights Commission published details of a new service to settle discrimination disputes called the Disability Conciliation Service.[10]

MALE MIDWIVES

Under the Sex Discrimination Act 1975 Section 20 the employment, training, promotion and transfer of men as midwives were restricted. These restrictions were brought to an end by Statutory Instrument 1983 No. 1202 and implemented from 1st January 1984. (Statutory Instrument 1983 No. 1841.) Health Authorities were notified that in implementing these changes they should make appropriate arrangements to ensure that women have freedom of choice to be attended by a female midwife and that where male midwives are employed provision is made for them to be chaperoned as necessary. In the statistics for 2000, 93 male midwives, out of a total of 33,291 practising midwives, were on the effective Register of the UKCC.

RIGHTS OF PART-TIME STAFF

On 1st July 2000 regulations came into force to prevent part-time workers being treated less favourably than full-time workers,[11] implementing the European Directive.[12] Paragraph 5 of these regulations gives the part-time worker:

'the right not to be treated by his employer less favourably than the employer treats a comparable full-time worker

– as regards the terms of his contract, or

– by being subjected to any other detriment by any act, or deliberate failure to act of his employer.'

Any worker who considers that his rights have been infringed can present a complaint to an employment tribunal within three months of the day of less favourable treatment or detriment taking place. This is subject to the right of the tribunal to consider out-of-time cases, if in all the circumstances it is just and equitable to do so.

THE WORKING TIME DIRECTIVE

A Directive had been adopted by the member states of the European Community on 23rd November 1996, but implementation in the UK was delayed until 1st October 1998 when the Working Time Regulations[13] came into force.[14] The fundamental provision is that a worker's working time, including overtime, should not exceed an average of 48 hours for each period of seven days over a specified period of 17 weeks. Regulations also specify provisions for rest breaks and annual leave. Night work should not normally exceed an average of 8 hours for each 24 hours.

Doctors in training, and civil protection services (ambulance) are specifically excluded from the Regulations. NMC practitioners are not specifically excluded.

However they come within the definition of the group

'where the worker's activities involve the need for continuity of service or production, as the case may be, in relation to:

– services relating to the reception, treatment or care provided by hospitals or similar establishments, residential institutions and prisons.'

The effect of this is that the Regulations on night work, daily rest, weekly rest period, and rest breaks do not apply to UKCC practitioners where there is a need for continuity of service. However, Regulation 24 requires that where a worker is required to work during a period which would otherwise be a rest period or rest break, the employer shall wherever possible allow her to take an equivalent period of compensatory rest and in exceptional cases, where this is not possible, the employer shall afford her such protection as may be appropriate in order to safeguard the worker's health and safety.

The General Whitley Council (GWC) has agreed the implementation of the Regulations for non-medical staff.[15] Section 44 of the GWC Handbook sets out the new provisions which apply to all non-medical staff.

Individual employees can if they wish agree to work more than the average of 48 hours a week. However this must be an individual decision.

WHISTLE BLOWING

This is the term which refers to a person (usually an employee) who draws attention to concerns which have health and safety implications. Because of a fear that persons, many of whom had a professional duty to draw attention to dangers and hazards, would be victimised as a result of their actions, the Department of Health issued a circular recommending that each trust and Authority should set up a procedure whereby an individual employee could draw these concerns to the management internally without being victimised and thus not needing to bring in the media or other external bodies.

The need to establish statutory protection for employees who raised concerns led to the passing of the Public Interest Disclosure Act 1998.

PUBLIC INTEREST DISCLOSURE ACT 1998

The Public Interest Disclosure Act received the royal assent on 2nd July 1998 and came into force on 2nd July 1999. It introduces amendments to the Employment Rights Act 1996. The explanatory memorandum envisages that the Act will protect workers who disclose information about certain types of matters from being dismissed or penalised by their employers as a result. The Act applies to specific disclosures:

- That a criminal offence has been committed, is being committed or is likely to be committed
- That a person has failed, is failing or is likely to fail to comply with any legal obligation to which he is subject
- That a miscarriage of justice has occurred, is occurring or is likely to occur
- That the health or safety of any individual has been, is being or is likely to be endangered
- That the environment has been, is being or is likely to be damaged, or
- That information tending to show any matter falling within any one of the preceding paragraphs has been, is being or is likely to be deliberately concealed.

To qualify for protection, the worker making the disclosure must:

- Make the disclosure to his employer or to another person to whom the failure relates or who has legal responsibility
- Be acting in good faith.

Protected disclosures include:

- Disclosures made to obtain legal advice
- Disclosures to a Minister of the Crown if the employee's employer is appointed by the Crown.

Any provision in an agreement between employer and worker is void if it purports to preclude the worker from making a protected disclosure.

Guidance has been issued by the Department of Health,[16] which requires every NHS trust and Health Authority to have in place local policies and procedures which comply with the provisions of the Act.

In one of the first cases to be reported after the coming into force of the Act, compensation of more than a quarter of a million pounds was awarded.

Box 22.11 Compensation for a whistle blower[17]

An accountant who was dismissed after blowing the whistle on his managing director's expenses claims was awarded compensation of £293,441 by an employment tribunal. The Tribunal held that he was victimised by his employers for raising genuine concerns.

CONCLUSIONS

Like many other areas of law, employment law is constantly changing as new Statutes, Directives and Regulations are introduced as a result of changes to the law in the European Community and the courts then determine how these statutory provisions are to be interpreted. In addition, the human rights set out in Schedule 1 of the Human Rights Act 1998 (see Appendix 1 of this book) apply to employees within the public sector or those working for organisations which exercise functions of a public nature. Employees will therefore be able to argue a breach of Article 3 if they are subjected to inhuman or degrading treatment or punishment or a breach of Article 6 if in the determination of their civil rights and obligations (which of course include rights under a contract of employment) they are not given a fair hearing.

QUESTIONS AND EXERCISES

1. Examine the written particulars of your contract and compare them with the list shown in Box 22.3. Are there any other terms which you consider should be included?

2. The trust has decided that in view of future uncertainties, midwives will be placed on fixed-term contracts. What are your rights in this situation?

3. A colleague is facing disciplinary action as a result of pointing out the need for improved staffing levels. Advise her on the legal situation. Refer also to Chapter 19 on health and safety.

References

1 Secretary of State for Employment v. ASLEF (No. 2) [1972] 2 All ER 949

2 ACAS. 2001. *The ACAS arbitration scheme for the resolution of unfair dismissal disputes: a guide to the scheme*; www.acas.org.uk/arbitration.htm

3 Tarnesby v. Kensington and Chelsea AHA [1981] IRLR 369

4 Council Directive 97/80 [1998] OJL 14/6

5 Sex Discrimination (Indirect Discrimination and the Burden of Proof) Regulations 2001 SI 2660

6 Royal College of Midwives. 1997. *Race case midwife awarded substantial compensation*. London: RCM

7 Royal College of Midwives. 2000. *Racism and the maternity services*. London: RCM

8 Royal College of Midwives. 2001. Know your rights 4: Racial harassment. *RCM Midwives Journal*, 4(5)

9 Department of Health. 1998. New plan to end racial harassment in the NHS. London: DoH
Department of Health. 1999. Tough action to tackle racism. London: DoH

10 Disability Rights Commission. 2001. Press release: New Service to settle discrimination disputes launched by the DRC

11 The Part-time Workers (Prevention of Less Favourable Treatment) Regulations 2000 SI No 1551 and SI 2001 No 1107

12 Directive 97/81/EC Part-time Work Directive as extended to the UK by Directive 98/23/EC

13 Working Time Regulations 1998 SI 1998 No 1833

14 NHS Executive. 1998. Working Time Regulations: Implementation in the NHS. Health Service Circular (98)204;
Department of Trade and Industry. *A Guide to the Working Time Regulations*. URN 1998/894

15 NHS Advance letter (GC) 3/98 18 November 1998

16 Department of Health. Public Interest Disclosure Act. Health Service Circular (99)198

17 Booth J. Man who shopped boss wins £290,000. *The Times*, 11 July 2000

Chapter 23

THE INDEPENDENT MIDWIFE AND PRIVATE MATERNITY HOSPITALS

This chapter explores the legal issues relating to the independent midwife. It also considers the legal situation of private maternity hospitals in which many midwives are employed.

INDEPENDENT MIDWIVES

In the last chapter we looked at the situation of employed midwives and the terms of the contract of employment. The vast majority of midwives are employed. As can be seen from Chapter 2, out of a total of 33,291 practising midwives in 2000-2001 only 63 are recorded in the UKCC figures as being self-employed in private practice. The employed midwives enjoy not only the contractual and statutory rights which are given to them by virtue of their employment, they also enjoy the indemnity of the employer who on the basis of his vicarious liability for the employee will pay out to those harmed by the negligence of the employee the compensation due (see Chapter 13). Here we look at the situation of the independent midwife.[1]

The independent midwife is self-employed. She has no employer and is comparable to a small business person. This section on independent midwives will look at those issues set out in Box 23.1.

Box 23.1 Legal issues and the private practitioner

Contract for services: not contract of employment

- No vicarious liability

- No indemnity by employer

- Contracts with trusts

- No employee rights

▶

- Personal liability for health and safety of self and others

- Liable for breach of contract.

In addition, since the independent midwife is a self-employed contractor she must ensure that she has an understanding of the topics set out in Box 23.2.

Box 23.2 The independent midwife and business law

- Inland revenue and VAT

- National insurance: self and employees

- Insurance and indemnity

- Health and safety regulations
  - personal accident cover

- Contracts for supplies and services

- Training and development

- Employment law

- Data protection regulations

- Pensions and sickness

- Formation of business

  - Type: Sole trader
           Partnership
           Limited company
           Co-operative

  - Name
  - Protection through patents

- Registering designs

- Premises
  Planning permission

▶ Building regulations
The lease

– Special trades
- Trading laws

– Sale of goods and services

– Trade description acts

– Unfair Contract Terms Act

– UKCC advisory paper on advertising
- Taxation and starting up

– Capital allowances

– Deciding on the tax year.

It is impossible in a work of this kind to look in detail at all the topics listed in Box 23.2. Advice on running a business is provided[2] and the independent midwife should refer to specialist books on the different areas. Helpful guidance on setting up in independent practice with details of the equipment she would require, money matters, marketing and other concerns is provided by the independent midwife Lesley Hobbs.[3] The independent midwife should also remember that like any employed midwife she is bound by the Midwives Rules and Codes and by the rules and code relating to supervision. She should also be aware that if she employs others, then as an employer she has statutory and contractual duties under health and safety legislation.

EMPLOYEES AND VICARIOUS LIABILITY

All employees are covered for indemnity payments by their employers provided that the unlawful or negligent acts which lead to compensation being payable take place during the 'course of employment'. This is discussed in full in Chapter 13.

Midwives who are employed by an NHS trust, whether acute or community, or for a Primary Care Trust, or who work in a private hospital are covered by the vicarious liability of the employer. Even if a midwife is personally sued, it would be the usual procedure for the employer to accept liability if it can be established that the negligent person was an employee. The employer could of course dispute that the act was carried out in the course of employment.

INDEPENDENT MIDWIVES

Independent midwives are self-employed. Even though they have to have a Supervisor of Midwives (or often supervisors), who may be a midwife manager in a nearby hospital, the fact of supervision does not make the supervisor liable for the negligence of the midwife, nor does it make the supervisor's employer vicariously liable for the negligence of the independent midwife.

Independent midwives therefore have to ensure that they have adequate insurance cover to protect them against the claims and which would cover not only their legal expenses but also the compensation payable. Such indemnity cover must be sufficient to cover the greatest sum likely to be awarded and be upgraded each year to cover any inflationary rises.

In August 1993 the RCM was advised that higher insurance premiums would be payable in respect of independent midwives who had previously enjoyed the same insurance cover as their employed colleagues via the RCM. An additional cost of almost £½ million was requested but it was made clear this would not be required if self-employed midwives were excluded from protection. After the failure of attempts to renegotiate the insurance cover, the RCM notified the self-employed midwives that their cover via the RCM would terminate on 31st March 1994. As a consequence independent midwives were required to pay £4,950 per annum premium for indemnity insurance.[4] In 1997 £10,000 premium was required by the MDU to provide insurance for an independent midwife. This led to many midwives giving up independent practice. Obtaining reasonable insurance cover for independent midwives to practise is still an on-going concern.

Compensation claims in relation to birth injuries are the highest risk area of insurance within healthcare. However since employed midwives are covered by the vicarious liability of the employer for compensation arising from negligent acts which have led to harm in the workplace, they are a lower financial risk to the RCM insurers than independent midwives who would have to pay out the full cost of any successful claim.

Insurance cover is also essential for the car, for any equipment used, for negligence by any employees employed by the independent midwife and for personal injuries. Insurance cover for any legal expenses is also useful.

EXCLUDING LIABILITY

Could the independent midwife ask the mother to agree to use her services on the understanding that the mother would accept all the risks and in the event of negligence occurring would not sue her?

Such an arrangement could constitute either an exclusion of liability by the midwife or a voluntary assumption of risk by the mother. The former is prohibited by the Unfair Contract Terms Act 1977 which prevents a person excluding herself from liability in the event of her negligence causing personal injury or death. The latter would only be valid if it can be shown that the person voluntarily assuming all the risks of negligence had all these risks spelt out and agreed not to sue in respect of these risks. Clearly if the kind of negligence which arose had not been contemplated by the parties it would be outside the agreement and the mother could bring a claim. Such a defence as voluntary assumption of risk would be fraught with difficulties in these circumstances and there may well be a view that it is not professionally acceptable for the midwife to reach such an agreement since it deprives the mother of a legitimate claim for compensation.

If the independent midwife were to take the risk and not pay for insurance cover and was sued successfully by a claimant, she would find that any assets which she owned (eg. house, car and other property) could be taken by bailiffs in satisfaction of any debt subject to the exclusion of certain statutory necessities (eg. bed and tools of her trade).

CONTRACTS WITH TRUSTS

When an independent midwife works in a hospital to take part in the delivery of her own patient, it is often customary to provide an honorary contract. An example of the content which might be included is shown in Box 23.3.

Box 23.3 Contents of an honorary contract

Names of parties

Duration of the contract

Duty of the midwife to take out indemnity insurance cover

Duty of midwife in arranging admission of patient

Procedure on arrival in hospital

Provisions for the subsequent care of the patient, covering such issues as:

- relationship between the independent midwife and the hospital midwives

- any procedures which the independent midwife may not perform in the hospital

- record keeping and documentation

▶

▶
- drugs

- equipment

- procedure following delivery

- subsequent care.

HONORARY CONTRACTS AND THE LAW

Honorary contracts have not, to the author's knowledge, been the subject of any court decision on their legality.

Contractual requirement for consideration

The honorary contract would not be considered valid as an agreement with binding contractual force unless there was an element of reciprocity. If the agreement simply said 'the independent midwife can use our facilities', what has the midwife done in return for this undertaking? An agreement where there is no consideration (i.e. some act/payment/token) is not a valid contract in law. To be binding, a promise to do/give/perform etc. where there is no consideration must be made under seal. Thus, if a wealthy grandfather were to sign a deed promising to pay money to his grandchild and it was made under seal then the grandchild could enforce the payment. Alternatively. the grandfather could promise to give money to his grandson provided 'he wore my tartan shirt once a week'. This element of reciprocity would then count as consideration and the promise could be enforced even though it were not under seal.

If it can be shown that the midwife does indeed perform some service for the trust then the honorary contract to permit her to use the premises and facilities might then be enforceable.

Accountability of the independent midwife remains

The honorary contract usually makes it clear that the independent midwife remains personally and professionally accountable for her care of the patient. However there could be considerable difficulties in determining liability.

Disputes over liability

What if the contract requires the independent midwife to use the equipment provided by the hospital, and the midwife alleges that harm occurred because this was defective? Such a claim is likely to be disputed by the hospital who might claim that any harm to the patient was entirely caused by the midwife. In addition the independent midwife will be working with a team of hospital midwives and doctors in the delivery suite and when harm occurs it is not always easy to pinpoint which person in the team caused the harm. The courts do not accept any principle of team liability and each and every member of the team is personally and professionally accountable for his/her actions.

If harm occurs where does the claimant stand?

If a mother or baby is harmed following delivery by an independent midwife in an NHS hospital working alongside NHS employees and there then follows a dispute over liability between the independent midwife and the others on the team who are employed by the trust, it is likely that the patient would bring a claim against the trust. The latter could then bring in the independent midwife as a third party and if found liable could claim an indemnity against the independent midwife. At the heart of the dispute would be the issue of causation and which of the many persons involved caused the harm and were in breach of their duty of care.

What if the independent midwife is injured?

The honorary contract should not affect the duty of care owed to the independent midwife as a visitor to the hospital. If she is injured on the premises, the same obligations would be owed to her under the Occupier's Liability Act 1957 as are owed to any other visitor. The occupier would be the NHS trust or the Primary Care Trust. It might be even be an independent contractor if the harm has occurred because of the negligence of one of its employees on site.

Would the independent midwife be regarded as an employee for the purposes of the employer's duty to care for the health and safety of his employees?

Whilst not an employee, the independent midwife is comparable to a volunteer coming onto the premises to assist in the working of the organisation. There are guidelines which suggest that volunteers should be the recipients of the same duty of care that the employer owes to his employees. Thus if the independent midwife is infected as a result of the negligence of an employee of the trust or Health Authority, she should be compensated by the employer. A duty of care would be owed to her in the law of negligence and she might be able to sue the NHS organisation for its direct responsibility in failing to take reasonable care of her safety or for its vicarious liability for the negligence of an employee. In addition under Section 3 of the Health and Safety at Work Act 1974 (see Chapter 19) an employer has a general duty to ensure the reasonable health and safety of the public at large which would include the independent midwife working in a hospital.

NO EMPLOYEE RIGHTS

The independent midwife cannot benefit from the statutory rights which the law gives to the employee (see Chapter 22). However, if she herself employs staff, she will have to ensure that she enables them to have the rights to which they are entitled.

PERSONAL LIABILITY FOR THE HEALTH AND SAFETY OF HERSELF AND OTHERS

In Chapter 19 the laws on health and safety were considered. Most of the duties under the Health and Safety at Work Act 1974 and the Regulations under it are binding on the self-employed person who employs others. The independent midwife is therefore required to ensure that she observes the Regulations. Ignorance of the law is no defence to a prosecution for breach of the regulations.

LIABILITY FOR BREACH OF CONTRACT

Box 23.4 shows some of the different parties with whom the independent midwife may contract.

Box 23.4 Contracting parties for the independent midwife

- Private patients

- NHS trusts

- Primary Care Trusts

- General Practitioners

- Private hospitals

- Agencies

- Charities and voluntary bodies

When the independent midwife agrees a contract with a client, that agreement would be subject to the same laws which bind any contract for the sale of goods and services. Should the midwife be in breach of that contract the client may be able to sue her for compensation.

If as a result of negligence the midwife causes harm to the client, unlike the NHS patient, the private patient has a remedy, not only in negligence (as the NHS patient has) but also has a remedy for breach of contract. This may not be of any significance since the contract is likely to require the same duty of care as required under the laws of negligence, however, it depends upon the nature of the alleged breach of contract.

Where a private practitioner or organisation has a contract with an NHS trust for the provision of health services the agreement for the provision of and payment for midwifery services would be enforceable in a court of law.

SUSPENSION FROM PRACTICE

Like any employed midwife the independent midwife could face suspension from practice by the Local Supervising Authority. Suspension from practice for the independent midwife means that she will immediately cease to be able to obtain income from her practice within the geographical area of that Local Supervising Authority. Where an employed midwife is suspended from practice, this would not necessarily mean that she is suspended from her contract of employment, and she may continue to receive her full pay even though she is unable to work within the geographical area of the LSA which has suspended her. Where she is suspended by the NMC, she could not of course continue to carry out those services she supplies as a registered practitioner.

CONCLUSION ON INDEPENDENT MIDWIFERY

Independent midwifery is fraught with financial and contractual problems, but it does provide, for those who can afford it, an alternative service which may meet their needs in a way in which the NHS is failing. The financial problems in obtaining reasonable insurance cover for the ever increasing value of claims following brain damage at birth is the biggest deterrent to midwives being prepared to undertake independent practice. Alice Coyle, an independent midwife interviewed in a journal[5] stated that one of the greatest pleasures of being an independent midwife, as opposed to an employed midwife was 'being in control of my clinical practice and the deep levels at which I am able to work with women.' She also stated: 'I think that it is very difficult for any midwife with a huge caseload to provide the necessary intensity of interaction with women. I cope by attending a maximum of 2-4 births a month with occasional gaps when I do other things.' Her ideal would be a central fund so that women could 'choose their care, a bit like the dreaded voucher system. This would enable women to vote with their feet, and services which weren't meeting their needs would be under-used and hopefully scrapped with popular services built on and funded properly such as caseload practices with realistic caseloads.'

It may be that the publication of the NSF for maternity and children's services (see Chapters 6 and 21) may suggest the support and positive promotion of women's choice including that of an independent midwife.

PRIVATE MATERNITY HOSPITALS

CARE STANDARDS ACT 2000

Many wealthy celebrities opt for obstetric and midwifery care outside the NHS. It has been estimated that £25,000 would in August 2001 cover the cost of a birth in a private hospital such as the Portland Hospital in London, a maternity nurse for 6 weeks, a doula for 5 hours a day for the next 3 months and a night nanny for 5 nights a week for 5 months.[6] (Doula comes from the Greek word for the most important female servant in the house. They are trained to provide practical and emotional support. A birth doula would attend labour providing support and encouragement. A post-birth doula provides general support and help for the mother.)

Private maternity homes have in the past come under the provisions of the Registered Homes Act 1984. This Act has now been repealed by the Care Standards Act 2000 which has established a new central registration body, known as the National Care Standards Commission, which is a new, independent regulatory body for social care and private and voluntary healthcare services. (The National Assembly for Wales has established a department/unit to be the regulatory body for such services in Wales.) The legislation follows a government report on the regulation of private and voluntary healthcare.[7] Under the Registered Homes Act 1984, individual Health Authorities had been the registration authorities for nursing homes and Local Authorities for residential care homes within their catchment areas. The emphasis is now on national standards set out by the Secretary of State and the National Assembly of Wales who have powers under the Act to make regulations and issue national minimum standards.

MIDWIVES IN AN INDEPENDENT HOSPITAL

The midwife may be employed to work in an independent hospital which is used in connection with maternity services so she needs to have an understanding of the registration provisions and how these affect the environment and standard of care. Of those registered in 2000 as practising midwives, 121 were practising in private institutions. 2099 were employed by a midwifery bank and 504 were employed by an agency: and some of these may work in the private sector.

Box 23.5 shows the definition of independent hospital for the purposes of the Care Standards Act 2000.

Box 23.5 Section 2 Care Standards Act 2000

(2) A hospital which is not a health service hospital is an independent hospital.

(3) 'Hospital' (except in the expression health service hospital) means

    a.   an establishment

        i. the main purpose of which is to provide medical or psychiatric treatment for illness or mental disorder or palliative care; or

        ii. in which (whether or not other services are also provided) any of the listed services are provided;

    b.   any other establishment in which treatment or nursing (or both) are provided for persons liable to be detained under the Mental Health Act 1983.

(4) 'Independent clinic' means an establishment of a prescribed kind (not being a hospital) in which services are provided by medical practitioners (whether or nor any services are also provided for the purposes of the establishment elsewhere).

But an establishment in which, or for the purposes of which, services are provided by medical practitioners in pursuance of the NHS Act 1977 is not an independent clinic.

(5) 'Independent medical agency'...

(6) ...

(7) In this section 'listed services' means:

    a.   Medical treatment under anaesthesia or sedation

    b.   Dental treatment under general anaesthesia

    c.   Obstetric services and in connection with childbirth, medical services

    d.   Termination of pregnancies

    e.   Cosmetic surgery

    f.   Treatment using prescribed techniques or prescribed technology.

These independent hospitals are regulated under the Care Standards Act 2000.

Care homes are defined as establishments providing accommodation, together with nursing or personal care for people who are or have been ill, persons who have or have had a mental disorder, persons who are disabled or infirm, persons who are or have been dependent on alcohol or drugs. However, an establishment is not a care home if it is a hospital, an independent clinic or a children's home (Section 3(3)). The old distinction in the Registered Homes Act 1984 between nursing and residential care home is thus abolished.

Most midwives working outside the NHS would be providing services in an independent hospital, but there may be some establishments providing post-convalescent nursing and personal care which would come under the definition of care home.

NATIONAL CARE STANDARDS COMMISSION

This body and its Welsh equivalent have the following functions (Section 7)

- To keep the Secretary of State informed about the provision in England of Part 2 services and in particular the availability of the provision and the quality of the services

- To encourage the improvement in the quality of Part 2 services

- To make information about Part 2 services available to the public

- To advise the Secretary of State

- To carry out functions specified in Regulations by the Secretary of State.

- To work with the Commission for Health Improvement. The CHI and the NCSC have the power to carry out each other's functions.

REGISTRATION

Box 23.6 shows a summary of the provisions of Part 2 of the Care Standards Act in so far as they are likely to affect midwifery.

Box 23.6 Provisions of Part 2 of the Care Standards Act 2000

Section 11 Requirements to register

Section 12 Application for registration

Section 13 Grant or refusal of registration

▶

Section 14 Cancellation of registration

Section 15 Application by registered persons

Section 16 Regulations about registration

Section 17 Notice of proposals

Section 18 Right to make representations

Section 19 Notice of decisions

Section 20 Urgent procedure for cancellation

Section 21 Appeals to the tribunal

Section 22 Regulations of establishments and agencies

Section 23 National minimum standards

Section 24 Offence of failure to comply with conditions

Section 25 Offence of contravention of regulations

Section 26 Offence of false descriptions of establishments and agencies

Section 27 Offence of false statements in applications

Section 28 Offence of failure to display certificate of registration

Section 29 Proceedings for offences

Section 30 Offences by bodies corporate

Section 31 Inspections by persons authorised by registration authority

Section 32 Inspections supplementary

Section 33 Annual returns

It is not the intention to go through each of these sections in detail but rather to give to the midwife who works in this area an understanding of the basic provisions and a knowledge of where she can seek further information.

It is an offence to carry on an unregistered independent hospital. Any independent hospital offering abortion facilities must obtain the prior approval of the Secretary of State under Section 1(3) of the Abortion Act 1967 (see Chapter 26).

Section 16 enables regulations to be made relating to registration. Section 22 enables the Secretary of State to make regulations which impose specific requirements on the establishment in relation to the persons who are fit to carry on or manage the establishment, the fitness of the premises, the numbers of persons working there. Under Section 23 national minimum standards can be prepared and published by the Minister. Regulations under Section 22 will give effect to these standards. Essential information required under the 1984 Regulations about the birth of a child is shown in Box 23.7.

Box 23.7 Particulars of child born

1. Details of the weight and condition of the child at birth.

2. A daily statement of the child's health.

3. If any paediatric examination is carried out involving any of the following procedures:

    a   examination for congenital abnormalities including congenital dislocation of the hip

    b. measurement of the circumference of the head of the child

    c. measurement of the length of the child

    d. screening for phenylketonuria

    details of each such examination.

BIRTH CENTRES

An example of a privately run birth centre is that of the Wessex Maternity Centre of which the parent company is Independent Maternity Centres Ltd (IMC Ltd). Kate Walmsley[8] described how it started as a pilot scheme, employing five midwives who work as autonomous practitioners in a non-hierarchical setting. It takes referrals from GPs who feel that particular women would benefit from the individualised care the midwives give. The centre provides indemnity cover for the midwives. The author, who is also a director of IMC Ltd, considers that this model of a midwifery service is one which would work well within the primary care sector.

Jilly Rosser and Tricia Anderson launched a project to encourage the establishment of small, community-based birth centres with the emphasis on normal birth.[9] Such centres could either be provided within the NHS or they could be part of the private sector but receive NHS funding like the Wessex Maternity Centre described above. (See also Chapter 24 and the midwifery management in a birth centre.)

CONCLUSION

Any midwife who works in an independent hospital or care home should make herself aware of the conditions for registration including the numbers of persons permitted to be cared for. She should ensure that she brings to the manager or the proprietor any conditions which would appear to be unacceptable in relation to both the registration of the hospital or home and also under the Code of Professional Conduct of the UKCC. The Scope of Professional Practice requires that even practitioners who are not employed as registered practitioners but who work for the personal social services departments of a Local Authority or in a care home should still be regarded as coming under the Code of Professional Conduct.

QUESTIONS AND EXERCISES

1. If you are an employed midwife, consider the advantages and disadvantages of becoming independent from the point of view of the client and from the point of view of the midwife.

2. What are the main legal differences between the situation of the employed midwife and that of the independent midwife?

3. What do you consider should be the minimum requirements of an agreement between a trust and an independent midwife for the latter to be able to deliver her clients in the trust hospital when necessary?

4. Make enquiries to ascertain the number and type of private maternity hospitals in your area and if possible obtain details of the registration provisions.

5. A client asks you for details of the differences between maternity hospitals provided within the NHS and those provided privately. Obtain the answers for her.

6. Obtain from the National Care Standards Commission (or the Welsh equivalent) a copy of the national minimum standards for private maternity homes and assess the extent to which you consider that they are in place in the organisation in which you work.

References

1 Hobbs L. 2000. *The Independent Midwife*. 2nd edition. Oxford: Books for Midwives Press

2 How to make your independent midwifery practice more business-like: key tips for lifting performance. 2000. *Communique*, 8(Autumn), 37-8

3 Hobbs L. 1993. Going Independent. *Nursing Times*, 89(20), 68-9

4 Independent Midwives Association. 1995. *Women lose their right to choose as midwives lose indemnity insurance cover*. Botley: Independent Midwives Association

5 Coyle A. 1999. Pleased to meet you. *Practising Midwife*, 2(4), 42

6 O'Driscoll E. 2001. Putting mothers and children first. *The Daily Telegraph* 17 August 2001

7 Department of Health. 1999. *Regulating Private and Voluntary Healthcare: a Consultation Document*. London: HMSO
Welsh Office. 1999. *Regulation and Inspection of Social and Healthcare Services in Wales – A Commission for Care Standards in Wales*. Cardiff: Welsh Office
Welsh Office. 1999. *Regulating Private and Voluntary Healthcare in Wales*. Cardiff: Welsh Office
Department of Health. 2000. *Regulating Private and Voluntary Healthcare: The Way Forward*. London: HMSO
Department of Health. 2001. *Regulating Private and Voluntary Healthcare: Developing The Way Forward*. London: HMSO

8 Walmsley K. 1999. The Wessex Maternity Centre. *Practising Midwife*, 2(8), 12-13

9 Rosser J and Anderson T. What next? Taking normal birth out of the labour ward. *Practising Midwife*, 3(4), 4-5

Chapter 24
MIDWIFERY MANAGEMENT

The management of a maternity department in a hospital, or a midwife-managed unit, or a community midwifery service, or a combination of all three, requires a high standard of management practice and a clear understanding of the laws which apply. In this chapter some of the specific laws which relate to management will be considered with references to chapters where some of the topics are considered in more detail.

The topics set out below will be considered:

- Delegation and supervision

- Difference between supervision as a Supervisor of Midwives (see Chapter 2) and line management supervision

- Standards of care

- Staffing levels and resource issues

- Audit and quality assurance

- Record keeping

- Employment and health and safety issues

- Primary Care Trusts and transfer of employment contracts

- Midwife-managed units.

DELEGATION AND SUPERVISION

It is the manager's responsibility to ensure that appropriate delegation and supervision is taking place in her department. A patient is entitled to the reasonable standard of care, whoever has provided that care. It is no defence to a patient to argue that harm occurred because a person of a lower grade or less experience undertook a particular activity. This means that where activities are being delegated to non-registered staff (NB attendance at a confinement cannot be so delegated), the delegator must ensure that the knowledge, experience and training of the person who is to carry out that activity is sufficient to ensure that the patient will receive a reasonable standard of care. The person delegating must also decide the level of supervision required. Initially probably a high level of close supervision will be required, but this could be reduced as confidence in the abilities of the person undertaking the activities grows. The situation should be constantly reviewed and monitored.

Where activities are safely and appropriately delegated and supervised, the manager would not be responsible if the person undertaking the activities acts negligently. Nor is there a concept of vicarious liability for the delegation of a senior to a junior. However where the delegator has delegated or supervised negligently, then there would be personal liability of the delegator, though in practice, the employer would be sued for its vicarious liability for the negligent employee.

The NHS Plan[1] envisages greater use of support staff to alleviate the chronic shortage of registered professionals across many different areas including midwifery. The use of support workers in maternity care is considered by Doug Charlton[2] who discusses the many concerns which arise including the vexed question of the supervision of support workers in the community, when they may not be under the direct supervision of the registered midwife, the education of support workers and the dangers of breaking the law relating to the attendance at childbirth of only the registered midwife, doctor or student of either. He suggests that 'the way ahead looks rocky and untried. Many of the issues raised in this article will need further debate before the profession launches headlong into accepting healthcare support workers as equal partners in maternity care.'

SUPERVISION AND LINE MANAGEMENT

There is a clear distinction between the role of the Supervisor of Midwives which is based on the statutory provisions and the role of a manager who as part of their management responsibilities has a line management responsibility. To add to the confusion sometimes the same person might hold both roles in relation to the midwife being supervised. The role of the Supervisor of Midwives is considered in Chapter 3. As a line manager, a midwife would have responsibilities to ensure that clear instructions were given over the delegation of responsibilities, that records were audited, that the employer's responsibilities to the midwife were carried out (eg. in the management of stress, see below) and in being accessible to any concerns which the midwife wishes to raise.

STANDARDS OF CARE

Whilst each individual practitioner is personally and professionally accountable for her own practice, a manager has an overall responsibility in ensuring that the unit she manages is meeting the reasonable standards of care to which the patient is entitled. Guidance published by the National Institute for Clinical Excellence, reports from the Audit Commission or from the Commission for Health Improvement, any relevant National Service Frameworks, criteria published by the Clinical Negligence Scheme for Trusts and any other information from Registration bodies or professional associations should, where appropriate, be incorporated within the standards of the department/unit (see Chapter 13). Guidance is provided by the NHS Executive on the role of the ward sister which would also apply to the midwife who is responsible for running a ward or maternity unit.[3] This guidance envisages that under the NHS Plan (see Chapter 21) senior nurses or charge nurses will have the authority and support they need to get the basics of care right. By April 2002 NHS trusts and Primary Care Trusts with wards are required to have identified matrons, each accountable for a group of wards. Supporting policies for these roles include:

- tackling standards of cleanliness

- improving the quality of hospital food

- introducing ward housekeepers

- patient forums and the Patient Advocacy and Liaison Service (PALS) (see Chapter 11 on complaints)

- ward environment budgets

- benchmarking the fundamental and essential aspects of care

- prevention and control of hospital acquired infection

- clinical leadership development

- ·the Chief Nursing Officer's ten key roles for nurses.

The implementation of the policy of hospital matrons requires the review of job descriptions and organisational structures, ensuring that adequate support is given to the ward sisters, reviewing staff establishments and skill mix, ensuring that Clinical Governance (see Chapter 21) is in place and ensuring that leadership development exists and there is investment in education and training.

STAFFING LEVELS AND RESOURCE ISSUES

The manager should be in a constant dialogue with senior management to ensure that the resources necessary to implement the identified standards are available. In addition the manager would have the responsibility of advising the trust board or employer if the level of staffing resources is such that a safe system of work cannot be guaranteed for mothers and babies. In some circumstances the scope of the service might have to be curtailed to ensure that priority was given to clinical need, in others arrangements may have to be agreed with neighbouring trusts to share workloads and staff. Failure to take such reasonable measures might if a mother or baby were harmed lead to a successful action either because of breach of the direct duty of care owed to the patient by the trust or because of its vicarious liability for negligence by an employee.

CASE LOAD

Midwives frequently ask 'what does the law say about the workload that any midwife should be undertaking?' Unfortunately laws, whether statute or case (common) law are rarely so precise as to give an answer to the question of how many clients any midwife should be responsible for. The circumstances are of course extremely wide. To compare the case load of a community midwife working in a rural area of the West Country with that of a midwife in an obstetric unit in a district hospital would be very difficult. Travelling time would not feature in the latter's working hours; it may be a significant feature in the former's. There are other differences depending upon whether the midwife in the obstetric unit would be working on the labour or antenatal wards. However even though there is no stated figure on workloads given by law, there must be an attempt at formulating what would or would not be reasonable. The mother may have to show, if she is seeking compensation for a brain-damaged baby, that there was not a reasonable number of staff allocated to her care; the midwives need to have clear evidence to place before managers if they are alleging that the lack of sufficient staff is placing patients at risk, and therefore they are in danger of breaking the Code of Professional Conduct. Particularly at this time, when there is a national shortage of midwifery staff, managers need to know what are recommended figures for staffing levels so that they can inform the trust board of the significance of the current situation.

The law requires the trust, its managers and staff to provide a reasonable standard of care for pregnant women. The National Health Service Act 1977 places a statutory duty upon the Secretary of State to provide a comprehensive service to such extent as he considers necessary to meet all reasonable requirements. The stipulated services include hospital and medical and nursing services and 'such other facilities for the care of expectant and nursing mothers and young children as he considers are appropriate as part of the health service' (see Chapter 21).

There is also a duty recognised in common law or case law for the staff of the hospital to act with reasonable care according to the standards of competent professional practice (i.e. the Bolam Test) (see Chapter 13). It is therefore no defence for a midwife to claim that she acted in error in caring for a mother because she was so pressured as a result of shortage of staff.

It could therefore be said that both statute and common law require a reasonable standard of care to be provided for the care of expectant women and their children. In addition the NMC will hold any registered midwife accountable if it can be shown that she is responsible for management failures resulting in patient harm. Thus it was reported that three midwives were cautioned by the UKCC (the predecessor of the NMC) when a baby died 10 days after birth partly as a result of inadequate staffing levels.[4]

REASONABLE WORKLOADS

How can the demands of a reasonable standard of care be translated into a reasonable workload for the midwife? Research has been undertaken in this area by Marie Washbrook and Jean Ball whose earlier research into assessing midwifery staffing requirements[5] for the Nuffield Centre for Health Services Studies and Trent Region Midwifery Manpower Project led to their textbook on the subject.[6] The book provides guidance to managers in assessing staffing required for antenatal clinic, delivery suite, hospital-based postnatal care and community care.

The Royal College of Obstetricians and Gynaecologists established a working party to identify minimum standards of care in labour.[7] The report sets out the basic standards of care required to provide a safe and pleasant childbirth experience and provides an assessment of staffing, facility and equipment levels in relation to the number and kind of deliveries. Various models for measuring workload in midwifery services have been applied including the GRASP systems workload methodology used by Hurley and Dickson in identifying staffing needs based on patient dependency levels on a labour ward.[8] The Clinical Negligence Scheme for Trusts has also given guidance on staffing figures (see Chapter 13).

Constant updating of such figures is essential to take account of new technologies,[9] new systems of working such as team midwifery,[10] how midwives work with nurses and General Practitioners[11] and the actual work that midwives undertake as shown by their diaries[12] or observation. The legal issues arising from inadequate staffing are considered by the author in an article.[13]

PERSONAL RESPONSIBILITY OF THE MIDWIFE

A midwife who believes that she is under too much pressure to provide a safe service is required by the Code of Professional Conduct to ensure that she brings this to the attention of the appropriate person. If this is not an isolated situation, then there are clear management failings in not providing a safe environment. There can be legal liability if managers, knowing that staff are suffering from stress to such extent that it amounts to a serious illness, fail to take reasonable steps to remedy the situation.[14] There would also be a duty on the manager to prevent any bullying (see Chapter 19).

AUDIT AND QUALITY ASSURANCE

The concept of Clinical Governance derives from Section 18 of the Health Act 1999 which imposes a duty of quality upon the trust board and Health Authority (see Chapter 21). This statutory duty requires the establishment of quality standards and their regular monitoring. In practice the trust board would delegate these responsibilities to the directorate managers and in turn to the departmental managers. Any manager would therefore have responsibilities in defining reasonable standards of practice and ensuring that arrangements were in place for their regular monitoring. Records should be kept of both the standards and the dates and results of the monitoring.

RECORD KEEPING

One of the main ways of ensuring that standards of records and record keeping are maintained is by carrying out regular internal audit. This could be undertaken in a non-confrontational, constructive manner within each department or ward, when a set of records are taken and then reviewed to identify the errors, omissions, ambiguities etc. (see Chapter 15) and to assess the extent to which they would be robust in defending professional practice in ten years' time in a court of law. A record could be made of the main ways in which standards could be improved and a similar audit carried out a few weeks later to see if improvements had been maintained.

EMPLOYMENT AND HEALTH AND SAFETY ISSUES

A manager has a responsibility for ensuring that the duties in the health and safety laws and employment rights are implemented on behalf of the employer. For example, if an employee is being subjected to unreasonable stress and reasonable action is not taken by the manager to secure the reasonable health and safety of the employee, then the employee may have grounds for suing for compensation (see Chapter 19). Many of the statutory duties placed upon the employer would in practice be delegated to the manager to ensure that they are implemented and that the processes are in place to ensure they are regularly implemented. Records maintained by the manager on health and safety audit, training, disciplinary action, counselling, complaints by staff would all be relevant in the event of any dispute arising. The manager would also have responsibility for ensuring that complaints were correctly recorded and the proper procedure followed in their investigation (see Chapter 11). In addition, the manager would have to ensure that the procedure drawn up by the trust under the Public Interest Disclosure Act 1998 ('whistle blowing charter') (see Chapter 22) is made known to the staff and is operating effectively.

PRIMARY CARE TRUSTS AND TRANSFER OF EMPLOYMENT CONTRACTS

As more midwives find that their contracts of employment are transferring to new Primary Care Trusts or Care Trusts, there are likely to be concerns about employment rights and the conditions of employment. The manager has a major responsibility to ensure that arrangements are made for staff to receive the appropriate advice and counselling.

MIDWIFE-MANAGED UNITS

'On the basis of what we have heard, this Committee must draw the conclusion that the policy of encouraging all women to give birth in hospitals cannot be justified on grounds of safety.'

These are the words of the Health Committee of the House of Commons which recommended that maternity services should be provided which gave women a greater choice in the maternity care which they received. At present the choice of home births or birth in small maternity units appear to be options which have been substantially withdrawn. For most women there is no choice. This does not appear to be in accordance with their wishes. In Chapter 6 we considered the implications of the House of Commons report on maternity services[15] and the Expert Committee Changing Childbirth[16] in relation to the choices that women should have. The UKCC position statement on supporting women to have a home birth is discussed in Chapter 6.

There are however considerable concerns felt by midwives about the implications of a midwife-managed service. A workshop was held to discuss the concerns of about 20 midwives who were being consulted on setting up such a unit. The unit would not have theatres or 24-hour obstetric cover and would be comparable to a domiciliary confinement. The group of midwives were asked to write down anonymously their worries and the legal implications of these were considered.

Box 24.1 illustrates the main areas which were raised.

Box 24.1 Principal areas of concern

- Risks

- Transfers from the unit to the District General Hospital

- Refusals by clients

- Indemnity/litigation/protection by management

- Prescribing, training and updating

RISKS

Risk management and assessment are considered in Chapter 19 as part of the health and safety regulations. However the same techniques can be used in planning the operational policy of a midwife-managed unit, in determining the client group and in deciding upon the equipment, supplies (drugs, blood etc.) and the staffing levels necessary to operate safely.

Box 24.2 sets out the type of risks which worried the midwives. Many of them cited the same risk.

Box 24.2 Risks mentioned by midwives

- What if a woman has a huge haemorrhage and we are unable to site an intravenous line to administer fluid and she dies? Or, in the same situation, the bleeding continues after the IV is set up? And, in the same situation, the mother is too ill to be transferred by ambulance? (Cited by many)

- What if there is a cord prolapse and the baby is stillborn? (Cited by many)

- What if something goes wrong when administering a pudendal block?

- What if an unbooked patient arrives on our doorstep, fully dilated with the baby only 28 weeks?

- What if the fetal heart is heard in second stage but the woman is delivered of a fresh stillbirth?

- What if there is retained placenta bleeding?

- What if the baby is flat at delivery and resuscitation and intubation is attempted but is unsuccessful?

- What if there is an unexpected stillbirth?

- What if the patient suddenly collapses and is too ill to be moved?

- What if the woman has a life-threatening problem such as a postpartum haemorrhage or is fitting and is too unstable to be transferred?

The risks cited are probably the same as those which would be cited by midwives who worked in a District General Hospital. The fear in a midwife-managed unit is whether there would be the resources necessary to cope and whether transfers could be effected in time. Worries over transfers are set out in Box 24.3.

Box 24.3 Fears relating to transfers

- What if the client delivers an abnormal baby who dies in transit? (The baby's abnormality might prevent our being able to resuscitate the baby.)

- What if there is a cord prolapse and the baby is lost during the transfer?

- What if the mother needs to be transferred because of postpartum haemorrhage but the District General Hospital has no empty beds and is unable to take the transfer, or harm occurs to the mother and baby whilst an empty bed is being sought?

- What if the registrar refuses to admit the mother following transfer?

- What if the mother refuses to be transferred? (Many cited this)

- What if the baby is stillborn following fetal distress during transfer?

- Is the midwife responsible for what happens in transit even after the medical staff are notified that it is taking place?

- If something goes wrong after transfer, will the medical staff blame the midwives for not acting quickly enough? If a doctor disagreed in retrospect with the midwife's decisions or some aspect of her care, after transfer to the doctor, what would the midwife's position be legally?

- What if a problem occurs during transfer by ambulance, eg. eclampsia or haemorrhage?

- If there is a GP booking and a problem occurs during labour and the GP asks us to transfer the care of the patient to a Consultant, what is the midwife's position?

- What if the baby is born in the ambulance and dies because of lack of facilities?

- What if there is no adequate 24-hour transport for emergency transfers?

- What if I am abused by the Consultant after the transfer of a baby with fetal distress and told 'I told you' so by the Consultant?

Many of the risks are foreseeable and the elimination of the risk does rely upon a high standard of screening at antenatal stage to identify those patients who should be delivered in a District General Hospital unit. However all accept that even with the most efficient screening it is possible there would still be emergency situations. Most of these concerned the possibility of unexpected haemorrhaging or prolapse of the cord. Plans can be made to deal with these emergencies. The preparations would include higher levels of training of midwives in the resuscitation of the newborn, in the siting of canulae and giving intravenous substances and in the administration of a wider range of medicines than those currently agreed.

As a result of the workshop and the identification of risks, several working parties were set up to draw up procedures, policies and preparations to meet these risks.

From the point of view of legal liability, if there is no reason discoverable at antenatal stage which suggests that the women should be delivered in a District General Hospital and if something goes wrong, provided all reasonable care is taken, all reasonable action is taken to meet reasonably foreseeable risks and the actions performed by the midwife accord with the Bolam Test[17] then there is unlikely to be a successful civil action. However, much depends upon the evidence which is given and the records of the midwife are extremely important.

TRANSFERS

The concerns expressed by midwives about problems relating to transfers are set out in Box 24.3. Much pre-planning on the transfers could allay the fears about the associated risks.

Transport services

Preparation would include the provision of ambulance transport with a paramedical team trained in obstetric emergencies, and especially equipped to cover all foreseeable emergencies. Training for midwives would have to include alertness as to when a transfer was likely to be necessary, what signs to watch for, and other indications. (However, such training is also required for domiciliary deliveries.)

Theatre services

Preparation would include the need to establish good liaison with theatre staff in the District General Hospital so that as soon as an obstetric emergency was apparent with the need to use theatres, the appropriate action could take place within the DGH to avoid delay. This would include the acceptance by DGH ward and theatre staff of instructions from the midwifery unit that an obstetric emergency was being transferred. Midwives were concerned that delays could result from red tape and requiring a particular person to permit the transfer. It was calculated that even when the confinement was taking place in the maternity unit within the DGH, there might be delay of as long as 30 minutes to prepare for a Caesarean section. Often obtaining an anaesthetist could take some time.

Liaison with obstetricians

It is essential that midwives managing a midwife unit have the cooperation and support of their obstetric colleagues and that any element of competition or conflict is removed. Some midwives feared that they would be criticised for their handling of the delivery by obstetricians in front of clients and that they would have little protection against such contempt. Every effort must be made to ensure joint planning between the professions including others such as pharmacists, physiotherapists etc. to ensure the highest standard of care for the client. Policies relating to the suitability of clients for the unit and the transfer of those at risk are essential before the unit can begin its operation.

REFUSALS BY CLIENTS

The philosophy behind the Cumberlege Report and the House of Commons Health Committee on childbirth is that the mother should have more choice and her wishes should be taken into account. This concept can however give rise to fear by midwives that the mothers might insist upon inappropriate treatment, care or place of confinement thus endangering the lives of both mother and child. Chapter 7 sets out the legal principles relating to the right of the mother to give or refuse consent. One of the hopes of a midwife-led service is that the contact between mother and midwife will be much improved with a named midwife seen regularly by the mother so that the latter develops respect for the judgement of the midwife and there is likely to be less conflict between the two. A birth plan can be agreed with the mother recognising when departure from the agreed plans are necessary.

Can the mother insist upon delivery in a midwife-managed unit even though she is assessed as being a high-risk case? The answer is no. The managers of the unit have the right to determine who will be admitted and could refuse admission to a mother who was a high risk. They could also enforce a policy that only those who have been booked into the unit by the midwives are entitled to be delivered there. This would prevent ambulances bringing inappropriate patients to the unit. The same principles would apply as those when hospitals with no accident and emergency facilities make it clear that they cannot take such cases.

Box 24.4 sets out some of the fears which result from the client refusing to follow the advice of the midwife.

Box 24.4 Client refusals

– What if a transfer were required, but the client refused to agree? (Several cited this concern)

– What if a high-risk mother came to the unit, who had not been booked in there, but who refused to be transferred to the DGH?

▶

▶
- What if the mother refuses to be transferred, and is delivered in the unit, and the baby is stillborn?

- What if during antenatal care, the mother needs to be transferred to Consultant care and she refuses?

- What if the client refuses fetal monitoring?

- What if she refuses to be transferred when there are problems in labour?

- What if a high-risk woman who is unsuitable for delivery in a midwifery-led unit insists on being delivered in the unit?

- What if a mother who requires obstetrical intervention refuses to be moved, and she and her partner want the flying squad to attend in the unit?

- What if a mother refuses syntometrine?

Since the DGH is seen as the safety net when obstetric problems occur, it is not surprising that one of the major fears of the midwives was the possibility that mothers would refuse to be transferred and would not accept the midwife's judgement that such a transfer was essential. Allied to this was the worry that some mothers would attempt to use the unit inappropriately, attempting to be delivered there even when the antenatal care had shown that they were in a high-risk category and required to be in the DGH.

INDEMNITY/LITIGATION/PROTECTION BY MANAGEMENT

Box 24.5 sets out these concerns.

There is a feeling that if the midwife follows the professional guidelines and does all she reasonably can to ensure that the mother and baby are safe, then she is entitled to receive the loyalty and protection of the management. At present we have a system of fault liability and unless the person bringing the action can show that there was fault (i.e. the defendant was in breach of the duty of care) litigation will not be successful. However this does not mean that the death or injury of a baby will not lead to litigation.

In practical legal terms, this would mean that if litigation is brought, then the midwife should be protected and indemnified by the management. This is actually what happens. Employed midwives are covered by the vicarious liability of the employer for any negligence of the midwife whilst acting in course of employment.

This means that even if a claim form initiating the legal action is issued personally against the midwife, the employer should assist the midwife in the defence and agree that if any compensation is payable then it will be the employer who pays. The Health Authorities have since 1948 accepted responsibility for the negligence of their non-medical and non-dental staff. Since January 1990 the Health Authority or NHS trust has accepted liability for doctors and dentists. This means that there is no need for the employed midwife to take out insurance cover for negligence which occurs whilst she is acting in the course of employment.

Midwives, however, would like to have this legal situation set out in writing in their contract of employment. In practice this is not necessary since it would be implied into the contract by law.

Even when there is no apparent negligence on the part of the midwife but she is facing a complaint or litigation, then she is entitled to receive the support of her employer particularly if the complaint has arisen because she is carrying out the instructions of the employer. This would mean that the NHS trust's solicitors should advise her on defending the claim, on making a statement and give her a briefing before any court hearing. The Kennedy report on the Bristol Paediatric cardiac surgery scandal (which is discussed in Chapter 21) recommends that staff should be given greater support.

Box 24.5 Concerns about indemnity/litigation etc.

– Do I have to take out medical insurance cover?

– What if parents take legal action after I have done everything which I should have done?

– Can we draw up new legal contracts to give us more cover when we do go midwifery-managed?

– What form of legal back-up would be provided by the Health Authority/trust? Would this be provided in writing to each midwife?

– What guarantees and protection would be given us by the Health Authority/NHS trust in court?

– As this is an innovative idea and one which is almost a pioneer in this country, would there be a specific, written cover for us in the event of a catastrophe, as long as we have acted according to the rules?

– If someone delivers a baby with an abnormality that could have been detected during the antenatal period with screening tests, can the family blame the midwife involved?

PRESCRIBING, TRAINING AND UPDATING

There was concern that the necessary additional training would not be given to ensure that midwives were competent for this enhanced role. There was also a fear that even if initial training were provided, there would not be an on-going commitment to ensure opportunities for regular updating. The statutory requirement for professional development to enable a midwife's name to be re-entered on the register should ensure that midwives should obtain regular professional updating and this could be built into the contract of employment.

CONCLUSIONS ON MIDWIFE-MANAGED UNITS

Any attempt to go along the path of midwife-managed units involves risks. Extensive detailed planning can eliminate most of those risks but at the end of the day there may be stillbirths and maternal deaths. These occur even when the confinement takes place in the DGH. Ultimately the decision must be given to the mother, after she has received full information, and if she meets the clinical criteria for admission. If it is clinically reasonable for a woman to be delivered at home or in a midwife-managed unit, then the choice should be there. Childbirth can be seen as a non-medical event except for those exceptional cases which require obstetric intervention. The Scope of Professional Practice of the UKCC[18] provides the principles for the professional development for the midwife to take responsibility in these units. The Cumberlege report makes clear the path which could be taken. NICE (see Chapter 21) may develop guidelines for the function of midwifery-managed services.

BIRTH CENTRES

Another variant of the midwife-managed unit which is becoming increasingly popular is a birth centre which is managed, staffed and run by midwives. They may be outside the NHS or contract with the NHS for the provision of their services (see Chapter 23), or they may be run within the NHS by an NHS trust or Primary Care Group. Details of the Edgware Birth Centre were given by Jane Walker to the All-Party Parliamentary Group on maternity at its meeting on 18th July 2001 as an example of a midwife-managed unit run by midwives and midwifery assistants funded by the NHS.[19] A comparison of its results since it opened in 1997 showed a significantly lower rate of inductions, interventions in labour, planned Caesarean sections, episiotomies and pharmacalogical analgesia than births in the local hospital. In the last 2 years, 50% of women at the Centre birthed in water compared with 2% in the UK, and 85% breast-fed.

Clearly the midwife manager of such a unit would require specific training in the necessary management skills and would also have responsibility for clarifying and enforcing the criteria for admission to ensure that only those women suitable for delivery in such a unit were admitted.[20]

CONCLUSIONS

It cannot be assumed that a midwife can become a manager without additional training. The management activities described in this chapter have serious implications for the professional accountability of the midwife manager. As in all other areas of midwifery practice, the midwife manager should ensure that she has the training, competence and experience to carry out her management functions satisfactorily. There are considerable challenges for the midwife manager including the implementation of Clinical Governance (see Chapter 21) and the increasing number of initiatives which the government is introducing to improve standards in the NHS, as set out in the NHS Plan. National Service Frameworks for midwifery services and children are to be published by 2004, with specific sections being implemented earlier. It will be the responsibility of the midwifery manager to ensure that the recommended standards are secured in their units.

QUESTIONS AND EXERCISES

1. Your NHS trust has suggested that you might like to apply for a senior midwifery management post and that you might like to write a job description for the post. How would you set about responding to this invitation? What would you put in the job description and what training would you consider was essential for such a position?

2. A midwife-managed unit is to be set up in your locality. Examine the factors which should be taken into account to ensure that risks to the mother and child are reduced to a minimum.

3. Discuss the suggestion that a specialist body of trained midwives should be capable of carrying out Caesarean operations.

4. Prepare a leaflet giving information to a client about a new midwife-managed unit which is to be established.

5. How would you distinguish between the roles of the Supervisor of Midwives (see Chapter 3) and the midwifery line manager?

References

1 Department of Health. 2000. *NHS Plan: A plan for investment, a plan for reform*. London: HMSO

2 Charlton D. 2001. Support workers in maternity care. *MIDIRS Midwifery Digest*, 11(3), 405-6

3 NHS Executive. 2001. Implementing the NHS Plan: Modern Matrons. *Health Service Circular* 2001/010

4 News item. 1998. UKCC cautions midwives. *Nursing Times*, 94(22), 11

5 Ball JA. 1992. *Birthrate: using clinical indicators to assess case mix, workload outcomes and staffing needs in intrapartum care and for predicting postnatal bed needs*. Oxford: Nuffield Centre for Health Care Studies Washbrook M. 1992. Assessing midwifery staffing requirements. *Nursing Standard*, 6(25), 39

6 Ball JA and Washbrook M. 1996. *Birthrate plus: a framework for workforce planning and decision making for midwifery services*. Oxford: Books for Midwives Press

7 Royal College of Obstetricians and Gynaecologists. 1994. *Minimum standards of care in labour*. London: RCOG

8 Hurley J and Dickson K. 1998. Assessing midwifery workload on a labour ward. *British Journal of Midwifery*, 6(7), 444-9

9 Mugford MA. 1998. Review of the economics of care for sick newborn infants. *Community Medicine*, 10(2), 99-111

10 Stock J. 1994. Continuity of care in maternity services – the implications for midwives. *Health Manpower Management*, 20(3), 30-6

11 Young D, Lees A, Twaddle S. 1997. The costs to the NHS of maternity care: midwife managed vs shared. *British Journal of Midwifery*, 5(8), 465-71

12 McCourt C. 1998. Working patterns of caseload midwives: a diary analysis. *British Journal of Midwifery*, 6(9), 580-5

13 Dimond B. 1998. Crisis in midwifery staffing: The legal aspects. *British Journal of Midwifery*, 6(12)

14 Dimond B. 1995. Stress at Work. *Modern Midwife*, 5(10), 32-4

15 1993. Second Report Session 1991-92. London: HMSO

16 Department of Health. 1993. *Changing Childbirth: Report of the Expert Maternity Group*. London: HMSO

17 This refers to the case of Bolam v. Friern Barnet Hospital Management Committee QBD 2957 2 All ER 118 where the judge applied the test of the reasonable professional acting in those same circumstances following the approved accepted practice.

18 UKCC. 1992. *The Scope of Professional Practice*. London: UKCC

19 For report of the meeting (and other meetings) contact Catherine Eden at the National Childbirth Trust 020 8992 2616; c_eden@national-childbirth-trust.co.uk

20 Rosser J. 2001. Birth Centres: the key to modernising the maternity services. *MIDIRS Midwifery Digest*, 11(s2), s22-6

SECTION E

STATUTORY PROVISIONS
AND CHILDBIRTH

This section considers certain statutory provisions which impact upon the work of the midwife. Chapter 25 sets out the legal duties placed upon midwives and others in relation to the confinement, the notification and registration of birth and the registration of death including stillbirths. Laws relating to the termination of pregnancy are then considered. The next chapter looks at the statutory provisions covering human fertilisation and embryology, followed by the provisions relating to vaccine damage compensation, infectious disease notification and the midwife's situation in relation to AIDS/HIV.

Chapter 25
CRIMINAL LAW AND CONFINEMENTS

Section 16 of the Nurses, Midwives and Health Visitors Act 1997 (re-enacting provision in the Midwives Act 1951 Section 9 and the Nurses, Midwives and Health Visitors Act 1979) made it a criminal offence for a person other than a registered midwife or a registered medical practitioner to attend at a childbirth. The Nursing and Midwifery Order[1] re-enacts this provision in Article 45. This is set out in full in Box 25.1.

Box 25.1 Criminal offence for unauthorised persons to attend at childbirth

Article 45 of the Nursing and Midwifery Order

(1) A person other than a registered midwife or registered medical practitioner shall not attend a woman in childbirth.

(2) Paragraph 1 does not apply:

  a. where the attention is given in a case of sudden or urgent necessity; or

  b. in the case of a person who, while undergoing training with a view to becoming a medical practitioner or to becoming a midwife, attends a woman in childbirth as part of a course of practical instruction in midwifery recognised by the Council or by the General Medical Council.

(3) A person who contravenes Paragraph shall be liable on summary conviction to a fine not exceeding level 5 on the standard scale.

The fact that an authorised person can be prosecuted for attending a woman in childbirth gives the midwife some powers in the situation where a husband or co-habitee or the mother herself is anxious that a midwife should not be present at the birth but that the partner should be in control. The midwife can make it clear that failure to summon the midwife in order that the partner can attend would be a criminal offence. She should report any such possibility to her Supervisor. If there are records that a written warning has been given to the couple it is less likely that a defence under Paragraph 2 would succeed.

There have been several convictions under this section. Brian Radley from Wolverhampton was charged with attending a woman in childbirth otherwise than under the direction and personal supervision of a duly qualified practitioner and was fined £100 (August 1983). If the charge were defended the midwife would of course be a key witness for the prosecution and her records would come under close scrutiny.

In October 2000 the UKCC reported that a nurse who delivered a baby despite having no midwifery qualification was found guilty of professional misconduct and removed from the UK Register. The offence took place in April 1999 when the registered nurse delivered a baby at a home in North London. It was said that she was a member of a religious group which banned members from attending hospitals or seeing midwives when they give birth. The UKCC Director of Professional Conduct stated that registered practitioners were entitled to hold strong religious beliefs and convictions. However, the nurse was not entitled to use these beliefs as a justification for breaking the law and endangering women and babies. Her belief that her religious views put her above the law meant that removing her from the Register was the only appropriate penalty to ensure the protection of the public.

REGISTRATION AND NOTIFICATION OF BIRTHS

Certain duties are placed upon the registered midwife in connection with the registration of births and stillbirths and she should therefore have a good understanding of her statutory duties in this respect. In addition she may be asked by the clients about the duties of registration, about changing the registered names or about the situation in relation to an illegitimate child. Full details are therefore given for reference. The statutory provisions governing this area are shown in Box 25.2.

Box 25.2 Statutory provisions for birth and death

Births and Deaths Registration Act 1953

Regulations of the Births, Deaths and Marriages Regulations Statutory Instrument 1968 No. 2049

Stillbirth Definition Act 1992

National Health Service Act 1977 Section 124

National Health Service (Notification of Births and Deaths) Regulations Statutory Instrument 1982 No. 286

Some of the main provisions of the 1953 Act are shown in Box 25.3.

Box 25.3 Births and Deaths Registration Act 1953

1(1)   ... the birth of every child born in England and Wales shall be registered by the registrar of births and deaths... by entering in a register kept for that sub-district such particulars concerning the birth as may be prescribed...

(2)   The following person shall be qualified to give information concerning a birth...

    a.   the father and mother of the child

    b.   the occupier of the house in which the child was to the knowledge of that occupier born

    c.   any person present at the birth

    d.   any person having charge of the child

    e.   in the case of a stillborn child found exposed, the person who found the child. (Added by Children Act 1975 Schedule 3 Para. 13(2).)

  2. In the case of every birth it shall be the duty

    a.   of the father and mother of the child; and

    b.   in the case of the death or inability of the father and mother, of each other qualified informant,

to give to the registrar, before the expiration of a period of forty-two days from the date of the birth, information of the particulars required to be registered concerning the birth, and in the presence of the registrar to sign the register:

Provided that

1. the giving of information and the signing of the register by any one qualified informant shall act as a discharge of any duty under this section of every other informant

▶

2. this section shall cease to apply if, before the expiration of the said period and before the birth has been registered, an inquest is held at which the child is found to have been stillborn

3. where any stillborn child is found exposed, it shall be the duty of the person finding the child... to give to the best of his knowledge and belief to the registrar, before the expiration of forty-two days from the date on which the child was found, such information of the particulars required to be registered concerning the birth of the child as the informant possesses, and in the presence of the registrar to sign the register.

3A.(1) Where the place and date of birth of a child who was abandoned are unknown to, and cannot be ascertained by, the person who has charge of the child, that person may apply to the Registrar General for the child's birth to be registered under this section.

The Registrar General's duties are detailed in the Act, but he shall not register a child's birth if he is satisfied that the child was not born in England or Wales, or has been adopted, or the birth is known to have been previously registered under this Act.

NOTIFICATION OF BIRTHS

There is a statutory duty on the midwife or doctor attending the woman in childbirth to give notification to the prescribed medical officer (the District Medical Officer) of the birth or stillbirth within 36 hours (Section 124 National Health Service Act 1977). The duty applies whether the birth is at home or in hospital.

REGISTRATION

There is a statutory duty placed upon certain informants for the birth to be registered with the registrar for births, marriages and deaths. Details of the duty are shown in Box 25.4.

Box 25.4 Duties of informants

Under the Births and Deaths Registration Act 1953 it is the duty of the mother or father to give information to the Registrar within 42 days of the birth or stillbirth and to sign the register. If either of them cannot, then there is a duty to do so on the occupier of the house, or any person present at the birth, or any person having charge of the child.

'House' is defined as including a public institution which covers a prison, lock-up or hospital, and such other public or charitable institution as may be prescribed. The occupier is defined in relation to a public institution as including a governor, keeper, master, matron, superintendent or other chief resident officer. The unit general manager or other person nominated by him would therefore have the responsibility for registering the birth. The nominated person might well be the midwife.

Powers of enforcement

If there is a failure to register within 42 days the Registrar can compel any qualified informant to attend to give information and sign the register. The Registrar must give 7 days notice in writing (Section 4 of 1953 Act). If the birth is registered within three months of the date of the birth, no registration fee is required.

There are additional powers if there is no registration after that date (Section 6). After twelve months since the date of the birth, the birth can only be registered with the written authority of the Registrar General. This does not apply to a stillbirth (Section 7(3)).

The Registrar shall if required by the informant give to the informant a certificate that he has registered the birth (Section 12).

Registration of the name of the child or alteration of the name (Section 13)

Where before the expiration of twelve months from the date of the birth of any child, the name by which it was registered is altered, or, if it was registered without a name, a name is given to the child, the registrar or superintendent registrar having custody of the register in which the birth was registered, upon delivery to him at any time of a certificate in the prescribed form signed:

a. if the name was altered or given in baptism, either by the person who performed the rite of baptism or by the person who has custody of the register, if any, in which the baptism is recorded, or

b. if a name has not been given to the child in baptism, by the father, mother or guardian of the child or other person procuring the name of the child to be altered or given...

shall without any erasure of the original entry, forthwith enter in the register the name mentioned in the certificate as having been given to the child, and, after stating upon the certificate the fact that the entry has been made, shall forthwith send the certificate to the Registrar General together with a certified copy of the entry of the birth with the name added under this subsection.

ILLEGITIMATE CHILDREN

Under Section 10, in the case of a child whose father and mother were not married to each other at the time of his birth, no person shall as father of the child be required to give information concerning the birth of the child, and the registrar shall not enter in the register the name of any person as father of the child unless certain specified exceptions apply. These exceptions include the joint request of the mother and the person acknowledging himself to be the father of the child (in which case that person shall sign the register together with the mother), or at the request of the mother or the putative father on production of specified declarations.

Under Section 10A where the birth of a child whose parents were not married at the time of its birth has been registered under this Act, but no person has been registered as the child's father, the registrar shall re-register the birth so as to show a person as the father at the joint request of the mother and that person; or at the request of the mother or of the putative father on production of specified documentation.

Re-registration of births of legitimated persons

Section 14 enables the Registrar General (subject to certain conditions) at any time to authorise the re-registration of a person's birth on the production of evidence which appears to him to be satisfactory that the person has become a legitimated person. Both parents must furnish the information for the re-registration.

REGISTRATION OF GENDER

The gender recorded on the birth certificate cannot be changed at the request of a person who wishes to change their sex. The Court of Appeal has held that even where a person had undergone gender reassignment surgery, the registration of the person at birth as male remained as such. This meant that the transsexual could not validly marry a man, since she was in law still male.[2]

REGISTRATION OF DEATH

If the baby is born alive and then dies, there must be a registration of both the birth and the death.

MATERNAL DEATH

In the rare event of a maternal death, the midwife should be conversant with the legal requirements for the certification and registration of the death and the requirements when the family request a cremation rather than a burial. She should also ensure that she is familiar with specific ethnic and religious requirements when appropriate.

STILLBIRTH

A stillbirth is defined as

'Where a child issues forth from its mother after the 24th week of pregnancy, and which did not at any time after being completely expelled from its mother breathe or show any signs of life'

(Section 41 of the 1953 Act as amended by Section 1 of the Stillbirth Act 1992.)

The stillbirth has to be registered as such and the informant has to deliver to the Registrar a written certificate that the child was not born alive. This must be signed by the registered medical practitioner or the registered midwife who was in attendance at the birth or who has examined the body. The certificate must state to the best of the knowledge and the belief of the person signing it, the cause of death and the estimated duration of the pregnancy (Section 11(1)(a)). Where the midwife is in sole attendance at the confinement, whether in a home or in a hospital, she must complete the certificate.

Alternatively a declaration in the prescribed form giving the reasons for the absence of a certificate and that the child was not born alive could be made (Section 11(1)(b)).

A stillbirth should be disposed of by burial in a burial ground or church yard or by cremation at an authorised crematorium.

The midwife must inform the Supervisor of Midwives of any maternal death, stillbirth or neonatal death occurring when she is the midwife responsible for the care of that mother and her baby (Midwife's Code of Practice Paragraph 39)[3]

Further guidance on her statutory duties is given in Paragraphs 44-50 of the Code of Practice.

A Health Authority should not dispose of a stillbirth without the consent of the parents. In October 1993 the manager at the Bishop Auckland General Hospital, Co. Durham, admitted causing distress to Tracey Turner for burying her stillborn baby without her permission. It was stated that there would be an investigation into how the mistake occurred.[4] (See below on the disposal of fetus and organs after post-mortems.)

Fetus of less than 24 weeks

If the fetus was delivered without any signs of life, then no registration is necessary. The fetus may be disposed of without formality in any way which does not constitute a nuisance or an affront to public decency. If the fetus shows signs of life and then dies, it would have to be treated as both a birth and a death.

Midwives should be sensitive to the fact that parents may suffer the same feelings of bereavement whatever the period of gestation and should therefore arrange for counselling and support as they would if the baby were full term.

The Human Fertilisation and Embryology Act 1990 Section 37 changed the law relating to abortion. It substituted a new section for the Abortion Act 1967 and apart from some exceptional circumstances the rule now is that the pregnancy must not have exceeded its 24th week and that the continuance of the pregnancy would involve a risk greater than if the pregnancy were terminated to the physical or mental health of the pregnant woman or any existing children of her family (see Chapter 26). However a stillbirth was defined as one where the pregnancy had lasted 28 weeks or more. This anomaly has now been redressed by the Stillbirth (Definition) Act 1992.

Live birth followed by death
A fetus of 24 weeks or more gestation which is born alive but subsequently dies is not a stillbirth but must be registered as a birth and a death.

An abortion after 24 weeks
What happens in the very exceptional circumstances when an abortion takes place after 24 weeks' gestation?

This is possible (under the amendments to the Abortion Act 1967 by the Human Fertilisation and Embryology Act 1990) in the circumstances set out in Chapter 26.

How is the length of gestation determined?
The midwife or doctor have to use their professional judgement in determining whether the fetus comes within the provisions of the stillbirth regulations. If the fetus is considered to be less than 24 weeks the parents could still arrange a ceremony and formal disposal of the body if they so wish.

Should the fetus survive a termination, every reasonable care should be taken of him (see Chapter 17).

Other implications of the Act
The change of time for the definition of stillbirth also affects the right of the mother to maternity allowances. The meaning of confinement for the purposes of benefits under the Social Security and Benefits Act 1992 will cover confinements of 24 or more weeks rather than 28 weeks (see Chapter 12).

OFFENCES UNDER THE 1953 ACT

Sections 35 to 38 create certain offences in relation to registration. These are shown in Box 25.5.

Box 25.5 Offences in relation to registration

Section 35 Offences in relation to failure by the registrar to register or in carelessly losing or injuring the register

Section 36 Penalties for failure to give information

Section 37 Penalty for forging or falsifying any certificate, declaration or order under the Act or knowingly using or giving, sending as genuine any false or forged certificate, document etc.

Section 38 Gives the power to the superintendent registrar to prosecute any person for an offence under this Act.

POST-MORTEMS AND INQUESTS

POST-MORTEM REQUESTED BY THE HOSPITAL

Post-mortem consent forms have to be signed by one of the parents where a post-mortem has been requested. They have the right of refusal and the post-mortem cannot be carried out against their wishes unless the case has been referred to the coroner who has the right to order a post-mortem.

Under Section 2(2) of the Human Tissue Act a post-mortem must be carried out by or under the instructions of a fully registered medical practitioner and must have the authority of the person lawfully in possession of the body.

CORONER'S POST-MORTEM AND INQUEST

Relatives cannot refuse to give consent where the coroner requires a post-mortem to be carried out in order to fulfil his statutory provisions. Special provisions in the Human Tissue Act 1961 and under the Coroners Rules apply. Section 1(5) of the Human Tissue Act 1961 states that

'Where a person has reason to believe that an inquest may be required to be held on any body or that a post-mortem examination of any body may be required by the coroner, he shall not, except with the consent of the coroner:

a. give an authority under this section in respect of the body, or

b. act on such an authority given by any other person.'

The Coroner's Rules require material removed from the body to be preserved for such period as the coroner thinks fit.[5]

Where death occurs in a hospital in circumstances where the patient is suffering from a condition which could lead to death if monitoring and treatment is omitted, then the coroner is required to hold an inquest unless he/she can say there are no grounds for suspecting that the omission was an effective cause of death. This was the ruling in a case[6] where a woman gave birth to twins by Caesarean section at 10.25pm on 6th February 1999. Her blood pressure was normal post-delivery but was not monitored between that time and 1.35am on 7th February 1999. It was then checked and discovered to be raised and treatment began. She suffered a left-sided intracerebral haemorrhage at 5.15am and died on 15th February 1999. The coroner accepted that the failure to monitor her blood pressure post-delivery was wholly inadequate but held that it was not a case in which the defects and human fault complained of rendered the death unnatural, and refused to hold an inquest. The High Court held that an inquest should be held unless there are no grounds for suspecting that the omission of monitoring and treatment was an effective cause of death. The Court of Appeal dismissed the coroner's appeal, since there was material evidence available to the coroner upon which he could not properly decide otherwise than that there was reasonable cause to suspect that her death was

a. at the least contributed to by neglect, and was thus

b. unnatural.

Stillbirth and the coroner

If it is found that the body was that of a stillborn child there can be no complete inquest since there has been no independent life and therefore no subsequent death. Accordingly in such cases the inquisition should be marked 'stillbirth' and not completed. It is usual for the coroner to fill in Part Three of the certificate for disposal after an inquest which relates to a stillbirth.

REMOVAL, RETENTION AND STORAGE OF ORGANS, BODY PARTS AND TISSUE

The Human Tissue Act does not explicitly permit the removal and retention of tissues, but it has been interpreted as implying that 'authorization of a post-mortem examination can be taken to include authorization for the removal and retention of some tissue'.[7]

The Department of Health and Social Security provided a 'Post-Mortem Declaration Form' to ensure that inquiries of relatives were made not only as to any relevant objection to the post-mortem examination itself, but also to the removal and retention of tissue.[8] The Royal College of Pathologists has issued a consensus statement on the use of human tissue in research, education and quality control[9] and also guidelines for the retention of tissues and organs at post-mortem examination.[10] In October 2000 the British Medical Association issued advice to its members that relatives should give informed consent to the retention of organs. It should also be made clear that relatives can refuse consent to a post-mortem examination, unless it has been ordered by a coroner.[11] In the 6th Annual Report of CESDI,[12] Appendix 4 gives guidance on fetal and infant post-mortems.

Following an outcry by parents about organs from their dead children having been removed and retained without their explicit consent, an Inquiry was set up to look at the removal, retention and storage of body parts at Alderhey Children's Hospital. The Report of the Royal Liverpool's Children's Inquiry (chaired by Michael Redfern QC)[13] on the retention of organs and body parts was published on 30th January 2001. Its publication coincided with three other publications:

- A report of a Census of Organs and Tissues Retained by Pathology Services in England carried out by the Chief Medical Officer[14]

- The Removal, Retention and use of Human Organs and Tissue from Post-Mortem Examination Advice from the Chief Medical Officer[15]

- Consent to Organ and Tissue Retention at Post-Mortem Examination and Disposal of Human Materials.[16]

The Inquiry found that thousands of children's body parts had been collected at the hospital, some going back to before 1973. Most however were retained after 1988 when Professor Richard Van Velzen was appointed to the Department of Pathology and there was a huge increase in the number of organs removed and retained. Between 1988 and the end of 1995 it was the practice to remove every organ from every child in a post-mortem.

RETAINED ORGANS COMMISSION

In response to the Redfern Report, the Secretary of State has set up a Retained Organs Commission under the Chairmanship of Professor Margaret Brazier. It is a special Health Authority with the following functions:

- Oversee the return of tissues and organs from collections around the country

- Ensure that collections are accurately catalogued

- Provide information on collections throughout the country

- Ensure that suitable counselling is available

- Act as an advocate for parents if problems arise

- Advise on good practice in this area

- Handle inquiries from families and the public.

In addition it advises Ministers, provides guidance to the NHS and universities, and monitors trusts to ensure that they deal properly with organ returns. It also provides a national help-line via NHS Direct for parents and relatives.

It is clear that at present parents do not always appreciate that by signing a consent form to a post-mortem they may be implicitly authorising doctors to remove and to retain children's organs. The law covering this area is the Human Tissue Act 1961. Section 1(1) covers the situation where a person wishes to donate their organs after death. Section 1(2) covers the situation where there has been no specific consent by the deceased but:

'the person lawfully in possession of the body of a deceased person may authorise the removal of any part from the body for use for the said purposes (i.e. therapeutic purposes, or the purposes of medical education or research) if, having made such reasonable enquiry as may be practicable, he has no reason to believe:

a. that the deceased had expressed an objection to his body being so dealt with after his death and had not withdrawn it; or

b. that the surviving spouse or any surviving relative of the deceased objects to the body being so dealt with.'

Section 1(4A) provides special provisions for the removal of an eye.

Future changes to the law on organ/body part removal and retention
The government's intention is to bring in legal changes to amend the Human Tissue Act, to make it an explicit requirement that the informed consent of the parents or relatives must be obtained for the post-mortem to be carried out and for the removal and retention of organs or tissues. The possibility of creating a criminal offence for failure to obey the laws is also being considered.

Disposal of fetal material following a termination is considered in Chapter 26.

CONCLUSION

The midwife should find that within the medical records department or general office of the trust, expertise is available to assist her on the forms which have to be completed and the notifications which must be carried out on a stillbirth, birth or death. She must ensure that the guidance relating to obtaining consent from parents before a hospital (as opposed to a coroner's) post-mortem is carried out and that the parents are notified and agree to any retention and storage of organs. Following the work of the Retained Organs Commission, there is likely to be further guidance in this area.

QUESTIONS AND EXERCISES

1. You are asked to prepare a booklet for your clients on information which they would require to have in the event of a stillbirth. What topics would you include?

2. A client who has a miscarriage at 15 weeks has asked you if she could have a service and burial. What is the legal situation?

3. You are involved in caring for a client, when the child is born alive but dies within minutes of delivery. What is the legal situation?

4. A pathologist in your hospital is undertaking research into neonatal deaths and has asked you to obtain the consent of the relevant mothers for a post-mortem to be undertaken. What laws apply and what procedures should be followed?

References

1 Nursing and Midwifery Order 2001 SI 2002 No 253

2 B v. B (validity for marriage: transsexual) [2001] EWCA Civ 1140; The Times August 15 2001

3 UKCC. 1998. *Midwives Rules and Code of Practice.* London: UKCC

4 *The Times*, 11 October 1993

5 Coroners Rules 1984 SI 1984 No 552 Rule 9

6 Her Majesty's Coroner for Inner London North ex parte Peter Francis v. Touche Lloyds Rep Med [2001] 327

7 Kennedy I and Grubb A. 2000. Medical Law. 3rd edition. London: Butterworths

8 Department of Health Post-Mortem Declaration Forms. *Health Service Circular* (77) 28

9 Royal College of Pathologists, Institute of Bio-Medical Science. 1999. *Consensus statement of recommended policies for uses of human tissue in research, education and quality control. With notes reflecting UK law and practices prepared by a working party of the Royal College of Pathologists and the Institute of Bio-medical Science.* London: RCPath

10 Royal College of Pathologists. 2000. *Guidelines for the retention of tissues and organs at post-mortem examination.* London: RCPath

11 British Medical Association. 2000. *Consent to organ retention.* London: BMA

12 Confidential Enquiry into Stillbirths and Deaths in Infancy. 1999. *6th Annual Report 1996-7.* London: Maternal and Child Health Research Consortium

13 Department of Health. 2001. *The Royal Liverpool's Children's Inquiry Report.* London: HMSO

14 Chief Medical Officer. 2001. A report of a Census of Organs and Tissues Retained by Pathology Services in England. London: HMSO

15 Department of Health. 2001. *The Removal, Retention and Use of Human Organs and Tissue from Post-Mortem Examination: Advice from the Chief Medical Officer.* London: HMSO

16 Department of Health. 2001. *Consent to organ and tissue retention at post-mortem examination and disposal of human materials.* London: HMSO

Chapter 26

TERMINATION OF PREGNANCY

In 2000, terminations of pregnancy accounted for approximately 20% of all conceptions, with a total of 175,139 abortions being performed on residents of England and Wales. The highest number of abortions (48%) are performed on women aged 20-29.[1]

ABORTION AND THE CRIMINAL LAW

The Abortion Act 1967, as amended by the Human Fertilisation and Embryology Act 1990 (see Box 26.1) provides a statutory defence to certain offences under the Offences Against The Person Act 1861 and the Infant Life Preservation Act 1929. To bring about the death of a fetus, either intentionally or as a result of gross negligence, is unlawful under Sections 58 and 59 of the Offences Against The Person Act 1861, unless the Abortion Act applies. The Infant Life Preservation Act 1929 makes it a criminal offence to destroy the life of a child capable of being born alive (see below). However the Abortion Act 1967 Section 5(1) makes it clear that 'no offence under the Infant Life (Preservation) Act shall be committed by a registered medical practitioner who terminates a pregnancy in accordance with the provisions of this Act'. (For further discussion on the rights of the fetus see Chapter 17.)

To avail oneself of the defence under the Abortion Act 1967 it must be shown that the requirements set out in Section 1 were present (see Box 26.1). It would be a question of fact and evidence as to whether this situation existed.

Box 26.1 Abortion Act 1967 (as amended by the Human Fertilisation and Embryology Act 1990)

1(1)   Subject to the provisions of this section, a person shall not be guilty of an offence under the law relating to abortion when a pregnancy is terminated by a registered medical practitioner, if two registered medical practitioners are of the opinion formed in good faith:

     a.   that the pregnancy has not exceed its twenty-fourth week and that the continuance of the pregnancy would involve risk, greater than if the pregnancy were terminated, of injury to the physical or mental health of the pregnant woman or any existing children of her family; or

b. that the termination is necessary to prevent grave permanent injury to the physical or mental health of the pregnant woman; or

c. that the continuance of the pregnancy would involve risk to the life of the pregnant woman, greater that if the pregnancy were terminated; or

d. that there is substantial risk that if the child were born it would suffer from such physical or mental abnormalities as to be seriously handicapped.

1(2) In determining whether the continuance of a pregnancy would involve such risk of injury to health as is mentioned in paragraph (a) or (b) of subsection (1) of this section, account may be taken of the pregnant woman's actual or reasonably foreseeable environment.

1(3) Except as provided by subsection (4) of this section, any treatment for the termination of pregnancy must be carried out in a hospital vested in the Minister of Health or the Secretary of State under the National Health Service Acts, or in a place for the time being approved for the purposes of this section by the said Minister or the Secretary of State.

a. The power under subsection (3) of this section to approve a place includes power, in relation to treatment consisting primarily in the use of such medicines as may be specified in the approval and carried out in such manner as may be so specified, to approve a class of places.

1(4) Subsection (3) of this section, and so much of subsection (1) as relates to the opinion of two registered medical practitioners, shall not apply to the termination of a pregnancy by a registered medical practitioner in a case where he is of the opinion, formed in good faith, that the termination is immediately necessary to save the life or to prevent grave permanent injury to the physical or mental health of the pregnant woman.

The Human Fertilisation and Embryology Act 1990 added a further amendment to the Abortion Act 1967 to cover the situation where one or more fetus(es) in a multiple pregnancy is terminated. The termination may be justified either to protect the health or life of the mother or where there is a substantial risk that if the child were born it would suffer from such physical or mental abnormalities as to be seriously handicapped (i.e. Section 1(1)(d)).

EMERGENCY SITUATION

In an emergency situation Section 1(1) does not apply, where a registered medical practitioner is of the opinion, formed in good faith, that the termination is immediately necessary to save the life or to prevent grave permanent injury to the physical or mental health of the pregnant woman (Section 1(4)) (see Box 26.1). Where an emergency situation as defined in this Section exists, the termination would not have to take place in an NHS hospital or one approved for the purposes of the Act by the Secretary of State. (See Sections 1(3) and 1(4)). Section 1(4) could also cover the situation where a surgeon who had no reasonable cause to believe that a woman was pregnant had no option but to continue with an operation even though this might result in a termination of pregnancy if the life of the mother was to be saved.

CAPABLE OF BEING BORN ALIVE AND THE INFANT LIFE PRESERVATION ACT 1929

Prior to the amendments to the Abortion Act 1967 (which came into force on 1st April 1991) it was an offence to terminate a pregnancy where the fetus was capable of being born alive. In the case of C v. S[2] it was argued by the father, who was trying to stop the termination taking place, that a doctor who attempted to terminate a pregnancy of 18 weeks would be committing an offence under the Infant Life Preservation Act 1929, since the fetus was capable of being born alive. The Court of Appeal held that there was no evidence that the fetus was capable of breathing and so was not a child capable of being born alive. The termination would not therefore be an offence under the 1929 Act. In a case in 1991[3] a claim was made by a woman who had a spina bifida baby against the Health Authority on the grounds that the defect could have been found on a scan and therefore she could have had a termination. The claim was lost because the defendants claimed that at 26 weeks the fetus was capable of being born alive and therefore termination would have been an offence under the 1929 Act. The law has now been changed.

The amendments to the Abortion Act 1967 (effected by the Human Fertilisation and Embryology Act) make it clear that

'no offence under the Infant Life (Preservation) Act shall be committed by a registered medical practitioner who terminates a pregnancy in accordance with the provisions of this Act.' (Section 5(1) Abortion Act 1967 as amended)

Viability of the fetus and the capacity to be born alive are not now concerns in the lawful termination of a pregnancy.

ABORTION RESULTING IN A LIVE BIRTH

As can be seen from Box 26.1 there can be an abortion after 24 weeks where the conditions set out in Section 1(1) b, c and d are present. Section 5(1) enables an abortion to be carried out at a later stage of pregnancy even though the child is capable of being born alive, providing that the conditions set out in Section 1 are met. However if following a lawful abortion the child were to be born alive, there is no right to kill the child. If the child were to be considerably disabled with a very poor prognosis, there is no duty to keep the child alive against all the odds (see Chapter 9). However, where the child is capable of surviving with a reasonable quality of life, there would be a duty of care to ensure that every reasonable means were taken to do so.

There are now very few abortions which take place after 24 weeks' gestation.

TERMINATION BY A REGISTERED MEDICAL PRACTITIONER

The Act requires a termination of pregnancy to be carried out by a registered medical practitioner.

The Royal College of Nursing challenged the lawfulness of the use of prostagladins to terminate a pregnancy, since the patient was cared for by nursing staff and therefore the termination was not being carried out by a registered medical practitioner. In a majority decision, the House of Lords[4] held that when prostaglandins are used to terminate a pregnancy, the termination is lawful provided that it is under the control of a registered medical practitioner. Lord Diplock stated the position as follows:

In the context of the Act what was required was that a registered medical practitioner – a doctor – should accept responsibility for all stages of the treatment for the termination of the pregnancy. The particular method to be used should be decided by the doctor in charge of that treatment; he should carry out any physical acts, forming part of the treatment, that in accordance with accepted medical practice were done only by qualified medical practitioners, and should give specific instructions as to the carrying out of such parts of the treatment as in accordance with accepted medical practice were carried out by nurses or other hospital staff without medical qualifications. To each of them the doctor or his substitute should be available to be consulted or called in for assistance from beginning to end of the treatment. In other words, the doctor need not do everything with his own hands; the subsection's requirements were satisfied when the treatment was one prescribed by a registered medical practitioner carried out in accordance with his directions and of which he remained in charge throughout.

Midwives might sometimes be asked to take part in prostaglandins abortions but they would be entitled to rely upon the right of conscientious refusal (see below).

PROVISIONS RELATING TO NOTIFICATION

The Secretary of State in respect of England and Wales, and the Secretary of State in respect of Scotland, is empowered to make regulations to provide:

a. for requiring any such opinion as is referred to in section 1 of this Act to be certified by the practitioners or practitioner concerned in such form and at such time as may be prescribed by the regulations, and for requiring the preservation and disposal of certificates made for the purposes of the regulations

b. for requiring any registered medical practitioner who terminates a pregnancy to give notice of the termination and such other information relating to the termination as may be so prescribed

c. for prohibiting the disclosure, except to such persons or for such purposes as may be so prescribed, of notices given or information furnished pursuant to the regulations.

2(2)   The information furnished in pursuance of regulations made by virtue of paragraph (b) of subsection (1) of this section shall be notified solely to the Chief Medical Officer of the Department of Health, or of the Welsh Office, or of the Scottish Home and Health Department.

2(3)   Any person who wilfully contravenes or wilfully fails to comply with requirements of regulations under subsection (1) of this section shall be liable on summary conviction to a fine not exceeding level 5 on the standard scale.

2(4)   Any statutory instrument made by virtue of this section shall be subject to annulment in pursuance of a resolution of either House of Parliament.

The Abortion Regulations 1991[5] cover

– the Certificate of Opinion

– the Notice of Termination of Pregnancy and information relating to the termination

– restrictions on disclosure of information.

CONSCIENTIOUS OBJECTION TO ABORTIONS

A statutory defence is given by the law to a person who refuses to take part in abortions under Section 4 of the Abortion Act. Section 4(1) of the Abortion Act 1967 permits conscientious objection to participation in treatment and is set out in Box 26.2.

Midwifery is about preparation for, and care during and after, birth. It is not surprising therefore that some midwives should consider that they have no part to play in the termination of pregnancy. However methods of termination such as the use of prostaglandins rely on the discharge of the fetus through the birth canal as in normal labour. Midwives may therefore sometimes be asked to assist or even take responsibility for the abortion under the supervision of the registered medical practitioner.

Box 26.2 Section 4 Abortion Act 1967

4(1)   Subject to subsection (2) of this section, no person shall be under any duty, whether by contract or by any statutory or other legal requirement, to participate in any treatment authorised by this Act to which he has a conscientious objection;

Provided that in any legal proceedings the burden of proof of conscientious objection shall rest on the person claiming to rely on it.

4(2)   Nothing in subsection (1) of this section shall effect any duty to participate in treatment which is necessary to save the life or to prevent grave permanent injury to the physical or mental health of a pregnant woman.

(A conscientious objection provision similar to Section 4 of the Abortion Act is provided by Section 38 of the Human Fertilisation and Embryology Act 1990 which is discussed in Chapter 27.)

MEANING AND EVIDENCE OF CONSCIENTIOUS OBJECTION

It can be seen from Box 26.2 that the burden would be on the midwife to prove that she had a conscientious objection. How does she do that? What is the meaning of conscientious objection? There is no statutory definition. Subsection 4(3) provides that in Scotland it is sufficient for a person to make a statement on oath, that she has a conscientious objection to participating in any treatment under the Act and that is then sufficient evidence to discharge the burden of proof. That subsection does not apply however in England and Wales.

It would clearly have to be a settled view based perhaps on religious grounds or some other evidence of a belief against abortion. There has been no judicial decision on the definition of the objection but there has on the extent of the defence.

Extent of the defence of conscientious objection
In the case of Janaway v. Salford AHA,[6] Mrs Janaway was a devout Roman Catholic

who was a secretary employed by the Health Authority. She refused to type abortion referral letters and was dismissed. She applied to the Industrial Tribunal claiming the dismissal was unfair in that she was protected from having to participate in such activities by reason of her conscientious objection and the defence under Section 4(1) of the Abortion Act 1967. The House of Lords held that she was fairly dismissed since the protection of Section 4(1) did not extend to typing letters. 'Participate' actually meant taking part in treatment designed to terminate a pregnancy.

This means that whilst the midwife would be protected by Section 4(1) in her refusal to take part in the abortion treatment, she could not refuse to give advice to clients about abortion facilities, amniocentesis and other information which may lead to an abortion taking place.

This clearly places the midwife who has a conscientious objection to abortion in a difficult position. If during antenatal care, for example, a mother became aware of a possible genetical abnormality in her child and the appropriate advice would be to inform her about the possibility and need for an amniocentesis, a midwife would have a duty of care to ensure that the mother received this information, which might result in an abortion taking place, even though the midwife conscientiously objected to abortions for whatever reason.

The implications are two fold:

– either the midwife refuses to give the advice in which case she faces the possibility of being disciplined and even dismissed. The midwife's refusal may also be contrary to the human rights of the woman as set out in the European Convention of Human Rights and enacted in the Human Rights Act 1998 (see Chapter 6 and Appendix 1 of this book); or

– the midwife gives the client the information, against her own principles and beliefs.

A possible compromise solution is for another midwife to take over the responsibility for the antenatal care at that stage, but this would be contrary to the philosophy of the Cumberlege Report, Changing Childbirth,[7] and the continuity of care provided by the named midwife. In addition it is recognised by the European Community Midwives Direction that included within the activities of a midwife are those shown in Box 26.3.

Box 26.3 Definition of a midwife in European Directive[8]

Member states shall ensure that midwives are at least entitled to take up and pursue the following activities:

22.1 To provide sound family planning information and advice.

The activity shown in Box 26.3 might include advice on contraception, including the post-coital pill, and the midwife could not claim protection from carrying out that task. It must not of course be assumed that because the midwife had a strongly held personal view against abortion, she would not be capable of giving impartial sound comprehensive advice. Unpublished research has shown that there was no difference in the uptake of serum screening for risk estimation of Down's Syndrome of women in the second trimester, between patients counselled by midwives who held a conscientious objection to abortions and those counselled by midwives who did not object to abortions, provided that there was adherence to a protocol.[9]

CONSCIENTIOUS OBJECTIONS AND AN EMERGENCY SITUATION

The right to refuse to participate given by Section 4(1) does not apply in the circumstances set out in Section 4(2) which are shown in Box 26.4.

Box 26.4 Section 4(2) Abortion Act 1967

Nothing in subsection (1) of this section shall effect any duty to participate in treatment which is necessary to save the life or to prevent grave permanent injury to the physical or mental health of a pregnant woman.

Where life is at stake or the possibility of grave permanent injury is present, the duty of care to the mother takes precedence over any conscientious objection held by the midwife.

CONSCIENTIOUS OBJECTION AND THE UKCC CODE OF PROFESSIONAL CONDUCT

Clause 8 of the revised Code of Professional Conduct[10] is set out in Box 26.5.

Box 26.5 Clause 8 Code of Professional Conduct

Report to an appropriate person or authority, at the earliest possible time, any conscientious objection which may be relevant to your professional practice.

To comply with the requirement shown in Box 26.5 the midwife would obviously have to declare her conscientious objections at the time of the interview for a post.

She may therefore face discrimination against her appointment, because of the possibility of the midwife having to give advice during the antenatal stage as discussed above. In this controversial area where the midwife might not wish to be involved in abortions, whether through the actual activity or in giving advice, there are two rights which have to be balanced: on the one hand, the right of the woman to make available to herself the opportunities provided within the law to have an abortion and the necessary information; on the other hand, the right of the midwife to be entitled to work within her principles and beliefs. Section 4(1) provides a compromise but inevitably it will not always satisfy both sides.

Should the midwife be asked for advice about procuring an abortion, she should make sure that the questioner is referred to the correct authority and should be very careful about giving any advice which could assist a person in carrying out an unlawful termination of pregnancy. To do so would be a criminal offence under the Offences Against The Person Act 1861.

POST-COITAL PILL AND THE INTRAUTERINE DEVICE

There has been some controversy over whether the above forms of family planning are properly regarded as contraception or abortion. They both aim at preventing the fertilised egg being implanted in the womb. In the case of R v. Price[11] a doctor was charged and convicted under Section 58 of the Offences Against The Person Act 1861 after fitting a woman with an intrauterine device. His conviction was quashed in the Court of Appeal. Crucial to his defence was the fact that he believed the woman not to be pregnant at the time, i.e. he was preventing an implantation not assisting a termination. The Medical Protection Society[12] cited four cases in 1983 which were referred to the Director of Public Prosecutions to consider criminal proceedings (2 were referred by LIFE) on grounds that the post-coital pill is procuring a miscarriage and that the requirements of the Abortion Act 1967 were not met and therefore there should be a prosecution under the Offences Against The Person Act 1861. In a written Parliamentary Reply the Attorney General announced that no proceedings would be taken.[13] The provisions of the Offences Against The Person Act 1861 Section 58 make it an offence for any woman being with child to unlawfully administer to herself any poison or noxious thing with intent to procure her miscarriage. Section 59 covers the situation of the supply or procurement whether or not she be with child. The Attorney General took the view that the word 'miscarriage' in its ordinary meaning is not apt to describe a failure to implant, whether spontaneous or not, and that it refers to a later stage of antenatal development than implantation and also that the phrase 'Procure a miscarriage' cannot be construed to include the prevention of implantation.

In a more recent case,[14] an anti-abortion group won an application to the High Court to proceed with a case to stop the supply of over-the-counter sales of the morning-after pill to women over 16 years. The drug Levonelle-2 had formerly only been available on prescription, but in January 2001 its classification was changed to enable it to be sold by pharmacists. The barrister representing the Council for the Society of the Protection of Unborn Children argued that the change of classification permitted the commission of a criminal offence – the administration or supply of poisons or instruments with the intent to procure a miscarriage under the Offences Against The Person Act 1861. The judge decided that an important issue of public policy arose which should be heard in the civil courts.

Securing a miscarriage through the use of menstrual extraction either mechanically or by induction through a drug such as mifepristone would have to be performed in compliance with the requirements of the Abortion Act 1967. Section 1(3) of the Abortion Act 1967 was amended by the Human Fertilisation and Embryology Act 1990 to give the Secretary of State power to approve centres where such treatment may be carried out (Section 1(3A)) (see Box 26.1).

OPPOSITION TO ABORTIONS

In the case C v. S discussed above, the father was not married to the mother. In an earlier case a husband, Mr Paton, tried to prevent his wife obtaining a termination.[15] He failed on the grounds that provided the requirements of the Abortion Act 1967 were satisfied the termination was lawful and the husband had no locus standi to bring an action to prevent a lawful termination proceeding.

Mr Paton then took the case to the European Commission of Human Rights in Strasbourg[16] claiming that as a result of Article 8 of the European Convention of Human Rights which gave a right to respect for family life (see Chapter 6 and Appendix 1 of this book) he had a right to stop the termination going ahead. He lost on the grounds that the Commissioner held the rights of the mother were protected under Paragraph 2 of Article 8.

In a more recent Scottish case, a father separated from his wife, attempted to prevent an abortion taking place in the name of the child.[17] The court held that there was in law no justification for recognising the rights of the unborn child against the mother's right to lawfully terminate the pregnancy. The legal status of the unborn child is considered in Chapter 17. In cases where the mother is refusing a Caesarean section which is vital to the survival of the fetus, the Court of Appeal has refused to accept the view that the unborn child has rights which are enforceable against the mother[18] (see Chapter 7).

In the Case Re P 1982,[19] parents opposed the abortion wanted by their daughter and offered to bring up the child. The judge decided that the abortion was in the best interests of the girl. For further discussion of this case see Chapter 7.

RIGHT TO SECURE A TERMINATION

There appears to be considerable variation across the country in the availability of NHS facilities for termination of pregnancy. An audit carried out by the Royal College of Obstetricians and Gynaecologists in 2001 found that 34% of abortion services failed to meet minimum targets for acceptable waiting periods. The RCOG guidelines suggest that a woman seeking a termination should see a gynaecologist within five days and that the procedure should take place within a week. The conclusion of the report was that some parts of the country appear to be providing a good service, although not always within the NHS.[20]

DISPOSAL OF FETAL TISSUE FROM TERMINATION

The Department of Health and the Welsh Office (WHC(91)96)[21] have issued a circular requiring Health Authorities to ensure that full account should be taken of any personal wishes that have been requested about the disposal of fetuses and fetal tissue. Unless there are other requirements, the material should be incinerated. The disposal is subject to the guidance on the handling and disposal of clinical waste. Maceration and sluicing as a method of disposal should be phased out. Compliance with this requirement by an approved place will be necessary for continued approval under the Abortion Act 1967.

ORGAN REMOVAL, RETENTION AND STORAGE

An Inquiry was held into organ removal, retention and storage at Alderhey Hospital.[22] Following the report the government set up a Retained Organ Commission under the chairmanship of Professor Margaret Brazier and made recommendations on improving standards in relation to obtaining the informed consent of parents to the removal and use of organs and other body parts and tissue. These recommendations should improve practice in relation to consent for the disposal or use of aborted fetuses. (See Chapter 25 on organ removal, retention and storage.)

CONFIDENTIALITY OF RECORDS RELATING TO ABORTION

The question arose in a recent criminal case over the disclosure of documents relating to abortions.[23]

The defendants jointly organised and participated in a protest outside a clinic run by the British Pregnancy Advice Service at which abortions were regularly performed. The protesters prevented patients and staff from leaving the clinic and failed to comply with police requests to leave the scene. Twenty-six people were arrested and charged under Section 5(1)(a) of the Public Order Act 1986 which makes it an offence to use threatening, abusive, or insulting words of behaviour... within the hearing or sight of a person likely to be caused harassment, alarm or distress thereby.

They were convicted and in their appeal claimed amongst other points that the Crown Court had erred in setting aside a witness summons served on an officer of the British Pregnancy Advice Centre which would have required him to produce all records relating to abortions which had taken place or were to have taken place at the clinic on the day of the protest. They also claimed that they believed illegal abortions were about to be performed at the clinic on the day of the protest and therefore they were protected by the Criminal Law Act 1967 in that they were using such force as is reasonable in the prevention of a crime. Neither of these grounds of appeal succeeded.

The Court of Appeal referred to the specific provisions of the Abortion Act 1967 and the 1968 Regulations which ensured the maintenance of a high degree of confidentiality in respect of documents relating to abortions carried out under the Act. The documents were not relevant to the defence raised by the defendants. The 1991 regulations, though they came into effect after the case, continued to emphasise the confidentiality of the records.

Nor did the defendants come within the protection of the Criminal Law Act 1967, since their actions were aggressive and prevented other people from exercising their legal rights and did not distinguish between legal and illegal abortions.

CONCLUSIONS

The changes effected in the Abortion Act 1967 by the Human Fertilisation and Embryology Act 1990 have enabled terminations of pregnancies to take place at a much later date than the previous laws, since the time limit of 24 weeks only applies to the first condition for termination. However in practice there are very few terminations after 24 weeks. In practice too, the method of ending a late gestation usually ensures the death of the fetus in the womb so that a living child is not the result of the termination. There will always be continual pressure for legislative change in this emotive area since the pro-life groups will continue to press for the criminalising of termination of pregnancy. There are also likely to be concerns over the availability of terminations within the NHS and guidance may be issued by NICE.

QUESTIONS AND EXERCISES

1. A mother with four children (the last one only twelve months old) tells you that she is pregnant and probably over 24 weeks. She is anxious to obtain an abortion. What is the legal position?

2. You have been asked to assist in the gynaecology ward in the termination of pregnancies. You are not happy taking part in this work, since you wished to work only as a midwife. What is your legal position and what assistance does the law and the Code of Professional Conduct give you?

3. A client tells you that her 14-year-old daughter is pregnant but wants to have an abortion. The client wishes to bring up the child herself and prevent the daughter having a termination. What is the legal position? (See Chapter 7.)

References

1 www.statistics.gov.uk

2 C v. S [1988] 1 All ER 1230

3 Rance v. Mid-Downs HA [1991] 1 All ER 801

4 Royal College of Nursing of the UK v. Department of Health and Social Security [1981] AC 800; [1981] 1 All ER 545

5 The Abortion Regulations 1991 Statutory Instrument 1991 No 499

6 Janaway v. Salford [1988] 3 All ER 1051

7 Department of Health. 1993. Changing Childbirth: Report of Expert Maternity Group. London: HMSO

8 European Community Midwives Directive 80/155 EEC Article 4 quoted in the Midwives Code of Practice paragraph 2.2

9 Jones G and Dawson A. 1992. University Hospital of Wales. (I am indebted to Gill Jones for this personal communication)

10 UKCC. 1992. Code of Professional Conduct. London: UKCC

11 R v. Price [1969] 1 QB 541

12 Medical Protection Society. 1983. Annual Report, page 18

13 House of Commons May 1983 42 Parl Deb HC 238

14 Gibb F. High Court Challenge to morning-after pill. *The Times*, 3 May 2001

15 Paton v. Trustees of the British Pregnancy Advisory Service [1978] 2 All ER 987

16 Paton v. United Kingdom [1980] 3 EHRR 408 (EcomHR)

17 Kelly v. Kelly [1997] SLT 896

18 St George's Healthcare NHS trust v. S; R. v. Collins ex parte S [1998] 44 BLMR 160

19 Re P (a minor) [1982] 80 Local Government Reports 301

20 Templeton A. 2001. *Audit of abortion services.* London: Royal College of Obstetricians and Gynaecologists

21 The Department of Health and the Welsh Office (WHC(91)96)

22 Department of Health. 2001. *The Royal Liverpool's Children's Inquiry Report.* London: HMSO

23 Morrow and others v. Director of Public Prosecutions High Court of Justice QBD [1993] 14 BMLR 54 (reported in Medical Law Review 1994 99)

Chapter 27

LEGAL ISSUES RELATING TO FERTILISATION, EMBRYOLOGY AND GENETICS

Estimates are given that at least one in ten couples are affected at some stage in their lives by infertility problems. The midwife is therefore quite likely to have clients who as a result of problems in conception and fertility may be involved with in vitro fertilisation (IVF) and/or surrogacy. This chapter considers the legal issues which arise and the framework which has been established by statute. It also considers recent developments in genetics and the legal implications.

HUMAN EMBRYOS AND IN VITRO FERTILISATION

The present law dates from the Warnock report which was published in 1984.[1] Many of its recommendations were subsequently incorporated into the Human Fertilisation and Embryology Act 1990. The Act covers the topics shown in Box 27.1.

Box 27.1 The Human Fertilisation and Embryology Act 1990

1. Establishes a statutory authority

2. Prohibits specific activities in connection with embryos and gametes

3. Enables licences to be issued by the authority

4. Defines mother and father

5. Regulates disclosure of information and confidentiality

6. Amends the Surrogacy Arrangements Act 1985

7. Amends the Abortion Act 1967 (see chapter 26)

8. Provides a defence of a conscientious objection

▶ 9. Gives powers of enforcement and creates offences

10. Makes provision in relation to the giving and withdrawal of consent.

HUMAN FERTILISATION AND EMBRYOLOGY AUTHORITY (HFEA)

This Authority is appointed by the Secretary of State as a statutory non-crown body. The Secretary of State also appoints the chairman and deputy chairman. Registered medical practitioners, those concerned with the keeping or using of gametes or embryos outside the body and any person concerned with commissioning or funding research are ineligible to be appointed as chairman or deputy chairman.

The functions of the HFEA are shown in Box 27.2.

Box 27.2 Functions of HFEA

1. Keep under review information about embryos and advise the Secretary of State

2. Publicise the services provided to the public by the Authority

3. Provide advice and information for person to whom licences apply or who are receiving treatment

4. Grant, vary, suspend and revoke licences through licence committees

5. Issue directions either generally or specifically

6. Maintain a code of practice giving guidance about the conduct of activities and treatment services

7. Maintain a register containing specified information.

UNAUTHORISED ACTIVITIES

The Act regulates activities in respect of embryos (i.e. a live human embryo where fertilisation is complete and an egg in the process of fertilisation) outside the human body and gametes (eggs or sperm). The activities shown in Box 27.3 and Box 27.4 are prohibited.

Box 27.3 Prohibited activities in relation to embryos

S.3(1) No person shall

a. bring about the creation of an embryo, or

b. keep or use an embryo,

except in pursuance of a licence.

S.3(2) No person shall place in a woman

a. a live embryo other than a human embryo, or

b. any live gametes other than human gametes.

S.3(3) A licence cannot authorise

a. keeping or using an embryo after the appearance of the primitive streak (i.e. not later than the end of 14 days beginning with the day when the gametes are mixed)

b. placing an embryo in any animal

c. keeping or using an embryo in any circumstances in which regulations prohibit its keeping or use, or

d. replacing a nucleus of a cell of an embryo with a nucleus taken from a cell of any person, embryo or subsequent development of an embryo.

In 1994 an amendment[2] was made to the 1990 Act which came into force on 10th April 1995. This added Section 3A to the Act:

'No person, shall, for the purpose of providing fertility services for any woman, use female germ cells taken or derived from an embryo or a fetus or use embryos created by using such cells.'

As a result of this Section it is a criminal offence to use fetal eggs or embryos derived therefrom in medically assisted reproduction. The statutory definition of female germ cells is 'cells of the female germ line and includes such cells at any stage of maturity including eggs'.

Box 27.4 Prohibited activities in relation to gametes

S.4(1)   No person shall

    a.   store any gametes, or

    b.   during treatment services, use the sperm of any man unless the services are being provided for the woman and the man together, or use the eggs of any other woman, or

    c.   mix gametes with the live gametes of any animal,

    except in pursuance of a licence.

S.4(2)   A licence cannot authorise storing or using gametes in any circumstances in which regulations prohibit their storage or use.

S.4(3)   No person shall place sperm and eggs in a woman in any circumstances specified in the regulations except in pursuance of a licence.

GRANTING OF LICENCES

The Authority can grant licences

– authorising activities in the course of providing treatment services

– authorising the storage of gametes and embryos

– authorising activities for the purpose of a project of research.

Conditions for the giving of licences are laid down in Sections 12, 13, 14 and 15 and Schedule 2. Sections 16-22 cover the granting, revocation and suspension of licences.

DEFINITION OF MOTHER AND FATHER

The definition of mother for the purposes of the Act is shown in Box 27.5 and the definition of father in Box 27.6.

Box 27.5 Definition of mother

S.27(1) The woman who is carrying or has carried a child as a result of the placing in her of an embryo or of sperm and eggs, and no other woman, is to be treated as the mother of the child.

▶ (This does not apply to adoption but applies whether the woman was in the UK ·or elsewhere at the time of the placing in her of an embryo or the sperm and eggs.)

Box 27.6 Definition of father

S.28(1) Where a child is being or has been carried by a woman as the result of the placing in her of any embryo or of sperm and eggs or her artificial insemination; if

a. at the time of the placing in her of the embryo or the sperm and eggs or of her insemination, the woman was a party to a marriage, and

b. the creation of the embryo carried by her was not brought about with the sperm of the other party to the marriage

the other party to the marriage shall be treated as the father of the child unless it is shown that he did not consent to the placing in her of the embryo or the sperm and eggs or to her insemination.

If the treatment services were provided for her and a man together, by a person to whom a licence applies, then he shall be treated as the father of the child.

Where the sperm of a man is given for the treatment of others under Paragraph 5 of Schedule 3, or the sperm of a man or any embryo created from his sperm is used after his death, he is not to be treated as the father of the child.

Under Section 30 the courts can make orders providing for a child to be treated in law as the child of the parties to the marriage in certain circumstances. Regulations under this Section apply certain provisions of the Adoption Act 1976 to parental orders under Section 30 of the 1990 Act.[3]

DISCLOSURE OF INFORMATION AND CONFIDENTIALITY

Section 33 prohibits any member or employee of a licensing authority disclosing information which is contained in the register so that an individual can be identified. However, the consent of the person(s) protected by these confidentiality provisions can release the person from the prohibition.

The Human Fertilisation and Embryology (Disclosure of Information) Act 1992 was passed to enable additional exceptions to the duty of confidentiality to be recognised. The bar on a doctor passing information direct to the patient's GP has ended. The 1992 Act enables the patient to give consent to disclosure to a specified person or to give general consent to disclosure within a wider circle of people where disclosure is necessary in connection with medical treatment, clinical audit or accounts audit. Before consent is given, reasonable steps must be taken to explain the implications of giving consent to the patient. Disclosure of information is also permissible in an emergency where the person disclosing is satisfied that the disclosure is necessary to avert imminent danger to the health of the patient and at the time it is not reasonably practicable to obtain the patient's consent. The clinician can also disclose information to his legal adviser where necessary for the purposes preliminary to or in connection with legal proceedings. The 1992 Act allows access to records of treatment to be given to personal representatives and those bringing litigation on behalf of the incapacitated patient.

Power is given for new regulations relating to additional exceptions to the principle of confidentiality to be made if necessary.

Disclosure in the interests of justice can be made under section 34 in proceedings before a court when the question of whether a person is or is not the parent of the child by virtue of the act falls to be determined.

Under the Congenital Disabilities (Civil Liability) Act 1976, the court can make an application to the Authority authorising it to disclose information kept in the register and relevant to the issue of parentage (see Chapter 17 on the 1976 Act).

SURROGACY

The Surrogacy Arrangements Act 1985 is amended and a new section 1A provided (see below).

ABORTION ACT 1967

Major amendments are made to the Abortion Act 1967 and these are discussed in Chapter 26.

CONSCIENTIOUS OBJECTION

Section 38 provides a similar provision to that contained in the Abortion Act 1967 to protect any person who has a conscientious objection to working in the field. Its provision is shown in Box 27.7. There is no statutory definition of what constitutes a conscientious objection and a similar interpretation of the clause in the Abortion Act 1967 can be expected. This did not protect a secretary who refused to type correspondence relating to abortions (see Chapter 26).

Box 27.7 Conscientious objection: Section 38

S.38(1) No person who has a conscientious objection to participating in any activity governed by this Act shall be under any duty, however arising, to do so.

S.38(2) In any legal proceedings the burden of proof of conscientious objection shall rest on the person claiming to rely on it.

ENFORCEMENT PROVISIONS AND OFFENCES

Any member or employee of the Authority on entering and inspecting premises has the right to:

– take possession of anything which he has reasonable grounds to believe may be required

– take steps to preserve anything or prevent interference with anything, and

– can obtain from a JP, if there are reasonable grounds for suspecting that an offence under this Act is being (or has been) committed, a warrant to enter premises, using such force as is necessary and to search premises.

Offences include:

– undertaking activities prohibited by Section 3(2) or 4(1)(c) without a licence or doing anything which cannot be authorised by a licence

– Providing false or misleading information for the purposes of a licence

– Disclosing information in contravention of the Act.

The consent of the Director of Public Prosecutions is required before proceedings can be commenced.

CONSENT TO TREATMENT

The principles of law relating to the giving of consent are covered in Chapter 7. The 1990 Act makes very detailed provisions relating to the giving and use of gametes and embryos and the Act requires counselling to be given before consent is obtained.

Schedule 3 covers the consent to the use of gametes or embryos. Consent has to be given in writing and effective consent means consent which has not been withdrawn.

The provisions of the Schedule are set out in Box 27.8.

Box 27.8 Consent provisions

A. Consent to the use of an embryo must specify one or more of the following purposes:

   i. use in providing treatment services to the person giving consent, or that person and another specified person together

   ii. use in providing treatment services to persons not including the person giving consent, or

   iii. use for the purposes of any project of research,

   and may specify conditions subject to which the embryo may be so used.

B. A consent to the storage of any gametes or embryos must:

   i. specify the maximum period of storage (if less than the statutory storage period), and

   ii. state what is to be done with the gametes or embryo if the person who gave the consent dies or is unable because of incapacity to vary the terms of the consent or to revoke it, and may specify conditions subject to which the gametes or embryo may remain in storage.

C. Other matters to be included in the consent can be specified by the Authority.

D. Procedure for giving consent:

   Before a person gives consent under this Schedule

   i. he must be given a suitable opportunity to receive proper counselling about the implications of taking the proposed steps, and

   ii. he must be provided with such relevant information as is proper

   iii. he must be informed of his right to withdraw consent or vary it at any time by notice given by the person who gave the consent to the person keeping the gametes or embryo to which the consent is relevant.

The terms of any consent to the use of any embryo cannot be varied, and such consent cannot be withdrawn, once the embryo has been used:

– in providing treatment services, or

– for the purposes of any project of research.

Use of gametes for the treatment of others
A person's gametes must not be used for the purposes of treatment services unless there is an effective consent by that person to their being so used and they are used in accordance with the terms of the consent.

A person's gametes must not be received for use for those purposes unless there is an effective consent by that person to their being so used. This does not apply to the use of a person's gametes for that person, or that person and another together, receiving treatment services.

In vitro fertilisation and subsequent use of embryo
A person's gametes must not be used to bring about creation of any embryo in vitro unless there is an effective consent by that person to any embryo the creation of which may be brought about with the use of those gametes being used for one or more of the purposes mentioned in paragraph 2(1) above.

Each person whose gametes were used for IVF must give an effective consent before the embryo can be received (see the case of Diane Blood below).

Embryos obtained by lavage
An embryo taken from a woman must not be used for any purpose unless there is an effective consent by her to the use of the embryo for that purpose and it is used in accordance with that consent.

Storage of gametes and embryos
There must be an effective consent by the person whose gametes are to be stored and storage must be in accordance with their consent.

The case of Diane Blood[4] illustrates how tight the rules on consent to the use of gametes are.

Box 27.9 No written consent: The use of sperm from a dead husband

Mr and Mrs Blood had been married for 3 years and were intending to start a family when Mr Blood contracted meningitis and went into a coma. Mrs Blood asked for sperm to be taken from her husband and he died shortly afterwards. She then applied to the Human Fertilisation and Embryology Authority for the sperm to be used for her artificial insemination. The Authority refused on the

▶

▶ grounds that the written consent of the donor was required under Section 4(1) and Schedule 3 of the Act. Her application to the High Court for judicial review failed and she appealed to the Court of Appeal. It held that the Act clearly required the written consent of the donor to storage of the sperm and the court could not give consent to her being treated. It held however that HFEA has not lawfully exercised its discretion under Sections 23 and 24 to allow export and Mrs Blood would be able to seek treatment abroad.

It was subsequently made known that she had given birth to a child following successful insemination with her husband's sperm abroad. In 2002 it was reported that she was expecting a second child conceived by using her dead husband's sperm.

Following the Blood case, the government set up a review of the law under the Chairmanship of Professor Sheila McLean and a report was published in 1998.[5] The report recommended that in exceptional circumstances the removal of gametes from an unconscious person if that were in the best interests of that person should be permitted. It also suggested that the 1990 Act should be amended to remove the need for written consent from the donor for storage. In August 2000 the government published its response to the McLean Report.[6] It accepted all the recommendations of the report and went further, suggesting a retrospective effect:

– The father's name should be allowed to appear on birth certificates where his sperm has been used after his death.

– The legal position on consent and removal of gametes should remain unchanged: gametes can be taken from an incapacitated person who is likely to recover, if the removal of gametes is in their best interests.

– The HFEA should have the power to permit the storage of gametes where consent has not been given, so long as the gametes have been lawfully removed. This will also benefit children who are about to undergo treatment which will affect their future fertility. (Legislation will be required to implement this.)

– Families will be able to make these birth certificate changes retrospectively.

– The best practice is for written consent to be obtained, since this most clearly constitutes effective consent. Where there is doubt over whether an effective consent has been obtained, this should be a matter for the courts.

Legislation to implement these changes is awaited.

CODE OF PRACTICE

The HFEA has published and amended a Code of Practice which licensed centres must follow. This covers such topics as the decisions over which persons can obtain IVF treatment.

ACCESS TO FERTILITY SERVICES

There is no legislation which gives a statutory right to access fertility services within the NHS. There are cases outside the NHS where unlikely persons have been given facility services. For example a French woman aged 62 was reported as receiving IVF treatment in America with an egg donated by another woman but fertilised by the French woman's brother.[7] It was reported[8] in 1991 that doctors in Johannesburg announced the successful delivery by Caesarean section of the first baby (a girl – 9lb 6oz) born to a human male. A fertilised egg was implanted within the man's abdominal cavity where it attached to the abdominal wall, developed a placenta and grew to maturity. Sperm and ova were taken from the couple. The wife, who had a five-year-old child, could not have a second child safely. The man received female hormonal injections throughout the pregnancy and went for regular check-ups.[9] Such events give rise to considerable debate or controversy. It was reported in 2001 that a French woman treated in a London clinic received an embryo created from a donor egg from a younger woman and her brother's sperm. The HFEA is reported to have stated that treating the woman did not contravene British guidelines.[10] There is no enforceable statutory right for an individual to be given IVF treatment and the Code of Practice gives advice to the Licensed Centres on which persons to treat.

There is a statutory duty to

'take account of the welfare of any child who may be born as a result of the treatment (including the need of that child for a father), and of any other child who may be affected by the birth' (1990 Act Section 13(5))

before a woman is provided with treatment services. In one case this Section was applied to a woman who had a criminal record including offences for prostitution.[11]

In the following case the woman, aged 37 years, brought an action because she had been turned down by the Health Authority when she sought IVF treatment.

Box 27.10 Refusal to provide IVF treatment[12]

The applicant was 37, and was refused IVF treatment by the Health Authority as 35 had been set as the upper limit for such treatment. The judge held that her application for judicial review of this decision must be refused. There was no law to prevent the Health Authority setting limits for its financial expenditure.

Since 2nd October 2000 and the coming into force of the Human Rights Act 1998 an application could be made under Article 8 of the European Convention (see Chapter 6 and Appendix 1), which gives a right to respect for private and family life. However, this argument failed when a prisoner sought the right of access to artificial insemination facilities for the purpose of inseminating his wife whilst he was in prison.[13] The Court of Appeal dismissed the prisoner's appeal saying that the refusal to agree to the request was not breach of the Convention, nor unlawful nor irrational.[14]

At the present time there is considerable variation across England: 28 out of 100 Health Authorities provide some form of free treatment, but 20 of these prohibit women over 35 receiving fertility treatment; only 21 treat women over the age of 38 years. In December 2000 the Government announced that it was asking the National Institute for Clinical Excellence (NICE) to draw up guidelines on access to fertility services within the NHS[15] (see Chapter 21). These guidelines will set the maximum age of women and the number of treatments they can have on the NHS as well as the methods and drugs which should be available.

SURROGACY

Surrogacy is the use of another person for the production of a child. The surrogate mother might have no genetic link with the child she carries, if an embryo is implanted in her. Or she may herself provide the egg and be inseminated with donor sperm or the sperm of the husband of the couple wishing to have the child. Until the passing of the Surrogacy Arrangements Act 1985 the only law which related to a surrogacy situation was Section 50 of the Adoption Act 1958 which prohibits any payment in connection with adoption. The application of this section to a surrogacy situation arose in the case Re A.[16]

Box 27.11 Re A (1987)[16]

In this case Mr and Mrs A were unable to have children and because of their age had been refused as adoptive parents. They entered into surrogacy arrangements with Mrs B. It was agreed that she would be paid £10,000 to give up her job and have the child. Eventually she accepted £5,000 which did not cover her financial losses. The couple applied to adopt the baby. The judge held that a payment to a mother in a surrogacy arrangement did not contravene the Adoption Act if payments made by those others to the natural mother did not include an element of profit or financial reward. Even if they were made for reward, the court had a discretion under the Act to authorise the payments retrospectively. The court granted the adoption order.

The public disquiet over the actions of commercial companies led to the passing of the 1985 Act.

SURROGACY ARRANGEMENTS ACT 1985

This defines 'surrogate mother' as:

'a woman who carries a child in pursuance of an arrangement

    a.   made before she began to carry the child, and

    b.   made with a view to any child carried in pursuance of it being handed over to, and the parental rights being exercised (so far as is practicable) by, another person or other persons'

Section 1(6) as amended by the 1990 Act states:

'a woman who carries a child is to be treated for the purposes of subsection (2)(a) above as beginning to carry it at the time of the insemination, or of the placing in her of an embryo, of an egg in the process of fertilisation or of sperm and eggs, as the case may be, that results in her carrying the child.'

The legal definition of a surrogacy arrangement in the Act is Section 1(3):

'An arrangement if, were a woman to whom the arrangement relates to carry a child in pursuance of it, she would be a surrogate mother.'

The Act prohibits the making of surrogacy arrangements on a commercial basis. No person on a commercial basis can

    a.   initiate or take part in any negotiations with a view to the making of a surrogacy arrangement,

    b.   offer or agree to negotiate the making of a surrogacy arrangement, or

    c.   compile any information with a view to its use in making, or negotiating the making of, surrogacy arrangement, and

    d.   no person shall in the UK knowingly cause another to do any of those acts on a commercial basis.

Commercial is defined in Section 2(3) in relation to the receipt of payment for oneself or another but payment does not include payment to or for the benefit of a surrogate mother or prospective surrogate mother. Offences are also introduced in relation to advertising of surrogacy arrangements (Section 3).

The Warnock Committee recommended that such any surrogacy arrangements, whether on a profit-making basis or not, should be enforceable. This was enacted by Section 36 of the Human Fertilisation and Embryology Act 1990. This adds a new Section 1A to the 1985 Act as follows:

'No surrogacy arrangement is enforceable by or against any of the persons making it.'

The effect of this Section is that if the surrogate mother were to refuse to hand over the baby following the birth, the couple who made the arrangements could not enforce the agreement in court.

If a midwife is told that one of her clients has entered into a surrogacy agreement and is pregnant as a result of this, she should ensure that her duty to the mother and the child comes before the interests of any person on whose account the mother is bearing the child. She should ensure that she is aware of the legal position and that her Supervisor is informed of the situation.

In 1997, the government set up a committee to review surrogacy arrangements in the UK under the chairmanship of Professor Margaret Brazier. Its report[17] recommended that the Surrogacy Arrangements Act 1985 and Section 30 of the 1990 Act (see above) should be replaced by new legislation. A Code of Practice on surrogacy should be drawn up by the Department of Health. At the time of writing legislation is awaited.

A recent Court of Appeal case has held that a woman is not entitled to the costs of making a surrogacy arrangement when she had been negligently deprived of the prospect of conceiving and bearing a child naturally.[18] The case is discussed in Chapter 16.

USE OF OVARIAN TISSUE IN EMBRYO RESEARCH AND ASSISTED CONCEPTION

Public concern was raised in 1993 at reports that cells from expelled fetuses were being used in the course of in vitro fertilisation. The Human Fertilisation and Embryology Authority produced a consultation document in January 1994, Donated Ovarian Tissue in Embryo Research and Assisted Conception. The document considered the social and ethical issues which arose from using ovarian tissue obtained from mature women, cadaveric tissue or aborted fetuses. There is a shortage of donated eggs, and the use of tissue from a wider field which could assist in conception would go far in meeting the shortage. The Ethics Committee of the Royal College of Midwives stated that:

– There should be increased public awareness of the need for donated eggs.

– Ovarian tissue could be used in research or for the treatment of infertility subject to a Code of Practice (such as that drawn up by the Polkinghorne Report on the use of fetus and fetal tissue) and subject to the consent of the woman.

– The use of eggs or ovarian tissue from cadavers or fetuses should only be permitted for research into genetic diseases and should not be permitted for research into infertility or for the treatment of infertility.

– The use of ovarian tissue from live donors should continue to be subject to the Code of Practice of the Polkinghorne Report.

– Eggs or ovarian tissue from cadavers or fetuses should not be used in treatment.

– Legislation should be provided to enforce these recommendations.

EMBRYO RESEARCH

The Human Genetics Advisory Commission and the Human Fertilisation and Embryology Authority published a report on Cloning Issues in Reproduction, Science and Medicine in 1998[19] and concluded that the 1990 Act had proved effective in dealing with new developments relating to human cloning. The Report recommended that:

1. The government might wish to consider the possibility of introducing legislation that would effectively ban human reproductive cloning regardless of the technique used, so that the full ban would not depend upon the decision of the Human Fertilisation and Embryology Authority (HFEA) but would be enshrined in statute.

2. The Secretary of State should consider specifying in regulations two further purposes for which HFEA might issue licences for research, so that potential benefits can clearly be explored:

   a. the development of methods of therapy for mitochondrial disease, and

   b. the development of therapeutic treatments for diseased or damaged tissues or organs.

3. Because of the pace of scientific advances in the area of human genetics, the issues are examined again in five years' time in the light of developments and public attitudes towards them.

The government in its response to the report took the view that the 1990 Act was effective in preventing all forms of human cloning[20] and supported the recommendations of HFEA and HGAC and announced the creation of an Advisory

Group under the Chief Medical Officer to examine further the potential benefits, risks and alternatives to therapeutic cloning.

The Chief Medical Officer's Expert Advisory Group on Therapeutic Cloning

The Group[21] concluded that:

– stem cells have enormous potential as a source of new tissue for therapeutic use

– the research was warranted across a range of sources of stem cells, including embryos created by in vitro fertilisation or cell nuclear replacement

– the existing statutory framework of the 1990 Act would provide the necessary safeguards for this new research.

The Advisory Group also recommended that:

'Research Councils fund research into stem cells, including alternative sources of stem cells, and to establish collections of embryonic stem cells to minimise the need for the use of embryos in this research and for the importation of stem cell lines.'

The recommendations of this group closely reflected the conclusions of the HFEA/HGAC report. The government responded to the Expert Advisory Group by accepting all its recommendations and undertaking to introduce the necessary regulations. The government emphasised that it would unequivocally ban reproductive cloning by the cell nuclear replacement technique.

NEW REGULATIONS

In December 2000 and January 2001, the House of Commons and the House of Lords passed secondary legislation legalising research on the stem cells of embryos. There was an emotional and heated debate in both Houses.[22] The Statutory Instrument[23] specifies the additional purposes for which the Human Fertilisation and Embryology Authority (HFEA) may grant licences for research involving embryos under the 1990 Act for the purposes of increasing knowledge about the development of embryos or about serious disease, and enabling such knowledge to be applied. This research will be subject to the overriding control and monitoring of the HFEA. The HFEA will have to ensure that there has been explicit consent from individuals whose eggs or sperm are used to create embryos which are subsequently used in research to derive stem cells.

In a report to the House of Lords Scientific Committee which investigated stem cell research, the Royal Society has recommended that there should be a world ban on human cloning.[24] The House of Lords Committee reported in February 2002 and stated that stem cell research using embryos should be permitted subject to strict guidelines. Within a few days of the House of Lords report licences were issued by HFEA for research to be carried out. A decision by the Court of Appeal overruled an earlier High Court decision and held that cell nuclear replacement organism was an embryo for the purposes of the 1990 Act and therefore were subject to the control of HFEA.[25]

Egg freezing

In its Annual Report for 2000, the HFEA stated that carefully controlled use of frozen eggs in fertility treatment can be allowed, but clinics, who must be licensed to offer this treatment, must inform patients of any risks involved and also give clear information about the success rate, which is currently very low. The HFEA has produced a patient leaflet about this procedure.

Egg sharing

This is an arrangement whereby a woman may receive free or subsidised IVF treatment in return for donating her surplus eggs. HFEA has agreed that this practice can take place but only on condition that strict guidelines issued by HFEA were followed to protect all those involved in such arrangements.

Preimplantation Genetic Diagnosis (PGD)

PGD is a technique which is used to detect whether an embryo created in vitro is carrying a genetic defect which will give rise to a serious inherited genetic disorder. HFEA and the Advisory Committee on Genetic Testing (ACGT) (now absorbed into the Human Genetics Commission) issued a consultation paper at the end of 1999 and are at the time of writing preparing recommendations in the light of the response. Licences have been issued in 2002 by HFEA for genetic screening and IVF treatment to take place to ensure that an embryo was a compatible donor for a sibling who suffered from a genetic disorder. In one case the sibling suffered from a rare blood disorder which could be treated by a suitable bone marrow transplant.[26]

GENE THERAPY

Concern relating to experimentation with genes which would not be covered by the Human Fertilisation and Embryology Act 1990 (except in so far as it prevented research taking place on embryos after the appearance of the primitive streak or 14th day after mixing) led the government to establish a non-statutory body, the Committee on the Ethics of Gene Therapy, chaired by Sir Cecil Clothier, in November 1989. Its terms of reference were to draw up ethical guidance for the medical profession on treatment of genetic disorders in adults and children by genetic modification of human body cells, to invite and consider proposals from doctors wishing to use such treatment on individual patients, and to provide advice to UK Health Ministers on scientific and medical developments which bear on the safety and efficacy of human gene modification. The Committee reported in January 1992 and its recommendations are shown in Box 27.9.

Box 27.9 Recommendations of the Clothier Committee on the Ethics of Gene Therapy

1. Research should continue but a distinction should be drawn between:

    a. Germ line gene therapy which affects future generations – gene modification of the human gene line should not be done

    b. Somatic cell gene therapy which is concerned only with that person

        i.   should be subject to the requirements for other human research

        ii. should initially be for life-threatening diseases or those which cause serious handicap and for which treatment is at present unavailable or unsatisfactory

        iii. should not yet be used for non-disease situations.

2. There should be a new expert/supervisory body to provide scientific and medical advice on matters germane to the safety and efficacy of human gene modification and its use.

3. The approval of local research ethics committees to research projects should be conditional on the approval of the proposed supervisory body. Arrangements for the working of the advisory body and its co-ordination with LRECs should be made speedily.

4. The attention of the Advisory Committee on Gene Manipulation should be drawn to this report.

5. There should be an effective means of control and discipline from the Local Research Ethics Committees who should bring failures to heed its recommendations to the notice of its appointing body, to the relevant NHS body and to the appropriate professional bodies (GMC etc). The supervisory body should bring the matter to the attention of the Ministers.

6. The supervisory body should be non-statutory funded by and under the aegis of the Department of Health.

7. Gene therapy work should be confined to a small number of approved centres.

Early proposals to be approved by the Clothier Committee included research into adenosine deaminase deficiency, cystic fibrosis and skin cancer.

The Gene Therapy Advisory Committee was set up to review all proposals for gene therapy in the UK. It is at present chaired by Professor Norman Neven, Professor of Medical Genetics at Belfast City Hospital, and includes lay people such as journalists and church representatives as well as doctors and scientists. Its aims are to consider and advise on:

– Acceptability of proposals for gene therapy on human subjects

– Working with other agencies with responsibilities in the field

– Advising Health Ministers on gene therapy research developments and their implications.

In its sixth Annual Report it stated that since the first gene therapy clinical trial was approved for a start in September 1990 more than 400 clinical protocols have been approved worldwide. It expressed concerns at the lack of provision for long-term follow-up of patients who have received gene therapy. It has provided updated guidance notes to those who wish to propose a gene therapy trial.

GENDER SELECTION

There has been publicity given to a business which claimed to be able to assist parents in having a child of a specified gender. It used methods which were not covered by the HFEA or the provisions relating to genetic screening. There are at present no laws to prevent the commercialisation of this. Only where the child is born through IVF or where embryos are involved would the activities come under the licensing authorities. The HFEA has licensed four centres to carry out Pre-implantation Genetic Diagnosis (PGD) (see above) which can be used to determine the sex of an embryo where a family is at risk of passing on a serious sex-linked disorder, such as Duchenne's Muscular Dystrophy. However, the guidelines of the HFEA do not allow couples to select the sex of their embryos for non-medical reasons. Such selection is available in the USA and there are reports of many couples flying to the States so that they can choose the sex of their babies.[27]

GENETIC SCREENING

A project was proposed by Robert Sinsheimer in California in 1984 to identify the protein building blocks which shape human life. Known as the Human Genome Project, it was completed in 2000. The fact of identification of genetic predispositions raise huge ethical and legal dilemmas which are only just being confronted. One of the issues is the right to screen genetically persons for insurance or employment purposes. On the one hand it could be argued that the employer or the insurance company is entitled to receive all relevant information which would affect their decision to take a person on as an employee or for the purposes of insurance cover. On the other hand, it can be seen that without statutory protection against unfair discrimination the person who presents a risk could be subjected to extremely unjust treatment when there is only a probability rather than a certainty that the particular genetic predisposition will materialise.

At present there is no legislation to prohibit an insurance company or employer requiring genetic testing before providing insurance cover or taking a person into employment. There is of course the common law right to refuse to give consent, but this may mean the loss of insurance cover or of employment. The Association of British Insurers has agreed a Code of Practice on insurance and genetic tests (see below).

REPORT BY THE NUFFIELD COUNCIL ON BIOETHICS ON GENETIC SCREENING

The Nuffield Council on Bioethics was established in 1991 to consider the ethical issues presented by advances in biomedical and biological research. The subject of its first report, produced in December 1993, was genetic screening (Nuffield Council on Bioethics 1993). It emphasised the four points shown in Box 27.13.

Box 27.13 Important features of the report on genetic screening

- The difficulty in assessing individual health risks exposed by genetic screening

- The increased complexity of the ethical aspects of confidentiality

- The demands made upon professional and health resources by the required ethical procedures

- The broad framework provided as a safeguard against potential eugenic abuse.

The main conclusions of the report are shown in Box 27.14.

Box 27.14 Conclusions of report on genetic screening

1. Adequately informed consent should be a requirement for all genetic screening programmes.

2. Counselling should be readily available for those being genetically screened, as well as for those being tested on account of a family history of a genetic disorder.

3. Health professionals should seek to persuade individuals, if persuasion should ▶

---

be necessary, to allow the disclosure of relevant genetic information to other family members.

4. Appropriate professional bodies should prepare guidelines to help with the difficult decisions over confidentiality and the passing on of information within the family.

5. The Department of Health should consider with Health Authorities and the appropriate professional bodies, effective arrangements for the preservation of confidentiality, particularly in relation to genetic registers, and should issue the necessary guidance.

6. The Department of Employment keeps under review the potential use of genetic screening by employers.

7. Genetic screening of employees for increased occupational risks ought only to be contemplated in specifically defined circumstances such as where there is strong evidence of a clear connection between the working environment and the development of the condition for which genetic screening can be conducted.

8. British insurance companies should adhere to their current policy of not requiring any genetic tests as a prerequisite of obtaining insurance.

9. There should be early discussions between the government and the British insurance industry about the future use of genetic data, and that pending the outcome, the companies should accept a temporary moratorium on requiring the disclosure of genetic data.

10. The need for improving public understanding of human genetics should be borne in mind in any review of the National Curriculum and in the work of all public bodies concerned with the public understanding of science.

11. Its recommendations on adequately informed consent, confidentiality and the central co-ordination and monitoring of genetic screening programmes are essential to the safeguards about eugenic abuse.

12. The Department of Health in consultation with the appropriate professional bodies should formulate detailed criteria for introducing genetic screening programmes, and establish a central co-ordinating body to review genetic screening programmes and monitor their implementation and outcome.

INSURERS' CODE OF PRACTICE

The Association of British Insurers published a Code of Practice in 1997. It made further revisions to it in 1999.[28] It is a voluntary code for insurers over genetic tests and gives the following guidance.

1. It should not require a person to take a genetic test in order to obtain insurance cover.

2. If the results of a genetic test are in a person's medical records they can only be taken into account if they apply to one of seven conditions for which the tests are deemed reliable (these conditions include breast cancer, Alzheimer's and Huntingdon's disease).

3. If the test is later found to be unreliable then the person is entitled to a refund of overpaid premiums and cheaper future payments.

4. A person is obliged to tell an insurance company if he has had a genetic test and disclose the results.

5. Any one refused insurance cover or who wishes to complain can contact the ABI.[29]

Some evidence is emerging that contrary to the spokesman of the ABI, some people are being refused insurance cover on the grounds that they have a genetic disorder.[30,31] It may be that either statutory intervention or some form of state insurance cover is necessary to protect those who are vulnerable.

In April 1999 a Genetics and Insurance Committee (GAIC)[32] was established by the Department of Health to develop and publish criteria for the evaluation of specific genetic tests, their application to particular conditions and their reliability and relevance to particular types of insurance. In October 2000 the GAIC recommended new guidelines[33] and suggested that the reliability and relevance of the genetic test for Huntingdon's Chorea is sufficient for insurance companies to use the result when assessing applications for life insurance. Insurers will not be able to require prospective clients to take the test, but they will be able to ask clients if they have taken tests for Huntingdon's Chorea, and to ask for the results to be given. The recommendations have been criticised, for example by the National Consumer Council, on the grounds that they will create a genetic underclass and will dissuade people from taking the tests.[34] In addition, scientists are fearful that potential volunteers to genetic tests will refuse to co-operate in this country, thus many scientists would have no option but to work outside this country, where potential research subjects would not have to disclose results to insurance companies.[35]

In its first Annual Report[36] the Genetics and Insurance Committee reported on its work in drawing up criteria and guidelines for insurance providers to submit information on genetic tests that were to be used for insurance purposes. A test must satisfy the three criteria of accuracy measurement of genetic information, clinical relevance and actuarial relevance to be approved by the GAIC for consideration by the insurance industry in setting premiums for insurance. The House of Commons Science and Technology Committee Report on Genetics[37] was concerned at the possibility of premiums rising sharply for applicants identified as being of higher risk. The Committee recommended that there should be a two year moratorium. In the light of the Committee's report, the Department of Health announced in October 2001 that there was an agreement between the government and the Association of British Insurers that there would be a five year moratorium on the use of genetic tests.[38] The Department of Health decided that more time is needed to assess the importance of genetic tests to insurance. For the immediate future, only consumers who want more than £500,000 worth of life insurance, or over £300,000 worth of critical illness, income protection and long-term care insurance will have to disclose genetic test results. There is to be a review of the financial limits after three years.

The Human Genetics Commission (HGC) in May 2001 recommended a moratorium on the use of genetic test information by insurance companies and is at the time of writing conducting a review of the legal framework protecting personal genetic information.

Dangers of reliance on DNA results

An example of the dangers of over-reliance on genetic testing is seen in the report[39] that the Court of Appeal had set aside the conviction of a person on a charge of rape where the main prosecution evidence was of DNA matching. It had been discovered that tests for DNA matching performed by a private laboratory between 1988 and 1990 were flawed and as a result dozens of convictions may be overthrown.

GENETIC DISORDERS AND THE MIDWIFE

The opportunity for genetic screening to take place raises major concerns for the midwife who may be involved in the decision as to whether screening should go ahead. The midwife requires training in this area so that she has the skills to give the appropriate advice to a mother who is contemplating being screened. The midwife should ensure that she is familiar with the ways in which the mother can receive counselling in relation to the disease and the risks in relation to any future pregnancy. She should ensure that:

- the confidentiality of the information received from the mother is protected

- the mother has full information

- the mother knows that she has the right to refuse any genetic testing, and

- the mother should be protected against any zealous researchers anxious to explore the genetics of the mother and child.

In addition it is foreseeable that a mother might seek advice and comfort from a midwife when told that her child is suffering from a genetic disorder. The midwife should ensure that the mother receives all the appropriate information in relation to that disorder and that the child receives the correct treatment and care. The midwife should protect the rights of the mother and child at a time when the mother is likely to be extremely vulnerable and also protect the mother from any attempt to compel her to allow disclosure of this genetic information to other members of the extended family until such time as the mother is able to make a clear reasoned decision on her own account.

MISUSE OF GENETIC INFORMATION

Whatever rules are implemented about screening and the use of genetic information there is always a danger that codes of practice and procedures are not always closely followed, even by the courts, as the following case shows.

The use of DNA, the unique identity marker of each human being, is subject to strict rules in criminal proceedings. Thus the DNA sample taken from an accused on his arrest must be destroyed when he is acquitted.[40] However, in December 2000, the House of Lords held that evidence based on DNA which had been unlawfully retained and not destroyed following the acquittal of an accused, was still admissible in court, subject to the discretion of the trial judge,[41] when the person was charged on a subsequent offence. There is therefore always a danger that if knowledge is available it will be used, despite any regulations to the contrary, on the basis that the ends justify the means.

CONCLUSIONS

The area of fertilisation and genetics is one where the law usually lags behind the scientific developments and is always trying to catch up. Each of the institutions mentioned in this chapter have websites and provide regular updates on their investigations and recommendations which are easily available to the midwife.

QUESTIONS AND EXERCISES

1. A client tells you that she has agreed to bear a child for her sister. How would this affect your work as a midwife?

2. Obtain a copy of the Code issued by the Human Fertilisation and Embryology Authority and discuss the implications for midwifery.

3. A pilot study is being launched for screening for a genetic disposition for coronary heart disease. A client has asked for your advice on whether she should take part with her children. What advice would you give?

4. In what circumstances do you consider that a child should have the right to refuse consent to a genetic screening test?

References

1 Department of Health. 1984. *Report of the Committee of Inquiry into Fertilisation and Embryology Cmnd 9314*. London: HMSO

2 S. 156 Criminal Justice and Public Order Act 1994

3 Parental Orders (Human Fertilisation and Embryology) Regulations 1994 SI 1994 No 2767

4 R. v Human Fertilisation and Embryology Authority, ex parte Blood [1997] 2 All ER 687 CA

5 McLean S. 1998. *Review of Common Law Provisions Relating to the Removal of Gametes and of the Consent Provisions in the Human Fertilisation and Embryology Act 1990*. London: HMSO

6 Department of Health. 2000. Press announcement 25 August 2000

7 Bremner C. 2001. French Woman aged 62 has brother's baby. *The Times* 21 June 2001; Pank P. 2001. Fertility clinic under attack over 'incest'. *The Times* 27 August 2001

8 News item. 1991. *Health Alert*, 7(123), 331

9 See *MIDIRS Midwifery Digest*, March 1993, page 107

10 Rogers L. 2001. Woman to have brother's IVF child. *The Sunday Times* 26 August 2001

11 R v. Ethical Committee of St Mary's Hospital (Manchester) ex parte H [1988] 1 FLR 512

12 R v. Sheffield Health Authority, ex parte Seale [1994] 25 BMLR 1 QBD

13 R v. Secretary of State ex parte Mellor. Times Law Report 5 September 2000

14 R v. Secretary of State ex parte Mellor. Times Law Report 1 May 2001

15 Charter D. 2000. Fertility treatment 'lottery' to be ended. *The Times* 1 December 2000

16 Re A (an adoption)(surrogacy) [1987] 2 All ER 826

17 Surrogacy: Review for Health Ministers of Current Arrangements for Payments and Regulation. CM 4068. 1998. London: DoH

18 Briody v. St Helens and Knowsley AHA (Claim for damages and costs) sub nom Briody v. St Helens and Knowsley AHA [2001] EWCA Civ 1010 [2001] 2 FCR 481 CA

19 *The Human Genetics Advisory Commission and the Human Fertilisation and Embryology Authority Report on Cloning Issues in Reproduction, Science and Medicine*. December 1998

20 *Government Response to the Report by the Human Genetics Advisory Commission and the Human Fertilisation and Embryology Authority on Cloning Issues in Reproduction, Science and Medicine. Cm 4387*. June 1999

21 Department of Health. 2000. *Chief Medical Officer's Expert Advisory Group on Therapeutic Cloning "Stem Cells: Medical Progress with Responsibility"*. London: HMSO

22 Dimond B. 2001. The law regarding embryo and stem cell research. *British Journal of Midwifery*, 9(2), 111-14

23 Human Fertilisation and Embryology (Research Purposes) Regulations 2001 SI 2001 188

24 Royal Society. 2001. Royal Society Report prepared by Professor Richard Gardener

25 R (Quintavallo) v. Secretary of State for Health. Times Law Report 25 January 2002

26 Hawkes N. Couple win right to create life-saving baby. *The Times*, 23 February 2002

27 Harlow J. Couples fly out for designer babies. *The Sunday Times*, 7 October 2001

28 Association of British Insurers. 1999. *Code of practice for genetic testing*

29 Association of British Insurers: 0207 600 3333

30 News item. 1998. Insurers ignore genetics code. *The Sunday Times,* 13 December 1998

31 Winnett R. 2000. Medical underclass fears insurance blacklisting. *The Sunday Times,* 26 March 2000

32 www.doh.gov.uk/genetics/gaic.htm

33 Department of Health. 2000. Committee on Genetics and Insurance Report

34 Henderson M. 2000. Insurers to check for genetic illness. *The Times,* 13 October 2000

35 Henderson M. 2000. Scientists attack gene test ruling. *The Times,* 27 November 2000

36 Genetics and Insurance Committee. 2000. First annual report April 1999-June 2000. London: DoH

37 House of Commons Science and Technology Committee. 2001. Genetics and Insurance

38 Department of Health. 2001. Press release 2001/0494 Health Minister welcomes five year moratorium on genetic tests and insurance

39 *Sunday Times,* 8 May 1994

40 S.64 (3B) Police and Criminal Evidence Act 1984

41 R v. B Attorney General's Reference No 3 of 1999. Times Law Report 14 December 2000

Chapter 28
VACCINE DAMAGE PAYMENTS

Our system of compensation by means of civil action for negligence involves establishing fault, i.e. a breach of the duty of care owed to the person injured. (For further details on the tort of negligence see Chapter 13.) This can be difficult to establish and may mean that many claims are either not brought or are abandoned at an early stage. Critics have demanded a system of no-fault liability such as pertains in New Zealand, Finland and Sweden where compensation is paid for untoward medical accidents without the need to establish that one or more persons is at fault. The present government has indicated that it is prepared to consider the introduction of major changes to our system for compensation including a no-fault system of compensation.[1] A White Paper is to be published 2002 (see Chapter 14).

We do have examples of compensation paid on a no-fault liability basis. One such is the payment for vaccine damage. Another statutory scheme for compensation is the criminal injury compensation scheme. The government announced on 26th October 2000 that it was preparing a scheme for compensation and a trust fund for those who have suffered from variant Creutzfeldt-Jacob Disease (CJD) from BSE and their families. In the past the government created a scheme for haemophiliacs who were infected by the AIDS virus to obtain compensation. The manufacturers of thalidomide, Distillers, established a fund to pay those who were its victims and this fund has been recently topped up.

COMPENSATION FOR VACCINE DAMAGE

It is in the public interest for as many children as possible to be vaccinated against infectious diseases. However it is recognised that on very rare occasions there can be side effects of a very crippling kind from vaccines. The Royal Commission on Civil Liability and Compensation for Personal Injuries (The Pearson Report) 1978[2] recommended that where vaccine damage could be proved to have followed from medical procedures recommended by the government, then those who suffered serious damage should be entitled to bring an action in tort against the government on the basis of strict liability. It did not recommend the abandonment of fault liability in other cases of personal injury arising from medical accident. In the light of the Pearson recommendations the government introduced the Vaccine Damage Payments Act 1979 to provide for payments to be made out of public funds in cases where severe disablement occurs as a result of vaccination against certain diseases or of contact with a person who has been vaccinated against any of those diseases. The sum payable was originally £10,000 but this has been increased over the years and since June 2000 stands at £100,000.[3]

The diseases to which the Act applies are shown in Box 28.1.

Box 28.1 Diseases covered by the Vaccine Damage Payments Act 1979

Diphtheria

Tetanus

Whooping cough

Poliomyelitis

Measles

Rubella

Tuberculosis

Small pox

And any other disease specified by the Secretary of State by statutory instrument.

Haemophilius Type B infection (hib) was added to the list in 1995[4]

Meningococcal Group C was added to the list in 2001[5]

Severe disability must be established and this is defined in the Act as shown in Box 28.2.

Box 28.2 Definition of severe disability for the purposes of the Vaccine Damage Payments Act

S.1(4) For the purposes of this Act, a person is severely disabled if he suffers disablement to the extent of 80% or more (reduced to 60%) assessed as for the purposes of Social Security legislation.

The Act also covers the situation where a person is severely disabled as the result of a vaccination given to his mother before he was born (1(3)).

The conditions of obtaining the payment are set out in Box 28.3.

Box 28.3 Conditions to obtain payment under Vaccine Damage Payments Act 1979

1. a. Vaccination was carried out in the UK or Isle of Man

   b. on or after 5th July 1948

   c. in the case of small pox before 1st August 1971.

2. a. (Except for poliomyelitis and rubella) the vaccination was given whilst the person was under 18 years or during an outbreak of that disease in the UK or Isle of Man.

3. The disabled person was over the age of two on the date when the claim was made or, if he died before that date, he died after 9th May 1978 and was over the age of two when he died.

Children up to the age of 18 years are now able to bring a claim, but where a claim is made in respect of a vaccination for Meningococcal Group C, the conditions that a person should be under 18 years at the date of the vaccination and that there should be an outbreak of the disease in the UK or Isle of Man do not apply.

Causation
It must be shown that the disablement is the result of the vaccine. Where such causation is in dispute, the Act provides that 'the question whether the severe disablement results from vaccination against any of the diseases shall be determined for the purposes of the Act on the balance of probability.'

Time limits
A claim for payment must be made within six years beginning on the latest of the following dates:

– date of the vaccination

– date on which the disabled person attained the age of two

– 9th May 1978.

Referral to medical tribunal
The Secretary of State can refer to a tribunal:

- the question of the extent of the disablement suffered by the disabled person

- the question whether he is, or, as the case may be, was immediately before his death disabled as a result of the vaccination to which the claim relates, and

- the question whether, if he is or was so disabled, the extent of his disability is or was such as to amount to severe disablement.

The Act also provides for the payments to or for the benefit of the disabled person and the holding of money by trustees where appropriate.

Offences under the Act

A person, who, for the purpose of obtaining a payment under the Act whether for himself or for another person, knowingly makes any false statement or representation or produces or furnishes or causes or knowingly allows to be produced or furnished any document or information which he knows to be false in a material particular, is liable to prosecution (Section 9(1)).

CIVIL CLAIMS

In comparison with the statutory fixed sum for severe disablement, the awards which are payable by civil action for negligence are much larger. However, as is shown in Chapter 13, all elements necessary to establish liability must be shown or accepted by the defendant. The person seeking compensation must therefore show that:

- a duty of care was owed

- this duty has been broken by a failure to follow the accepted standard of care, and

- as a reasonably foreseeable consequence of this breach,

- harm has occurred.

Severe disablement does not have to be shown to recover compensation in the civil courts.

What happens if payment has already been paid out under the Vaccine Damage Payment Act 1979? Does this prevent a civil action taking place? The answer is no. Section 6(4) states that the making of a claim for, or the receipt of, a payment under the Act does not prejudice the right of any person to institute or carry on proceedings in respect of disablement suffered as a result of vaccination against any disease to which the Act applies. However, the fact that a payment has been made under the Act must be taken into account by the court in any civil proceedings where compensation in respect of such disablement is awarded.

Box 28.4 Loveday v. Renton (1988)[6]

Mrs Loveday claimed damages on behalf of her daughter Susan, then 17 years, for permanent brain damage after a whooping cough vaccine given in 1970 and 1971. The claim was brought against the Wellcome Foundation, who made the vaccine, and against the doctor who had administered it. The claim was dismissed because she had failed to show on a balance of probabilities that pertussis vaccine could cause permanent brain damage in young children. It thus failed on the issue of causation. The judge stated that if the case had not failed on the issue of causation, 'any plaintiff would face insuperable difficulties in establishing negligence on the part of the doctor or nurse who had administered the vaccine'. Such a claim would have to be based on the ground that the vaccination had been given in spite of the presence of certain contraindications.

In contrast to the Loveday case, a claim against the Wellcome Foundation succeeded in an Irish case in 1992 (Best v. Wellcome Foundation).[7]

The High Court had dismissed the plaintiff's claim because of the lack of proof of causation. However the Irish Supreme Court held that the Wellcome Foundation was liable for the negligent manufacture and release of a particular batch of triple vaccine and that the brain damage was caused as a result. It referred the case back to the High Court on the amount of compensation. On May 11th 1993 the High Court approved an award of £2.75 million as compensation for the brain damage sustained in September 1969.

It remains to be seen if there will be any further successful cases brought in the civil courts for vaccine damage. It must be stressed that in the Best case, there was evidence that the particular batch of vaccine was below standard and should not be released onto the market. However, the contrast between the sums available if fault and causation can be established in the civil courts is clear. The Association of Parents of Vaccine-Damaged Children has been formed to give advice and support to parents.

CONSUMER PROTECTION ACT 1987

If it can be established that a person has been injured as a result of a defect in a product, then there may be a claim under the Consumer Protection Act 1987. In this case it is not necessary to establish fault, merely that there was a defect (see Chapter 18). It has recently been held that a claim can be brought under the Consumer Protection Act 1987 where the claimant was infected with hepatitis through contaminated blood transfusions.[8] This could be used as a precedent for claims in relation to defective vaccines (see Chapter 19).

DISPUTES OVER THE SAFETY OF THE TRIPLE VACCINE

There has been considerable media concern about the triple vaccine (MMR) for mumps, measles and rubella. Two years ago a report suggested that the measles vaccine was linked with autism. There was growing evidence of parents choosing not to allow their babies to have the triple vaccine. In March 1999 it was reported that there is a growing danger of an epidemic of babies being born with rubella because the proportion of infants being immunised against the disease has been falling for more than four years.[9] Only five months later reports were published of a fear of a measles epidemic.[10] It is said that the figures (only 87% of babies are receiving the triple vaccine) are so alarming that doctors are being to ask whether vaccination should be made compulsory. Subsequently the government has said[11] that single doses are not available, since there was evidence that the single-dose mumps vaccine was not effective in protecting children. The government is hoping that banning single dose vaccines will increase the take-up of the triple vaccine. However, this may not prove to be correct. Ann Coote of Justice Awareness Basic Support which campaigns against the MMR vaccine says their helpline has been inundated with calls from fearful parents. A parent's choice now is either the complete triple vaccine or nothing at all. According to the standard medical advice at present, the triple vaccine should be given in the best interests of the child, i.e. it is in the welfare of the child to have that vaccine. However if a parent refuses to give consent for the child to have it, the right of the parent is respected, even though the child's welfare is placed at risk. If the situation continues to deteriorate then the government may well consider introducing legislation to compel vaccination. The Committee on the Safety of Medicines issued a statement to show that new research showed no link between MMR and autism or bowel disease (13 February 2002). However there is evidence that an increasing failure to take up the MMR vaccine is leading to increasing number of cases of measles.

Another scare relating to the possibility that autism has arisen from mercury being used in vaccines is highlighted in the press.[12]

As a consequence of these alarms, there is evidence of a lower take-up of the vaccinations and therefore a danger of outbreaks of these dangerous illnesses. Midwives are likely to be consulted by mothers over what is best practice for their children and they must ensure that they fulfil their duty of care in providing such information.

CONCLUSIONS

There is on-going research into the safety of vaccines and since midwives are likely to be consulted by mothers, they need to ensure that they are up-to-date. The Department of Health is considering (see Chapter 14) introducing a no-fault liability scheme for clinical compensation and this may be comparable to the present Vaccine Damages Payment Act.

QUESTIONS AND EXERCISES

1. A client asks for your advice on whether she should ensure that her children receive the triple vaccine. What advice do you give?

2. What differences are there between a claim for compensation under the Vaccine Damage Payments Act, a claim for compensation under the laws of negligence and a claim under the Consumer Protection Act 1987?

3. Are there any other injuries or disabilities which you consider should be covered by a statutory right to compensation comparable to the Vaccine Damage Payments Act?

References

1 Department of Health. 2001. Press release 2001/0313 New Clinical Compensation Scheme for the NHS

2 The Royal Commission on Civil Liability and Compensation for Personal Injuries (The Pearson Report) Cmnd. 7054 1978

3 Vaccine Damages Payments Statutory Instrument 2000 SI 1983

4 SI 1995 No 1164

5 Vaccine Damages Payment (Specified Disease) Order 2001 SI 1652

6 Loveday v. Renton The Times 31 March 1988 QBD

7 Best v. Wellcome Foundation, Dr O'Keefe, the Southern Health Board, the Minister for Health of Ireland and the Attorney General [1994] 5 Med LR; also discussed in *Medico Legal Journal,* 61(3), 178

8 A v. National Blood Authority sub nom Hepatitis C Litigation. *The Times,* 4 April 2001

9 Murray I. Rubella fears grow with fall in vaccination. *The Times,* 19 March 1999

10 Murray I. Doctors fear measles epidemic by 2000. *The Times,* 17 August 1999

11 Rumbelow H. Government bans parents' alternative to the measles jab. *The Times,* 28 August 1999

12 Waterhouse R. New autism doubt on mercury in vaccines. *The Sunday Times,* 22 July 2001

Chapter 29

INFECTIOUS DISEASES AND THE MIDWIFE

The midwife has both a duty to ensure that she does not pass on infections to her clients and also a duty to ensure that she notifies the appropriate authorities in accordance with her duties under the public health legislation. This chapter deals with both these areas and also looks in detail at the midwife and AIDS patients, and fear of contracting AIDS. Reference should also be made to Chapter 19 on health and safety.

THE MIDWIFE'S HEALTH

Rule 39 requires the midwife to be medically examined:

'A practising midwife shall, if the Local Supervising Authority deems it necessary for preventing the spread of infection, undergo medical examination by a registered medical practitioner.'

The Local Supervising Authority is the Regional Health Authority in England and Wales and the District Health Authority in Wales, in Scotland Health Boards and in Northern Ireland, Health and Social Services Boards (see Chapter 3).

In addition, it may possibly be implied into a contract of employment that a midwife has a duty to submit herself to an independent medical examination if it is feared that she is not capable, physically or mentally of being at work (see Chapter 22 on employment law).

Under the statutory duties relating to health and safety, and also under her common law duty of care to her patients, the midwife would have a wider duty in relation to the prevention of cross infection between patients and she should therefore follow a procedure which would ensure the highest standards of hygiene and infection control.

NOTIFIABLE DISEASES

Certain diseases are defined as notifiable and if the midwife is aware that one of her mothers, or relatives, is infected with such a disease she would have a duty to report it.

Diseases which are notifiable are shown in Box 29.1.

Box 29.1 Notifiable diseases

A. Cholera, plague, relapsing fever, smallpox, typhus

B. Acquired immune deficiency syndrome (AIDS), acute encephalitis, acute poliomyelitis, meningitis, meningococcal septicaemia, anthrax, diphtheria, dysentery, paratyphoid fever, typhoid fever, viral hepatitis, leprosy, leptospirosis, measles, mumps, rubella, whooping cough, malaria, tetanus, yellow fever, ophthalmia neonatorum, scarlet fever, tuberculosis, rabies and viral haemorrhagic fever

Those diseases under category A are covered by the duties under the Public Health (Control of Disease) Act 1984.

Those diseases under category B are covered by Regulation 3 of the Public Health (Infectious Diseases) Regulations 1988 and the 1984 Act only applies to the extent set out in column 2 of Schedule 1 of the 1988 Act.

Under Section 11 of the 1984 Act a registered medical practitioner has a duty to notify the proper office of the local authority if he becomes aware, or suspects, that a patient whom he is attending within the district of a local authority is suffering from a notifiable disease or from food poisoning. The duty does not apply if he believes, and has reasonable grounds for believing, that some other registered medical practitioner has complied.

WHAT INFORMATION MUST BE NOTIFIED?

Box 29.2 shows the information which must be notified.

Box 29.2 Information which must be given

– Name, age and sex of the patient and the address of the premises where the patient is

– The disease or, as the case may be, particulars of the poisoning from which the patient is, or is suspected to be, suffering and the date or approximate date of its onset, and

► – If the premises are a hospital, the day on which the patient was admitted, the address of the premises from which he came there and whether or not, in the opinion of the person giving the certificate, the disease or poisoning from which the patient is, or is suspected to be, suffering was contracted in hospital.

POWERS OF THE JUSTICE OF THE PEACE

Under Section 37 of the Public Health (Control of Disease) Act 1984, if the justice of the peace is satisfied that a person is suffering from a notifiable disease, and

a. that his circumstances are such that proper precautions to prevent the spread of infection cannot be taken or that such precautions are not being taken, and

b. that serious risk of infection is thereby caused to other persons, and

c. that accommodation is available in a suitable hospital...

then the JP can consult with the Health Authority in whose district the area lies and order the person to be removed to it.

Under Section 38 the JP can order the detention of a person suffering from a notifiable disease in a hospital for infectious diseases.

OTHER PROVISIONS OF THE PUBLIC HEALTH (CONTROL OF DISEASE) ACT 1984

Section 13 gives the Secretary of State power to make regulations to prevent the spread of notifiable diseases and preventing dangers from the arrival or departure of aircraft or vessels.

Section 43 enables the registered medical practitioner to take precautions in order to prevent the spread of infection where a person suffering from a notifiable disease dies in hospital.

Section 44 requires the person in charge of the premises where a person with a notifiable disease has died to take precautions to prevent anyone coming into contact with the body.

Section 47 of the Act enables the Secretary of State to make regulations relating to the disposal of dead bodies.

Section 48 enables the JP to make an order for the removal of a body and for burial within a specified time to prevent the lives of others being endangered.

Role of the midwife

If a midwife knows or suspects that one of her clients may be suffering from an infectious disease or food poisoning she should ensure that the General Practitioner of the patient is notified. Alternatively she could herself notify the local authority.

Duty of local authority

The local authority must notify the appropriate Health Authority within 48 hours of the receipt of a certificate of notification.

HIV/AIDS INFECTIONS

The notification provisions described above do not apply to AIDS/HIV infections. These come under the AIDS (Control) Act 1987 which requires periodical reports to be furnished to RHAs and the Secretary of State. The information required includes:

- the number of persons known to be persons with AIDS and the timing of the diagnosis

- the particulars of facilities and services provided by each authority

- the numbers of persons employed by the authority in providing such facilities

- future provision over the next 12 months

- action taken to educate members of the public in relation to AIDS and HIV, to provide training for testing for AIDS, and for the treatment, counselling and care or persons with AIDS or infected with HIV.

The AIDS (Control) (Contents of Reports) Order 1988 has extended the above required information to include that relating to HIV positive persons.

This information is required to enable the appropriate resources to be allocated and plans to be made. Over 3,500 new diagnoses of HIV infection have been reported for the UK for 2000, the highest annual total ever. The major routes of infection were: 39% homosexual contact; 49% heterosexual contact; 2.6% IDU; 2.5% mother to baby.

Under the Public Health (Infectious Diseases) Regulations 1985 local authorities have the power to apply to a Justice of the Peace for the removal of an AIDS sufferer to hospital to be detained there. The JP is also given the power to make an order for a person believed to be suffering from AIDS to be medically examined. There are also powers in relation to the disposal of the body of an AIDS sufferer.

AIDS/HIV AND THE MIDWIFE

The problem of AIDS/HIV gives rise to two different issues:

- In the first place the midwife as a health professional needs to know her rights and duties in relation to the care of the AIDS/HIV positive pregnant woman and the risk of infection to the midwife during the confinement.

- Secondly the midwife herself may contract AIDS or become infected by the HIV virus. What are her rights in employment law? Does she have to disclose this information to her employers? Could she be automatically dismissed?

The UKCC has issued some guidance for practitioners[1] in relation to AIDS/HIV but there appears to have been no guidance specifically for the midwife. The Royal College of Midwives has published a position paper on AIDS/HIV.[2] The Department of Health has issued guidance on AIDS/HIV infected healthcare workers.[3]

THE AIDS/HIV PATIENT

The midwife could not refuse to care for a pregnant woman who is suffering from AIDS or is HIV positive. This is not surprising and has been emphasised by the UKCC. A survey of attitudes of practitioners to HIV/AIDS patients reported that 37% specifically argued that nurses should be allowed to refuse to care for a patient who had developed AIDS.[4] Professional practice, and also legal duty, would however not permit a midwife to refuse. She could be dismissed from a job, removed from the Register and possibly sued by a mother who suffered harm.

Nor could the midwife insist that a person suspected of being an AIDS/HIV carrier should be compulsorily tested. This is not necessarily a disadvantage to the midwife since it is possible to have false negatives and if the person has only recently picked up the infection it may not show up on testing yet they could still transmit the disease. In addition a recent conference on AIDS highlighted the cases of eight people suffering from full blown AIDS who did not test positive for HIV. This finding has raised great concerns in relation to testing, blood transfusions, breast milk banks etc.

How, therefore, can the midwife protect herself against the possibility of being infected? Some deliveries can result in a lot of spilt blood and the midwife is extremely vulnerable.

As an employee she entitled to all reasonable care being taken for her safety against reasonably foreseeable risks and dangers (see Chapter 19). The fear of AIDS/HIV infection is one which could be regarded as reasonably foreseeable. This means her employer must take all reasonable care in terms of ensuring that a safe system of work is followed, that staff are trained and competent and that equipment, facilities, buildings and the working environment are safe. The employer's duty derives both from the contract of employment and from the criminal law and the laws relating to health and safety at work.

Any guidance offered by professional groups on what equipment the midwife should use to be reasonably safe should be followed. If the appropriate facilities are not available the midwife should draw the manager's attention to the deficiencies and ensure that the appropriate steps are taken. If necessary the midwife could use the whistle blowing procedures (see Chapter 22).

WHAT ARE THE REMEDIES IF NO ACTION IS TAKEN?

The criminal law

A breach of the Health and Safety at Work laws could result in the prosecution of the employer. The Health and Safety Inspectorate has the duty of enforcing the provisions of these laws and making regular inspections of health service premises to ensure that the duties are being observed. If the equipment provided to midwives for home deliveries is inadequate this could also be brought to the attention of the Inspectorate. Obviously all steps should be taken to ensure that management is made aware of the problems and has the opportunity to remedy them before external assistance is brought in.

The civil law

Since it is an implied term of the contract of employment that the employer should take all reasonable care for the safety of the employee, failure by the employer to provide reasonable standards of safety would be a breach of the contract of employment. In serious cases, breach of contract gives the innocent party the right to see the contract as at an end. Thus if the midwife was guilty of gross misconduct she could be dismissed instantly without notice. Similarly where the employer is in breach by failing to take reasonable steps to ensure the midwife's safety, the midwife could see the contract as terminated by his conduct and if she has worked for one year or more continuously, she could bring an action for unfair dismissal in the employment tribunal. She would be alleging that there has been a constructive dismissal by virtue of the employer's failures towards her. If she is to take this latter step she must be sure that she has good legal advice and the stages are well documented in writing.

Because it is unknown which mothers are likely to be a danger to the midwife it is important that every pregnant woman is treated as a potential source of infection and the same high standards are followed for every case. (For further information on health and safety law see Chapter 19.)

DUTY TO THE AIDS/HIV CLIENT

If the midwife knows that one of her clients is actually suffering from AIDS or is HIV positive, what action should she take? Hopefully her standards of care and safety are such that she would not have to take any additional precautions. However she should ensure that she has the knowledge to answer the client's questions and advise her on breastfeeding and the problems of infecting the baby with infected milk, if the baby has not already been infected during gestation. The fact that the mother is an HIV carrier or sufferer from AIDS in no way reduces the duty of care that the midwife owes to her. Indeed in some ways it is higher because of the additional information that the midwife should be passing on.

THE HIV POSITIVE CHILD

Where a baby is thought to have contracted the AIDS virus then 'the welfare of the child is the paramount consideration' (see Chapter 32) is the fundamental principle. This was at the heart of a judge's recent decision when he ruled that a baby could be tested for the HIV virus despite the opposition of her parents.[5]

The facts of the case are shown in Box 29.3.

Box 29.3 Facts of case of HIV test on baby

The mother was HIV positive but refused to allow her four-month-old baby to be tested for the HIV virus. Both parents believed that HIV does not cause AIDS and that the conventional medical treatment of the virus did more harm than good. Judge Wilson noted that both parents were devoted to the baby and that they were knowledgeable and concerned about HIV. However the judge accepted the current medical view that HIV could lead to AIDS and that drug therapy could be given to minimise the effect of the virus. The mother had refused to accept medical advice to have her baby delivered via a Caesarean and not to breastfeed the baby. Instead she arranged for a home delivery and was breastfeeding the baby.

The case in Box 29.3 came to light when a GP carrying out a routine check-up read in the mother's notes that she was HIV positive and raised the issue with Camden Borough Council which brought the case under the Children Act 1989. The British Medical Association and the Terence Higgins Trust supported the ruling because of the advances made in the treatment of HIV. The National Aids Trust said it was extremely regrettable that court intervention was thought necessary. However the government policy announced on 13th August 1999[6] by Minister of Health Tessa Jowell for all pregnant women to be encouraged to have a routine HIV test is likely to increase the numbers of babies found to be infected and therefore the potential for parental disputes over the babies being tested. 2.5% of the newly reported HIV cases in 2000 were mother-to-baby infections. Midwives need to have the necessary training to advise women on HIV testing, to ensure that they are given the appropriate counselling prior to having the test.

The case illustrates one of the most difficult dilemmas facing midwives, i.e. when should they seek to intervene against the wishes of the parents, in particular the mother, in order to protect the child. In the case itself, the judge ruled that an HIV test could be carried out, yet he did not rule that the mother should stop breastfeeding the child. Breastfeeding the baby by an HIV positive mother is considered to double the chance of the baby contracting the disease.

If the child's welfare was paramount it could be argued that the risk of contracting the disease through breastfeeding was so great that unless the mother agreed not to feed the baby, then the baby should be taken into care. Yet the judge did not rule on the breastfeeding.

THE MIDWIFE AS THE AIDS/HIV CARRIER

Liability of the midwife

As has been seen above, the midwife is one of the few professionals subject to a statutory duty to agree to a medical examination.[7] This means that if the midwife is suspected of being AIDS/HIV infected then her employers or Supervisor could quite legitimately request the Local Supervising Authority to arrange for a test to be taken. The midwife would also have a professional duty to notify the Registration body and also her employer that she was suffering from AIDS or was HIV positive. The Court of Appeal ordered a former dentist who was suffering from AIDS to hand over his records so that his patients could be contacted. However it barred the publication of his name and the name of the Health Authority for whom he worked.[8]

There would probably be civil liability if the midwife gave blood failing to disclose that she was a carrier of AIDS/HIV. If she gave blood deliberately knowing that she could infect others, then as well as being a civil wrong under a principle established in a 19th century case,[9] she could also be guilty of a criminal offence. Stephen Kelly, who was convicted of knowingly infecting a lover with HIV, was jailed for 5 years.[10] He was prosecuted under the Scottish common law. In February 2002 a carjacker was imprisoned for 15 years after he threatened victims with an HIV infected syringe.[11]

Protection of the midwife

She may have protection under the Disability Discrimination Act 1995, but the employer would be entitled to take reasonable measures to ensure that her patients were protected from the risk of cross infection. We do not have an AIDS/HIV discrimination act so any employee suffering from AIDS or who was HIV positive would have to claim protection from other legislation including the statutory protection from unfair dismissal and the Human Rights Act 1998 and Appendix 1 to this book. A case in 1988 protected the confidentiality of the names of the health professionals who are found to be AIDS/HIV positive against public disclosure.[12]

To remedy the lack of protection for those who are AIDS/HIV sufferers, various organisations have published charters to protect their rights. For example, Marks and Spencer joined with other employers to protect the interests of those who were infected.[13] A charter was drawn up by charities including the Terence Higgins Trust.[14] However, these charters do not in themselves have the force of law.

National strategy for sexual health and HIV services

In July 2001[15] the Department of Health announced a national strategy on sexual health and HIV services aimed to prevent the spread of sexually transmitted diseases and improve the care and treatment of those who need it, together with a new national information campaign to promote safe sex.

CROSS INFECTION AND HOSPITAL ACQUIRED INFECTIONS

In the care of pregnant and newborn babies, high standards of infection control are vital. In the sixth Annual Report of CESDI[16] it was found that 5% of the deaths analysed were the result of infection: 2 stillbirths and 6 neonatal deaths.

A recent report by the National Audit Office[17] has raised major concerns about the level of hospital acquired infection (HAI). The report suggested that HAI could be the main or a contributory cause in 20,000 or 4% of deaths a year in the UK and that there are about 100,000 cases of HAI with an estimated cost to the NHS of £1 billion. The NAO drew conclusions on the strategic management of HAI, surveillance and the extent and cost of HAI, and the effectiveness of prevention, detection and control measures. Its recommendations include reviewing the following:

– The value of using an Infection Control Manual

– The 1995 Guidance on Infection Control

– Cost effectiveness of screening patients and staff and isolation of patients together with standards and guidelines

– The policies on provision of education and training

– The arrangements for monitoring hospital hygiene and hospital practices

– Ensure advice on hand washing is implemented

– Clinical audit arrangements, to ensure infection control is covered

– Isolation facilities

– Guidance on management of HAI outbreaks

Following this report the government announced a multi-pronged initiative to tackle hospital-acquired infections. Amongst the initiatives planned is an antimicrobial strategy including a clampdown on inappropriate antibiotic use and better infection control measures.[18] In addition there will be independent inspection of hospitals by the Audit Commission and Commission for Health Improvement. The government has stated that the Commission for Health Improvement and the Audit Commission would conduct ward inspections and be given the right to seek information on HAI and to publish it.[19] The Report on the NHS commissioned by the government from Virgin Group reported that it found grubby wards, litter-strewn entrances and dirty casualty departments throughout the NHS. On 31st July 2000 the Health Minister, Lord Hunt, announced that NHS hospitals were to be given £150,000 each to clean up their wards and disinfect bathrooms as part of a £31 million campaign. The money could be used for extra cleaning staff, materials, equipment and new towels and linen. Patient Environment Action Teams would make unannounced inspections every six months and those hospitals that failed to meet standards would be 'named and shamed'. National standards for cleanliness would form part of performance assessment guidelines for hospitals. In September 2000, eight NHS hospitals were identified by the Department of Health as models for others. They were to assist in drawing up standards for a national action plan for cleanliness.

CONCLUSIONS

Central to the safety of the mother and child are high standards of infection control and implementation of the laws relating to notification of infectious diseases and the guidance on AIDS/HIV infected healthcare professionals. The midwife should also be aware of the rules relating to confidentiality which are considered in Chapter 10.

QUESTIONS AND EXERCISES

1. You visit a client and discover that she has been suffering from food poisoning since visiting a restaurant the night before. What action do you take?

2. A client tells you that her husband has just been diagnosed as HIV positive. In what ways, if any, will this affect your practice as a midwife in relation to the client?

3. In the case cited in question 2, which persons, if any, would you inform of the situation?

4. How can standards of cross infection control be improved in your own department and in the community?

References

1 UKCC. 1992. Registrars letter 8/1992 replacing circular PC/89/02 November 1989; UKCC. PC/89/01 Anonymous testing for the prevalence of the Human Imnunodeficiency Virus (HIV)

2 Royal College of Midwives. 1998. *HIV and AIDS position paper.* London: RCM

3 Department of Health. 1999. *AIDS/HIV Infected Health Care Workers: Guidance on the Management of Infected Health Care Workers and Patient Notification.* London: HMSO

4 Akinsanya J and Rouse P. 1992. Who will care? A survey of the knowledge and attitudes of hospital nurses to people with HIV/AIDS. *Journal of Advanced Nursing,* 17, 400-1

5 Rumbelow H. Judge orders mother to test baby for HIV. *The Times,* 4 September 1999

6 Baldwin T and Murray I. All pregnant women must test for Aids. *The Times,* 13 August 1999

7 UKCC. 1998. Midwives Rules and Code of Practice, Rule 39. London: UKCC

8 Horsnall M. Patients to be told of HIV dentist. *The Times,* 28 February 2002

9 Wilkinson v. Downton [1987] 2 QB 57

10 Harris G. Five years for the reckless lover who passed on HIV. *The Times,* 17 March 2001

11 de Bruxelles S. Carjacker held HIV syringe to victims' necks. *The Times,* 9 February 2002

12 X v. Y and others [1988] 2 All ER 648

13 Ashworth J. 1992. Charter launched by Sir Evelyn de Rothschild. *The Times,* 10 July 1992

14 UK Declaration Working Group August 1991

15 Department of Health. 2001. Press release 2001/0354 National Strategy for sexual health and HIV services

16 Confidential Enquiry into Stillbirths and Deaths in Infancy. 1999. *6th Annual Report 1996-7.* London: Maternal and Child Health Research Consortium

17 National Audit Office. 2000. The Management and Control of Hospital Acquired Infection in Acute NHS Trusts in England. London: HMSO

18 www.doh.gov.uk/arbstrat.htm

19 Department of Health. 2000. Press release 12 June 2000; Sherman J. 2000. Infections caught in hospital to be exposed. *The Times,* 13 June 2000

SPECIFIC SITUATIONS

This final section of the book looks at specific areas of midwifery practice and client groups including the midwife lecturer, researcher and the law relating to the special needs of children and those suffering from mental illness. Finally the legal issues arising from the practice of complementary therapies are considered.

Chapter 30

MIDWIFE TEACHERS, CLINICAL INSTRUCTORS, PRECEPTORS AND MENTORS

Most midwives are in some way involved in the instruction and support of others. Increasingly this role is likely to be formalised and become part of the contract of employment. Even those who are not employed in a teaching capacity might find that their job description includes responsibilities for the training and mentoring of others. April 2001 marked the end of the transition period for midwives to take on the requirements of post-registration education and practice (PREP) of the UKCC. The adoption of the UKCC PREP proposals and the requirement for preceptors should result in more midwives being involved in the role of instructor or preceptor (see Chapter 2 on educational requirements). For the most part this is unlikely to give rise to many legal issues. However, in some cases, an awareness of potential dangers and problems could prove to be of considerable advantage. Further information on the legal issues arising in the teaching and assessment process can be seen in the author's chapter in Partners in Learning by Ian Walsh and Caron Swann.[1] Following the UKCC's Education Commission report, Fitness for Practice,[2] the UKCC published revised standards for the preparation of teachers of nursing, midwifery and health visiting.[3] These standards also cover those for preceptors and for mentors and came into force in September 2001.

Reference should also be made to Chapter 31 on research.

TERMINOLOGY

First, what activities are we considering? Box 30.1 sets out some of the terminology used in the instruction and support of others.

Box 30.1 Terms used in instructing and supporting others

- Teacher

- Lecturer

- Clinical instructor

- Preceptor

- Mentor

- Supervisor

- Assessor

- Project manager

- Counsellor

To make discussion easier, the person who is subject to the instruction, mentorship etc. will be referred to as the student, even though the person may well be a registered practitioner.

PRECEPTOR

The definition given by the UKCC within the PREP guidelines is

'a role model and support for about the first four months of practice as a registered practitioner to:

- provide guidance
- be a member of the same team
- judge the appropriate level of responsibility
- agree objectives and outcomes for the period of support
- who may recommend an extension of time.'

MENTOR

Where a (usually) older and more experienced person acts in the nature of a protector for the other for a longer time than would normally be associated with preceptorship, and where the more experienced person provides guidance, support and a concern for the other's advancement and general progress.

TEACHER/INSTRUCTOR/LECTURER

This person would usually be based in a college of education and provide education and training for the student. Normally she would also have duties to instruct and assess in the workplace and assess the student's progress.

SUPERVISOR

A Supervisor of Midwives has a distinct role set by statute and this role is considered in Chapter 3. The Supervisor of Midwives might, of course, also be a mentor, preceptor or any of the other roles considered in this chapter. Clinical supervision, a form of reflective practice, has been recommended by the UKCC[4] for registered nurses, but, presumably because of the statutory form of supervision, has not been used in midwifery practice.

The legal areas which will be discussed in relation to all types of supporters/ instructors are shown in Box 30.2.

Box 30.2 Legal areas to be considered

- Statutory requirements

- Duty of care: Liability for negligent advice, delegation and supervision

- Appeals process

- Confidentiality and access to information

- Whistle blowing

- Contracts of employment

- Health and safety

- NHS agreements

- Giving references

STATUTORY FRAMEWORK

The NMC has the duty of setting the educational requirements for entry onto the Register for its practitioners. This would necessitate keeping in touch with European Directives on changes to the content of professional training. Box 30.3 shows the amended requirements of the European Community for the practical and clinical aspects of midwifery programmes.

Box 30.3 Article 27 of the EC Directive 89/594/EEC

(See UKCC Registrar's letter dated 12 April 1990 2/1990.)

This training is to be dispensed under appropriate supervision:

1. Advising pregnant women, involving at least 100 pre-natal examinations

2. Supervision and care of at least 40 women in labour

3. The student should personally carry out at least 40 deliveries

4. Active participation with breech deliveries. Where this is not possible because of lack of breech deliveries, practice may be in a simulated situation

5. Performance of episiotomy and initiation into suturing. Initiation shall include theoretical instruction and clinical practice. The practice of suturing includes the suturing of the wound following an episiotomy and a simple perineal laceration. This may be in a simulated situation if absolutely necessary

6. Supervision and care of 40 women at risk in pregnancy, or labour or postnatal period

7. Supervision and care (including examination) of at least 100 postnatal women and healthy newborn infants

8. Observation and care of the newborn requiring special care including those born pre-term, post-term, underweight or ill

9. Care of women with pathological conditions in the fields of gynaecology and obstetrics

10. Initiation into care in the field of medicine and surgery. Initiation shall include theoretical instruction and clinical practice.

The UKCC's requirements for pre-registration midwifery programmes[5] are set out in Chapter 2.

It is also a requirement that in order to be placed on the Register the applicant must satisfy the Council that she is of good character as well as having the appropriate professional qualifications. If, therefore, the lecturer becomes aware of evidence about a student which makes it clear that she is not of good character, and therefore should not be placed on the Register, then the lecturer would have a duty to inform the appropriate person. (Where evidence comes to light that a practitioner should not remain on the Register, then this should be reported to the NMC under the professional conduct jurisdiction which is considered in Chapter 4.)

DUTY OF CARE

It is essential to establish the extent of the duty of care owed to the student/trainee. Rarely is the instructor in a line management relationship with the student but there may be a responsibility when it can be seen that harm may occur to the student or to someone else if no action is taken by the instructor. Reference should be made to Chapter 13 on negligence and the basic elements to be established before a successful action can be brought.

The following principles emerge:

– There is no concept recognised in law of team liability

– There is no concept that a superior is vicariously liable for the wrongs of a junior. The superior must be shown to be personally and directly liable. (This is discussed further in Chapter 24 on the legal aspects of management.)

– Standards can differ (see the Bolam Test and Maynards Case)

– Liability can exist for negligent advice

– Liability can also exist for negligent delegations where the instructor is aware that the student has inadequate experience to undertake a particular activity (see Chapter 24)

– Liability can also exist for negligent supervision if the limited experience of the student indicates that a specific level of supervision is required in order to ensure that the client, the student and others are safe.

The extent of the duty of care

One area in which the teacher would be expected to show competence and have a duty of care, would be in ensuring that students were educated in the appropriate areas to obtain registration. The duty is placed upon the lecturer to ensure that the syllabus covered by the student and the standard of teaching, combined with due diligence from the student, is sufficient to enable the student to obtain the necessary qualifications for Registration and practice. The lecturer must therefore ensure that she keeps up-to-date with the statutory requirements for registration.

Incompetent or dangerous students

If it is known that the student is likely to refuse or ignore any advice which is offered and if this refusal was likely to endanger clients, then the teacher would have a responsibility to take the appropriate action to prevent harm. In serious situations this might involve reporting the midwife to the Supervisor of Midwives and/or line manager. In less serious circumstances, and depending upon whether the student is registered or not, it might necessitate warning the student that if the advice is ignored then further action will be taken. Should the instructor take the view that it is not her concern and harm befalls a client, a defence of 'it was not my business' might not prevail in a hearing before the NMC since the instructor would herself be a registered practitioner and therefore subject to the Code of Professional Conduct.

A similar situation would arise if the instructor forms the view that the student is too dangerous to practise. In such circumstances the instructor would have a clear professional responsibility to take any action which is necessary to protect the clients. This would also apply if the instructor fears that the student is mentally disordered. The dangers of such a situation are apparent from the Beverly Allitt case, though there it was not known that the nurse was mentally ill until several children had been murdered.

Where the instructor knows that the student is practising outside her sphere of competence she should ensure that her managers are notified and the necessary training is given to the student to enable her to practise safely.

Sometimes, however, the student might confide in the instructor about confidential matters. For example, the student might confess to the instructor that she is disclosing information which has been entrusted to her in confidence. She might tell the instructor that she has passed on to the mother information relating to the unborn child, contrary to the wishes of the Consultant who had wanted to keep that information from the mother for the time being. In such a situation the instructor should ensure that the manager of the midwife is informed and that the mother is receiving all the necessary support. Where the instructor might agree that the student may have been right in her approach, she should be careful not to intervene in a clinical situation for which she is in no way responsible. However, if it appears that the student is in danger of becoming a victim of whistle blowing, she should ensure that she obtains the required support (see below).

Where the student tells the instructor information about herself in confidence, for example that she is HIV positive, or that she has a drink problem or a criminal record, the instructor should make it clear that she cannot keep silent about such facts and advise the student to notify the Supervisor and her manager and if she fails to do so, then the instructor would be bound to take the necessary action. Where such information is given to the instructor anonymously the instructor would still have a duty to confront the student and take any necessary action.

Criticisms might also come to the instructor from the ward manager or others about the student's conduct. In such circumstances the instructor would have a duty to give the student advice and counselling and if necessary advise the head of school.

Students may criticise practice to the instructor. For example, a student might inform the instructor that a doctor is incompetent. In such a case, the instructor would have a responsibility to ensure that the student was supported in taking this further, so that appropriate investigations could be carried out by those with managerial responsibility.

APPEALS PROCESSES

Each education or training institution must ensure that there is a robust, equitable, accessible and just system of appeals. Article 6 of the European Convention on Human Rights (see Appendix 1 of this book) is of particular importance in the assessment process, since it gives a right to a fair trial and is therefore fundamental to any appeals process where results of the assessment or the actual carrying out of an assessment is challenged. Assessors should ensure that if there is a challenge to their assessment, they ensure that an independent person reviews the situation and the appropriate appeals machinery is enacted. The principles of natural justice would require that any person involved in hearing an appeal is independent and impartial, hears the evidence from the appellant and ensures that the decision made is in accordance with the evidence received. The decision of an appeals hearing could be challenged in the High Court by way of judicial review if there is an allegation that the principles of natural justice have not been followed or if there is an alleged breach of Article 6. The Appeals process should also cover the timing of assessments and examinations. For example, if an assessor fails to carry out an assessment in time to give the student an opportunity for rectifying any shortcomings, and such an opportunity should have been made available to the student, then the student may well have grounds for appeal.

CONFIDENTIALITY AND ACCESS TO INFORMATION

Since the instructor will not necessarily be professionally concerned with the care of the patient, what right in law does the instructor have to receive information which the student has received in confidence about the patient? It could be argued that the passing on of such information is in the interests of the mother. However, this is very indirect, and it would have to be shown that unless the instructor had this confidential information harm could arise to the mother or child. An alternative strategy, and one which would be far more open, is for the patient to be told about the situation relating to the instructor/student role and her/his consent obtained to relevant information being passed between them both for the education of the student and for the protection of the patient.

Where the student is concerned about a hazardous situation on the ward which involves confidential information about a patient, notifying the instructor for advice could be seen as an exception to the duty of confidentiality which is in the best interests of the patient or in the public interest. (See Chapter 10 for further discussion on confidentiality.)

WHISTLE BLOWING

The student should be guided in relation to the procedure for alerting management of any hazardous situations and the instructor should ensure that she is given the appropriate support. Advice should be given on record keeping and letters which are sent to management and copies should be kept (see Chapter 22).

CONTRACTUAL ASPECTS

Midwives employed by trusts

Where a midwife is appointed as an instructor she should ensure that her job description and her terms of service reflect her enlarged duties. Where she is employed by a trust and not by an educational establishment, but is carrying out responsibilities in relation to the latter, she should ensure that her employer is aware of and has agreed to these additional duties and any likely area of conflict is resolved before the agreement is made. If she has any liability towards the educational establishment this should be clarified. She should also have access to the agreement drawn up between the college and the NHS trust in relation to the practical education of the midwives and their preceptoring or mentoring and any provisions relating to liability.

Midwives employed by colleges of education

These midwives should ensure that their duties in relation to the clinical placements are spelt out in writing and they should ensure that they have an input into any agreement drawn up between the college and the trust over the clinical training of midwives and continuing education and preceptoring or mentoring. The agreement should establish clearly responsibility for any harm to the midwife whilst she is supervising the student on the clinical placement and which organisation is vicariously liable should the midwife cause harm through her negligence.

Consideration for additional duties

It is unlikely that extra payments would be made for midwives to take on the tasks of being mentors or preceptors. However, if certain inducements are offered, the midwife should ensure that these are put in writing.

HEALTH AND SAFETY ASPECTS

Depending on the circumstances of the relationship of instructor to student, the duty of care probably includes duties in relation to health and safety at work. Clearly where the instructor notes that the student is failing to observe instructions in relation to health and safety then she would have a duty in law to inform the student of the dangers and ensure that those who were supervising the student in the workplace were aware of the situation. (Refer to Chapter 19 for details of health and safety law.)

NHS AGREEMENTS

Agreements for NHS services are increasingly likely to set out the training and educational functions which are expected of the providers. Those who are involved in the instructing/mentoring of others should ensure that the standards both in terms of quantity and quality are detailed in the agreement so that the necessary resources are made available and that this function is specifically itemised for provision by the NHS trust. PREP responsibilities should be clarified so that continuing education and training is provided. Whilst midwives (and all other registered practitioners since the implementation of the PREP provisions) have a statutory duty to undertake refresher courses, the resourcing for this is not always apparent, nor is the provision of paid time off work for study leave. It could be argued that since the employer owes a duty (both under the contract of employment and as part of the duty owed to patients under the law of negligence) to ensure the provision of competent staff, then there is an implied term that the employer will, at its expense, ensure that the competence of professional staff is maintained and that standards of care are improved.

If such duties are built into the agreements for the provision of midwifery services, then this will strengthen midwives' entitlement to receive regular updating and professional development within their paid hours of work. However, ultimately, the duty is on the practitioner to ensure that she keeps up-to-date and receives the necessary study, whatever the policy of the employer in relation to paid study leave.

REFERENCES

Liability can arise when a midwife is asked to write a reference. If a reference is written negligently then liability can arise both to the recipient of the reference, if in reliance upon that reference he has suffered harm,[6] and also to the person who is the subject of the reference.

Box 30.4 Providing a reference

A midwife is asked to provide a reference for a student who has had a warning at work for coming into work in a dishevelled state. The midwife student asks the midwife not to refer to this incident, assuring her that she now takes considerable care over her appearance and cleanliness. What is the position if the midwife gives the reference without mentioning this warning, and the student obtains the post, and then the employer blames the midwife for an inaccurate reference?

If there is evidence that the student midwife is completely reformed then it would probably not be necessary to mention this in the reference, but much depends upon the questions which are asked. If inaccurate information is given then the person providing the reference could be liable for negligent advice. The recipient of the reference would have to show that harm had occurred as a result of reliance upon the reference. If a person asks for information to be withheld in a reference, the midwife would have to tell the student that she could not give a reference without mentioning specific information. There can also be liability to the person on whose behalf the reference is given, if the reference is written without reasonable care and if harm occurs to the subject of the reference as a result of potential employers relying upon the reference.[7] In one case[8] Sun Alliance Life Ltd appealed against a decision that it had been negligent in its provision of an unfavourable reference in relation to C, a former employee. The Court of Appeal dismissed the appeal, holding that an employer owed a duty of care in providing a reference in respect of a former employee. Sun Alliance had failed to take reasonable care to be fair or accurate with regard to the reference supplied. The reference had inaccurately implied that C had been suspended for serious matters of dishonesty and that the matters had been thoroughly investigated. However, no charges of dishonesty had ever been put to C, let alone investigated.

Every care should be taken to ensure that a reference is written accurately in the light of the facts available.

If a reference is given with due care but is defamatory of the individual, the writer of the reference should be protected from any successful action of defamation whether the comments are correct or they are incorrect, if they were given in a qualified privileged situation without malice by the writer.

CONCLUSION

More and more pressure is placed upon teaching staff, and also those midwives who, although they are not teachers, are expected to fulfil the role of preceptor or mentor or undertake a similar activity. Such activities inevitably carry additional legal responsibilities and midwives must ensure that they have an understanding of the legal implications of any such activity they are asked to undertake. As always, clear and comprehensive documentation of how the activity is carried out is essential.

In October 2001 the Department of Health announced the publication of a prospectus for the NHS University.[9] It is the intention that everyone in the NHS will begin their career with the NHS University through induction courses and direct training. This University will inevitably have a major impact on the current role of nurse lecturers at other institutions and may pave the way towards a more centralised curriculum and assessments for pre-registration and post-registration courses.

QUESTIONS AND EXERCISES

1. As a lecturer of midwives, you have been told by a student that a fellow student is acting very oddly and appears to be mentally ill. What action would you take?

2. You are employed by an educational institution but have responsibilities within the field of clinical practice. In the event of your being negligent and causing harm to a client, who would be liable: the educational institution or the trust? How would you find out the answer?

3. In litigation, proof of the instruction which has been given is of increasing importance as a defence. Examine your own record keeping in relation to what you teach or mentor.

References

1 Dimond B. 2002. Chapter 5. In: *Partners in Learning*. Walsh I and Swann C. Abingdon: Radcliffe Medical Press

2 UKCC. 1999. *Fitness for Practice*. London: UKCC

3 UKCC. 1999. *Standards for the preparation of teachers of nursing, midwifery and health visiting*. London: UKCC

4 UKCC. 1996. *Position Statement on Clinical Supervision*. London: UKCC

5 UKCC. 2000. Requirements for pre-registration midwifery programmes. Registrar's Letter 35/2000

6 Hedley Byrne v. Heller and Partners Ltd House of Lords [1963] 2 All ER 575

7 Spring v. Guardian Assurance plc and others. Times Law Report 8 July 1994; [1995] 2 AC 296

8 Cox v. Sun Alliance Life Ltd [2001] EWCA Civ 649; [2001] IRLR 448 CA

9 Department of Health. 2001. Press Release 2001/480 Introducing the NHS University

Chapter 31
MIDWIFERY RESEARCH

The midwife may be involved in research in three ways:

– she may be undertaking it herself as part of her own professional development

– she may be the project manager for someone else's research

– she may be caring for mothers or responsible for staff who are the subjects of a research investigation.

A useful introductory guide to research for midwives has been written by Colin Rees.[1] In addition, since midwifery should be a research-based profession,[2] it is important for the midwife to know when the research results should be incorporated into her standards of practice. Increasingly, the publications of NICE should bring to the attention of practitioners the results of research into midwifery and obstetric practice (see Chapter 21). The necessity for midwifery to be a research-based profession was emphasised by the Advisory Committee on the Training of Midwives of the Commission of the European Communities in its report and recommendations adopted at its meeting on 14th and 15th January 1992. The Committee's recommendations are shown in Box 31.1.

> **Box 31.1 Recommendations of the Committee on the Training of Midwives of the EC**
>
> 1. Research should be included in the curriculum for basic midwifery training. A curriculum should as a minimum include:
>
>   – principles of research
>
>   – elementary research methods including statistics and epidemiology
>
>   – analysis and interpretation of research findings
>
>   – library use
>
>   – ethical and moral implications of research
>
>   – practical application of research findings.

▶ 2.2 The member states should promote the aspects of research in the exercise of the profession of midwifery.

2.3 All research achieved or undertaken by midwives should be entered into a database in the member states.

The issues to be considered in this chapter are shown in Box 31.2.

Box 31.2 Legal issues arising in research

- Consent

- Local Research Ethics Committees

- Confidentiality

- Injuries to the research subject

- Health and safety and the researcher

- Project management

- Research results and the standards of care

- International codes protecting human rights

CONSENT

Consent in relation to treatment and care is considered in Chapters 7 and 8. Chapter 7 looks at the issues relating to trespass to the person and the giving of consent. Chapter 8 looks at the information which must be provided to prevent an action for breach of the duty of care owed in negligence arising. This section builds on these two chapters and considers consent in relation to research.

Box 31.3 illustrates the issues which must be considered in relation to consent to research.

Box 31.3 Issues arising in consent to research

- Nature of the consent

- How consent should be given

- The capacity of the person giving consent

- The information to be given

- Payment and voluntary consent

- Risk of harm to the fetus

- Role of the midwife

- Consent and a records search.

A personal anecdote might be of interest.

In preparation for the birth of my first child, I had undergone the intensive course on psychoprophylaxis and felt well prepared. An obstetric registrar was undertaking research into anaesthetic gases during confinement and asked me for some blood soon after admission, which I was happy to give him. He told me nothing else. At a later stage he returned and asked me to take some gas mixture he brought. I did not wish to have this as I was coping well with the breathing according to the training. He was fairly insistent and my capability to refuse was much reduced. His visits became more and more frequent over the next 12 hours. I am not sure how often blood samples were taken but I know that I was given a lot of gas which I had not wanted and did not think I needed as I had been coping well through the breathing. There was also a clash between the questions I was being asked by the registrar on the impact of the gas and the techniques of psychoprophylaxis. For three days after the birth the registrar returned to take blood samples. The baby was drowsy to the point of being comatose. I asked him if she could be suffering from the effects of the gas and he said most probably and took a sample of blood from her too.

This incident illustrates several important points about consent and research:

- My consent was never explicitly obtained.

- I was never given full information about the research, its aims, methods and my choices.

- There was a confusion as to whether the research was therapeutic and part of my care or whether it was non-therapeutic. I was not aware, for example, of the status of the registrar: was he on my Consultant's junior medical team or not?

- The effects of the research on the baby were never explained to me or evaluated in advance.

- No account was taken of my inability, because of mental and physical fatigue, to refuse to participate.

WHAT IS THE NATURE OF CONSENT WHICH IS REQUIRED?

It is essential that the fully informed voluntary consent of the research subject should be obtained before the research progresses. The consent should be given without compulsion and must be given by an adult who has the mental capacity to give consent. The form should explain to the research subject that refusal to participate in the research project will not lead to any prejudice in the care and treatment which is given. Clearly there are advantages in obtaining the mother's consent to participate in a research project about labour, well before labour commences.

SHOULD THE CONSENT BE IN WRITING?

Whilst in practice both written and spoken consent would be defences against an action for trespass to the person, it is easier to prove that consent has been given where it is in writing and the Local Research Ethics Committee (LREC) (see below) would normally require a written consent.

Consent should preferably be obtained both in writing and by word of mouth. The research project should have been before the Local Research Ethics Committee (see below) which would look at the information to be given to the subject and the consent form which is signed.

A research project looking at consent forms for research protocols[3] found that

'consent forms for research were more difficult to read than newspaper editorials. Poor readability was caused by the use of long paragraphs and long sentences, not by the excessive use of long words.'

HOW SHOULD THE COMPETENCE OF THE MOTHER TO GIVE CONSENT BE DETERMINED?

Consent should be given at a time when the mother is capable of giving it. It would not be appropriate to request consent when the mother is part way through labour and does not have the capacity to give consent. The midwife could have an important role in ensuring that consent is not obtained from the mother at a time when she does not have the capacity to make a valid decision. If there are concerns over whether or not the mother has the capacity to give consent, it would be wise to bring in a health professional who is not involved in the research project to make an assessment of the mother's competence and record it in writing.

HOW MUCH INFORMATION SHOULD BE GIVEN TO THE RESEARCH SUBJECT?

Whilst the courts have held that the doctrine of informed consent is not recognised when consent is given for treatment where research is being carried out which has no direct therapeutic benefit for the patient, a higher standard of information giving would probably be required (see Chapter 8 and the Sidaway case). All risks should be explained beforehand. It is doubtful too, if the mother could give consent to a risk of harm to the fetus, unless the risk was so insignificant and the benefits to be obtained by the research outweighed these insignificant risks.

PAYMENT AND VOLUNTARY CONSENT

The general principle is that if the payment is such as to materially to affect the patient's attitude, and in a sense buy that consent, there would be concern at the voluntary nature of the consent. Much would of course depend upon the economic circumstances of the mother. Payment of out-of-pocket expenses – travelling if the mother is required to visit the hospital/research centre – would probably not come within the category of a payment which affected the mother's voluntary agreement to participate.

CONSENT AND RISKS TO THE FETUS

What if the mother gives consent to a research project which harms the fetus: could the child when born bring an action against the mother? (This is quite separate from an action against the researcher which might also exist.) Such an action against the mother would not be possible under the Congenital Disabilities (Civil Liability) Act 1976 since under that Act the mother can only be sued if her negligence, which led to the congenital disabilities, occurred when she was driving a car (see Chapter 17). The right of action at common law[4] is no longer available since the implementation of the Congenital Disabilities (Civil Liability) Act 1976.

If the mother gives a valid consent to the research taking place but harm subsequently occurs to the fetus who is born disabled, since the child's right derives from the action in negligence which the mother has, the consent of the mother may well prevent the action from the child succeeding (see Section 6 of the Congenital Disabilities Act 1976).

THE ROLE OF THE MIDWIFE

Where the midwife is aware that researchers are wishing mothers to take part in research projects, she should ensure as protector of the mother that full information is given to the mother, and that the research proceeds only if the mother's consent has been given. If she is not satisfied on these facts the midwife should be prepared to take up these points with the researchers. She should also make sure that she herself is fully informed about the research. The same principles apply when any medication is being given as part of a research project. If it is an unlicensed medicine which is given on the basis of a personal license to the doctor for a named patient the midwife should ensure that the mother is fully informed of the situation. If this does not appear to be the case, she should ask the doctor to explain the situation fully to the mother and obtain her full consent.

CONSENT AND RECORDS SEARCH

The giving of consent by the research subject provides a defence against an action for trespass to the person. However, where the nature of the research is the gathering of information from case records, is consent necessary? The answer is yes, since the disclosure of confidential information would be protected by the patient's right to sue for breach of confidentiality by the holder of records in giving access to the researcher. The Data Protection Act 1998 applies to both computerised and manually-held records and there would therefore have to be registration for the additional purpose of research. The consent of the LREC (see below) to undertake the research would also be required. Usually it would be sufficient to assure the mother that there would be no disclosure of personal information relating to her and that in any research publication the research subjects would not be identifiable.

LOCAL RESEARCH ETHICS COMMITTEES

The issues to be discussed here can be seen in Box 31.4.

Box 31.4 Local Research Ethics Committees

- Function and constitution

- Powers and sanctions (if any)

- Role in multi-centre trials

- Financial situation: charging for their services and the legal significance of this.

FUNCTION AND CONSTITUTION

In 1991 the NHS Management Executive issued a booklet entitled Local Research Ethics Committees, which gave detailed guidance on the establishment and function of LRECs, and the administrative framework within which they work, the ethical principles to which LRECs should have regard and particular groups of research subjects.[5] It was clearly stated that the responsibility for deciding whether a research project should proceed, within the NHS, lies with the NHS body under whose auspices the research would take place.

Any NHS body asked to agree a research proposal falling within its sphere of responsibility has to ensure that it has been submitted to the appropriate LREC for research ethics approval.

The role of the LREC is defined as being 'to consider the ethics of proposed research projects which will involve human subjects' and to advise the NHS body concerned. It is the NHS body which has the responsibility of deciding whether or not the project should go ahead, taking into account the ethical advice of the LREC. They are not 'in any sense management arms of the District Health Authority'.

NHS bodies include Special Health Authorities, NHS trusts and District Health Authorities.

Jurisdiction
The guidelines require the LREC to be consulted for any proposal shown in Box 31.5.

Box 31.5 Jurisdiction of LREC

LRECs should be consulted on any proposal which involves:

– NHS patients including those private sector patients treated under contract

– fetal material and IVF involving NHS patients

– the recently dead, in NHS premises

– access to the records of past or present NHS patients

– the use of, or potential access to, NHS premises or facilities.

The LREC MUST be consulted but the NHS body must also give permission before the project can proceed.

Constitution

Each District Health Authority should establish an LREC and provide it with administrative support but the LREC should be independent of the DHA.

It should have 8 to 12 members drawn from:

– hospital medical staff

– nursing staff

– General Practitioners

– two or more lay persons

and be drawn from both sexes and a wide age range.

The members are not to be representatives of the groups from which they are drawn but are 'appointed in their own right, to participate in the work of the LREC as individuals of sound judgement and relevant experience'. It is therefore envisaged that the meetings should be held in private and minutes taken which are confidential to the committee. This should enable the members to discuss the proposals freely.

The HA should consult with various professional groups before making the appointments and appointing a chairman and vice-chairman.

Members serve for terms of 3 to 5 years. They can be renewed but usually only once.

The LREC has the power to obtain advice from specialists or co-opt members to the committee to cover any relevant area of a research proposal on which the committee lacks expertise.

Working procedures

Decisions should be recorded, including the reasons given when research proposals are rejected, and these should be disclosed to the applicants. A register should be kept of all the proposals which come before it and should include the information shown in Box 31.6.

Box 31.6 Contents of Register kept by LREC

– Name and address of organisation carrying out the research

– Names and qualifications of the research team

– Details of the premises in which the research will be conducted

▶
- Medical support and other facilities available

- A brief description of what is required of the research subjects

- Confirmation of compliance with any other guidelines.

The register would not normally be open to the public but could be open to the NHS body for management purposes.

The researcher is required to notify the LREC of any significant deviation from the original protocol.

An Annual Report is required to be submitted to the relevant NHS body and Community Health Council. When CHCs are abolished the report will probably have to be submitted to the Patients' Forum (see Chapter 11). The report should contain the information shown in Box 31.7.

Box 31.7 Contents of Annual Report of LREC

- Names of committee members

- Number of meetings held

- List of proposals considered indicating approval, approval after amendment, rejection or withdrawal

The Annual Report should be available to public inspection.

POWERS AND SANCTIONS

The LREC has the power to give advice to the health service body on the approval of the project, the approval subject to modifications in the research protocol or the rejection of the project. Sometimes it might be advised that the researcher withdraws his project from the scrutiny of the LREC until a later (unspecified) time. It could object if the NHS body does not refer projects which come within its jurisdiction to it for approval. However it has no other powers.

ROLE IN MULTI-CENTRED TRIALS

The guidelines emphasise that each LREC is free to arrive at its own decision when considering a proposal which is planned to take place in more than one area. However it recommends that the committee should arrive at a voluntary arrangement under which one LREC is nominated to consider the issue on behalf of them all. It suggests that Health Authorities should encourage such networking.

FUNDING OF LREC AND THE MEMBERS

The guidelines assume that membership is voluntary and unpaid and that most of the members would be employees and therefore would be carrying out this work on behalf of their employers. The midwife might well be asked to be a member of an LREC or to be co-opted onto it to provide specific expertise, and she should therefore be aware of its functions and constitution and obtain a copy of the booklet from the Department of Health.[5]

CONFIDENTIALITY

Exactly the same principles apply in relation to the duty to recognise and keep confidential information obtained during research as apply in the treatment and care of patients. Reference should therefore be made to Chapter 10. Probably the same exceptions would also exist. However, these have not been tested in court. Disclosure in the public interest is likely to cause some difficulties and reference should therefore be made to the UKCC guidelines on professional practice.[6]

INJURIES TO THE SUBJECT OF THE RESEARCH

At the present time there has been no implementation of the suggestion made in the Royal Commission on Personal Injuries (The Pearson Report 1978)[7] that those persons who have been injured or harmed as a result of participation in a research project should receive compensation without proof of fault. Any such person must therefore prove that there has been negligence which has caused the harm which he has suffered. However, many research companies and particular drug companies offer compensation without the need to establish that there has been fault. An indemnity is offered both to the researchers and to the subjects when the research is agreed. If the midwife is involved in a research project, whatever her role, she should find out the details of any indemnity provision. The LREC will check the indemnity provisions before agreeing to a research project funded by a pharmaceutical company. The Department of Health at the time of writing is considering a new scheme for compensation for clinical negligence which may include a no-fault liability scheme. If this is implemented, those persons injured during a research project should receive compensation without proving negligence (see Chapter 14).

HEALTH AND SAFETY LAW

The researcher must be aware of all those laws relating to the health and safety of his colleagues and the general public before embarking on any research project. Reference should be made to Chapter 19.

PROJECT MANAGEMENT

Where the midwife is asked to be responsible for a research project she should be aware of the issues shown in Box 31.8.

Box 31.8 Issues arising in research project management

- Negligent advice

- Liability for supervising

- LRECs

- Contracts of employment

- Patients' rights

- Consent

- Data protection

- Confidentiality

- Access to records

- Health and safety

- External funding

Many of these topics are covered in earlier chapters. In this section emphasis will be placed upon the authorisation of the research project.

It is essential before research is commenced to consider who has the right to control the publication of results and to exercise any censorship over it. Control might vary according to who is funding the research and whether or not it is part of a contract of employment. Box 31.9 illustrates the different forms of projects from the perspective of funding and contracts. Box 31.10 looks at different projects from the perspective of their methods.

Box 31.9 Different forms of funding and control

1. As part of a contract of employment

   - funded externally without the employer's support

   - funded externally with the employer's support

   - for career development eg. for higher degree etc. with the financial support of the employer

   - for career development without the financial support of the employer.

2. Outside the contract of employment

   - with external funding

   - with no funding.

Box 31.10 Types of project

- Non-invasive

- Invasive

- Using financial resources

- With no financial resources

- Statistical

▶

▶
- Data collection

- Questionnaires

- Observations eg. case study

- Action linked

- Paper/library search

The midwife's role as a supervisor of research is shown in Box 31.11.

Box 31.11 Midwife's role as a supervisor of research

- Co-ordination

- Commissioning

- Conduct

- Counselling/advising

Areas of potential liability as a supervisor are shown in Box 31.12.

Box 31.12 Areas of potential liability

- Negligent delegation

- Negligent advice

- Failure to support the student

- Failure to obtain funding

- Failure to complete

- Ignorance of earlier research and activities

Before beginning the research project management, the midwife should ensure that she has obtained the relevant permissions to embark on the research. As has been seen this would include not only the approval of the Local Research Ethical Committee but also the approval of the Health Authority or NHS trust.

It is advisable to ensure that there is agreement over who has control over publications and editing the research outcomes.

During the project the project manager should ensure that the rules relating to consent are implemented and that the other legal pitfalls mentioned in this chapter are taken into account.

STANDARDS OF CARE AND THE RESULTS OF RESEARCH

One of the most difficult issues is knowing when research results are ready to be incorporated into the standards of care expected of the midwife. Some results are, for example, still of only an exploratory nature and too uncertain to affect current standards of care. An example is the debate over the administration of vitamin K, following research which seemed to suggest that if given intramuscularly it could cause side effects to babies (see Chapter 14).

This is an area where the midwife should keep alert to any changes in the standards which are required of her and take an immediate note of any instructions from the Committee for the Safety of Medicines and other authorities.

INTERNATIONAL CODES OF HUMAN RIGHTS

The midwife should be aware of those international codes which attempt to protect the human subject from abuses in research. Any LREC should take into account the principles relating to humane conduct of research. Codes such as the Declaration of Helsinki have not yet been incorporated into English law. However they are enforceable through the International Court of Human Rights. The Declaration of Helsinki was amended in Edinburgh in 2000. The European Convention on Human Rights which has been incorporated into the laws of the UK (see Chapter 6 and Appendix 1) will also be relevant in ensuring that research practice respects basic human rights.

CONCLUSION

The emphasis on practice which is research-based will mean that the midwife will be increasingly be required to ensure that her practice is in accordance with clinically effective standards which are based on reputable practice. In addition she will have responsibilities to ensure that the rights of the women she cares for, and who are asked to become research subjects, are respected. Useful databases for midwifery research are MIRIAD[8] and the NHS database known as the National Research Register (NRR).[9]

QUESTIONS AND EXERCISES

1. An obstetrician is researching on pain in childbirth and wants to send a research assistant to accompany you in your work in the community. What questions would you ask about the project and whose responsibility would it be to obtain the consent of the client?

2. You have been told by your manager that a midwifery student has to undertake a research project and you are asked to supervise it. What initial preparations would you make?

3. A client complains that she has just discovered that she has been prescribed a drug which is not generally approved for general use. What action do you take?

References

1 Rees C. 1997. *Introduction to Research for Midwives*. Oxford: Books for Midwives Press

2 See Phillips R. 1994. The need for research based midwifery practice. *British Journal of Midwifery*, 2(7), 335-8

3 Priestley KA, Campbell C, Valentine CB et al. 1992. Consent forms for research protocols. *British Medical Journal*, 305(6864), 1263-4. Reported in *MIDIRS Midwifery Digest*, March 1993 3:1

4 Burton v. Islington Health Authority [1992] 3 All ER 833 Court of Appeal

5 Department of Health. 1991. Local Research Ethics Committees. *Health Service Circular* (91)5

6 UKCC. 1998. *Guidelines on Professional Practice*. London: UKCC

7 Royal Commission on Civil Liability and Compensation for Personal Injury. 1978. Chaired by Lord Pearson Cmnd 7054. London: HMSO

8 www.leeds.ac.uk/miru/miriad.htm

9 www.doh.gov.uk/research/nrr.htm

Chapter 32
CHILD PROTECTION

Midwives may become involved in issues relating to child protection. It may be for example that other children of the pregnant woman have to be taken into care, or the midwife might be concerned about the health or safety of the unborn child immediately following delivery. It is essential that the midwife has an understanding of the relevant laws and knows the action which she must take. The law relating to consent by a child or young person under 18 years is considered in Chapter 7.

The Children Act 1989 brought into place a new framework for the law relating to children and whilst not repealing all previous legislation on children introduced significant new provisions. The main areas covered by the Act are shown in Box 32.1.

Box 32.1 Provisions of the Children Act 1989

1. General principles

2. Orders with respect to children in family proceedings

3. Local authority support for children and families

4. Care and supervision

5. Protection of children

6. Community homes

7. Voluntary homes and voluntary organisations

8. Registered children's homes

9. Private arrangements for fostering children

10. Child minding and day care for young children

11. Secretary of State's supervisory functions and responsibilities

12. Miscellaneous and general

In this chapter we shall consider the principles established by the Children Act 1989 and the law relating to child protection. The status of the fetus is considered in Chapter 17. The basic principle is that an unborn child lacks a legal personality and cannot be taken into care, nor made a ward of court.[1]

THE CHILDREN ACT 1989

PART 1: BASIC PRINCIPLES

Part 1 of the Act sets out the basic principles which are to apply in the law relating to children.

They are shown in Box 32.2. Of significance is the fact that the Act places the emphasis upon the duties and responsibilities of the parent rather than the rights of the parent. Even where the child is not living with the parent, this does not remove from the parent his/her responsibilities to the child.

Box 32.2 Principles in the Children Act 1989

1. Welfare of the child:

    i.   When a court determines any question in relation to the upbringing of a child or the administration of a child's property and the income from it, the child's welfare shall be the court's paramount consideration.

    ii. In any proceedings relating to the upbringing of the child, the court must have regard to the general principle that any delay in determining the question is likely to prejudice the welfare of the child.

    iii. The court shall have regard in particular to:

        a. the ascertainable wishes and feelings of the child concerned (considered in the light of his age and understanding)

        b. his physical, emotional and educational needs

        c. the likely effect on him of any change in his circumstances

        d. his age, sex, background and any characteristics of his which the court considers relevant

▶

▶

e.   any harm which he has suffered or is at risk of suffering

f.   how capable each of his parents, and any other person in relation to whom the court considers the question to be relevant, is of meeting his needs

g.   the range of powers available to the court under this Act in the proceedings in question.

PART 2: PARENTAL RESPONSIBILITY FOR CHILDREN

– Where a child's father and mother were married to each other at the time of his birth, they shall each have parental responsibility for the child.

– Where they were not married at the time of his birth, the mother shall have responsibility for the child; the father shall not have parental responsibility for the child unless he acquires it in accordance with the Act.

   (Provisions as to how parental responsibility can be acquired are laid down in the Act. See also Chapter 25 of this book.)

– More than one person may have parental responsibility for the same child at the same time.

– Where more than one person has parental responsibility for a child, each of them may act alone and without the other (or others) in meeting that responsibility.

PART 3: MEANING OF PARENTAL RESPONSIBILITY

Parental responsibility is defined as:

'all rights, duties, powers and responsibilities and authority which by law a parent of a child has in relation to the child and his property.'

Parents who fail to take reasonable care for the health and welfare of their children could be guilty of a criminal offence (see below and Chapter 7).

PART 4: ACQUISITION OF PARENTAL RESPONSIBILITY BY FATHER

The court has the power to provide for the father to have parental responsibility where the couple were not married at the time of the child's birth.

PART 5: POWERS OF NON-PARENT

The Children Act 1989 gives power to a person who does not have parental responsibility to make decisions on behalf of the child. The Children Act 1989 Section 3(5) provides that a person who (a) does not have parental responsibility for a particular child, but (b) has care of the child, may (subject to the provision of this Act) do what is reasonable in all the circumstances of the case for the purpose of safeguarding or promoting the child's welfare. This would probably include giving consent to necessary emergency treatment in the absence of the parents. In addition, professional staff would have a duty of care to take action to save life in such circumstances.

CHILD PROTECTION

Where the midwife has reasonable cause to suspect that a child in the family of a client is being abused she must take the appropriate action. To make a diagnosis of suspected child abuse is a weighty matter. As the guidelines on inter-agency co-operation (Paragraph 1.13) stated:[2]

'The difficulties of assessing the risk of harm to a child should not be underestimated. It is imperative that everyone who deals with allegations and suspicions of abuse maintains an open and inquiring mind.'

PROCEDURE FOR THE MANAGEMENT OF CHILD ABUSE

There should be in existence an agreed procedure for the management of child abuse cases and the midwife should be acquainted with this. The procedure should specifically refer to the role of the midwifery department if child abuse is suspected. This would require any professional staff working in the department who suspect that there is a possibility of ill-treatment, serious neglect, sexual or emotional abuse of a child, to inform the senior midwife or Consultant in charge of the department who should contact a Consultant paediatrician. If he confirms this possibility, then he should inform the Social Services Department immediately.

INTER-AGENCY CO-OPERATION

Working Together to Safeguard Children[3] is a guide to inter-agency working to safeguard and promote the welfare of children, which replaces the publication Working Together Under The Children Act 1989 published in 1991. It highlights the duties in the Children Act 1989 which require inter-agency co-operation.

There should be in existence in each local authority area, a forum to ensure co-operation between all the agencies involved in the protection of children at risk. This forum is known as the Area Child Protection Committee (ACPC). On this forum there should be representatives of the medical and nursing services. This representation should be at a senior level and there should be a designated senior professional for child protection within the hospital or community unit.

The ACPC has the tasks set out in Box 32.3.

Box 32.3 Tasks of Area Child Protection Committee (ACPC)

a. Establishing, maintaining and reviewing inter-agency guidelines on procedures to be followed in individual cases

b. Monitoring the implementation of legal procedures

c. Identifying significant issues arising from the handling of cases and reports from inquiries

d. Scrutinising arrangements to provide treatment, expert advice and inter-agency liaison and making recommendations to the responsible agencies

e. Scrutinising progress on work to prevent child abuse and making recommendations to the responsible agencies

f. Scrutinising the work related to inter-agency training and making recommendations to the responsible agencies

g. Conducting reviews required under Part 8 of the Guide

h. Publishing an Annual Report about local child protection matters.

Midwifery departments which serve a large catchment area might have to liaise with more than one ACPC.

What if the doctor disagrees with the midwife?
The midwife should ensure that her concerns are made known to a senior member of the midwifery staff who should decide whether it is appropriate to bring the Consultant in to see the child.

What about the midwife's duty of confidentiality?
Reference to the UKCC Guidelines on Professional Practice which cover confidentiality[4] will show that the registration body accepts that there are

circumstances when a breach of confidentiality is justified in the public interest. This would include any suspicion of child abuse. Such information could be passed onto the appropriate agencies without fear of a successful action for breach of confidentiality by the parents (see Chapter 10).

If a suspected case is reported to the police, social services, or NSPCC and it turns out that the suspicions are unfounded, the parents have no right to be given the name of the person reporting them. The House of Lords has held that it is not in the public interest for such information to be disclosed to the parents.[5]

CHILD PROTECTION REGISTER

Each local authority must maintain a Child Protection Register. The purpose of the Register is set out in Box 32.4.

Box 32.4 Purpose of Child Protection Register

- To provide a record of all children in the area who are currently the subject of a Child Protection Plan and to ensure that the plans are formally reviewed at least every six months

- To provide a central point of speedy inquiry for professional staff who are worried about a child and want to know whether the child is the subject of a Child Protection Plan

- To provide statistical information about current trends in the area.

Access to the Child Protection Register would be permitted to an agreed list of personnel which would include senior medical staff or paediatric social workers in the local hospital departments.

WHAT IF THE CHILD IS NOT ON THE REGISTER AND ABUSE IS NOT CERTAIN?

If the Consultant is not able to confirm that this is a case of suspected child abuse, and there were no medical grounds for requiring the child to be detained in hospital, then the parent could not be stopped from taking the child home. However there should be arrangements in place for all such concerns to be notified to the appropriate health visitor or school nurse and also to the appropriate General Practitioner.

WHAT IF SUSPECTED CHILD ABUSE IS CONFIRMED BY THE CONSULTANT PAEDIATRICIAN?

The agreed procedures and the inter-agency arrangements should be followed immediately. The provisions of the Children Act 1989 enable the orders set out in Boxes 32.5, 32.6 and 32.7 to be made.

Box 32.5 Child assessment order (Section 43)

This is available where the court is satisfied that the applicant has reasonable cause to suspect that the child is suffering or likely to suffer significant harm. An assessment is required to determine whether or not the child is suffering or is likely to suffer significant harm, and it is unlikely that an assessment can be carried out without an order being made.

Notice must be given of an application for a child assessment order to the child's parents, any person, not the parent, but who has parental responsibility for him, any other person caring for the child and others who have a contact order.

The child assessment order cannot not be made if the court is satisfied that there are grounds for making an emergency protection order and that it ought to make that order rather than an assessment order. The order must specify the date by which the assessment is to begin and the period for which it will have effect, such period not exceeding 7 days beginning with the date specified in the order. The effect of the order is that it authorises any person carrying out the assessment or any part of the assessment, to do so in accordance with the terms of the order (Section 43(7)). The child has the right (Section 43(8)), if he is of sufficient understanding to make an informed decision, to refuse to submit to a medical or psychiatric examination or other assessment.

Box 32.6 Emergency protection order (Section 44)

If the court is satisfied that there is reasonable cause to believe (in the case of an application by a person) that the child is likely to suffer significant harm if:

a. he is not removed to accommodation provided by or on behalf of the applicant; or

b. he does not remain in the place in which he is then being accommodated;

then the court can order that an emergency protection order be made.

▶

▶ Where the applicant is a local authority it must show that enquiries are being made under Section 47(1)(b) (local authority's duty to investigate) and these enquiries are being frustrated by access to the child being unreasonably refused, and the applicant has reasonable cause to believe that access to the child is required as a matter of urgency (Section 44(1)(b)). An application may also be made by the NSPCC as an authorised person.

Box 32.7 Removal and accommodation of children by police in cases of emergency

This section enables the child to be taken into police protection. Where a constable believes that a child would be likely to suffer significant harm he may remove the child to suitable accommodation and keep him there. He may also take reasonable steps to ensure that the child's removal from hospital, or other place in which he is being accommodated, is prevented. The section lasts a maximum of 72 hours.

For further details of the sections shown in Boxes 32.5, 32.6 and 32.7 and the other provisions of the Children Act 1989 reference should be made to the Department of Health guides to the Children Act 1989.[6]

PROTECTION OF VULNERABLE ADULTS AND CHILDREN

Various measures have been taken in law to prevent those who are likely to abuse children from having contact with them. The Protection of Children Act 1999, the Sexual Offenders Act 1997 and the Care Standards Act 2000 enable employers to establish if there are grounds for not employing prospective employees.

THE PROTECTION OF CHILDREN ACT 1999

The Protection of Children Act 1999 makes statutory the Department of Health's Consultancy Service Index list and it requires childcare organisations to refer the names of individuals considered unsuitable to work with children for inclusion on the list. It also provides rights of appeal against inclusion and requires regulated childcare organisations to check the names of anyone they propose to employ in posts involving regular contact with children with the list and not to employ them if listed. Finally it amends Part V of the Police Act 1997 to allow the Criminal Records Bureau to act as a central access point for criminal records information, List 99[7] and the new Department of Health list. In other words, the Criminal Records Bureau will act as a one stop shop in the carrying out of checks.

The effect of the legislation is that organisations such as health trusts who work with children have a statutory duty from October 2000 to vet prospective employees, paid or unpaid, for work involving contact with children. From October 2000 organisations who have registered with the DoH will be able to check names from their own computers via the internet. In October 2000 there were about 1000 names on the DoH Consultancy Service Index,[8] who had been notified to the DoH because they had been dismissed from childcare posts or who have left such a post in circumstances where the employer considered that a child would be at risk of harm from them.

THE SEXUAL OFFENDERS ACT 1997

The Sexual Offenders Act 1997 was passed in order to ensure that once a sex offender had served his sentence and was about to be released, he would still be subject to some form of supervision to protect persons against the risk of his re-offending. Part 1 of the Act requires the notification of information to the police by persons who have committed certain sexual offences.

SEXUAL OFFENCES (AMENDMENT) ACT 2000

Under this Act the age at which certain sexual acts (for example homosexual acts in private) are lawful is reduced to 16 years and a new defence is available so that when one party to homosexual activity is below the age of 16 and the other over 16, the younger one does not commit any offence. However a new offence is introduced for a person 'A' over 18 years to have sexual intercourse with a person or engage in any other sexual activity with another person 'B' if A is in a position of trust in relation to B. 'Position of trust' is defined in Section 4 where B is detained in an institution or resident in a home, or cared for in a hospital, residential care home or nursing home, where A is looking after such persons, or A looks after persons under 18 who are receiving full-time education at an educational institution and B is receiving such education.

CARE STANDARDS ACT 2000

Under Part VII of the Care Standards Act statutory provision is made for setting up a list of individuals who are considered unsuitable to work with vulnerable adults. There is to be a single list established for both England and Wales and it will operate in a similar way to the list established under the Protection of Children Act 1999.

TRAINING

It is essential that all midwives should be given the opportunity to be trained in the local child protection procedure and the role and function of the ACPC and its procedures. It is essential that in this emotive area the midwife should feel confident in her knowledge of the policy and procedures which should be followed. The training should also include an understanding of the provisions of the Children Act 1989 and the recommendations of the reports of inquiries into the handling of child abuse cases, such as the Cleveland report.

RECORD KEEPING

Whether or not child abuse is confirmed at the time of the visit, the records of the midwife relating to that visit could be extremely significant evidence in the future. If there is a case conference and a court case, the midwife might well be required to give evidence of her meeting with the parent and child and the examination which she carried out. Since this might take place at an uncertain date in the future, she will be extremely reliant upon the comprehensiveness and clarity of her records.

DISPUTES WITH PARENTS

Parents may not always take the best course for their children and the question arises at what stage would a midwife be justified in intervening. For example, in Chapter 29 a case is discussed when the judge ordered an HIV test to be carried out on a baby, contrary to the wishes of the mother. The situation in relation to triple vaccine gives rise to similar issues (see Chapter 28).

CRIMINAL OFFENCE

In some circumstances the failure of a parent to take approved medical advice for their child can result in criminal proceedings. A Rastafarian couple who had refused on religious grounds to allow their diabetic daughter who was nine years old to be given insulin were convicted of manslaughter on October 28th 1993 in Nottingham. The father was given a sentence of imprisonment and the mother a suspended sentence.[9] They believed in using homeopathic medicine.[10] This is, of course, an extreme circumstance. In 2001 parents[11] who had fed their baby daughter a fruit-only diet pleaded guilty of cruelty to a child, when she died of a chest infection brought on by malnutrition. A manslaughter charge was left on the file.

APPROVED MEDICAL OPINION

As in the HIV case, in almost all cases where parents have disputed medical recommendations about treatment for their patients, the courts have supported the doctors' views. One significant case where this did not happen was where parents refused to permit a liver transplant to take place on their toddler. The Court of Appeal held that in the very specific circumstances of the case (the parents lived abroad and as health professionals they believed the transplant not to be in the best interests of the child) the transplant would not be ordered against their wishes.[12] In contrast, there are several cases where the courts have ordered blood transfusions to be given to children of Jehovah's Witnesses[13] (see Chapter 7).

PARENTAL RIGHTS AND RESPONSIBILITIES

The Children Act 1989 placed the emphasis on parental responsibilities rather than parental rights. Such responsibilities remain after divorce and care orders and will only cease with the death of the parent or the death or adoption of the child. Gradually, however, the room for manoeuvre of decision making of the parents is reducing. A decision of the European Court of Human Rights ruled that it was unlawful for a parent to use corporal punishment on a child (see Chapter 6). A father was given an admonishment after he was found guilty of smacking his child in a dentist's waiting room.[14] It is illegal for corporal punishment to be used by teachers in schools in this country. The government has provided advice to parents on how only limited corporal punishment can be used by parents. For example they should not smack the child above the neck and an instrument should not be used.

Could the parents have access to the midwife's and other professionals' records?

The Provisions of the Data Protection Act 1998 apply to both computerised and manually-held records. Where the patient is a child, an application for access can be made by a person having parental responsibility for the patient. However, access can be denied if the holder of the record is satisfied either

a. that the patient has consented (this would not be possible in the case of a very young child), or

b. that the patient is incapable of understanding the nature of the application and the giving of access would be in his best interests.

In addition, partial access must be refused by the holder to any part of the record which in the opinion of the holder of the record, would disclose

a. information provided by the patient in the expectation that it would not be disclosed to the applicant, or

b. information obtained as a result of any examination or investigation to which the patient consented in the expectation that the information would not be so disclosed. (Section 5(3)) (see Chapter 10)

CONCLUSIONS

Midwives may become involved in child protection cases or care proceedings. They should take advice from senior management or from lawyers to the trust. Their documentation is likely to come under close scrutiny in any conflict (see Chapter 15). Legal problems arising from teenage pregnancies have been considered by the author.[15]

QUESTIONS AND EXERCISES

1. A 15-year-old is expecting a child and an internal examination is necessary. The client is considered too young to give a valid consent. Could consent be given by an aunt who is accompanying her?

2. There is concern about the possibility of a client abusing her two-year-old child, and about the future safety of the unborn child. What action should the midwife take?

3. A 13-year-old girl who is expecting a baby is considered to be in need of care, what should the midwife do?

References

1 Re F (in utero) [1988] 2 All ER 193

2 Home Office, Department of Health, Department of Education and Science, Welsh Office. 1991. *Working Together Under the Children Act 1989: a guide to arrangements for inter-agency co-operation for the protection of children from abuse.* London: HMSO

3 Department of Health, Home Office, Department for Education and Employment, the National Assembly for Wales. 1999. *Working together to safeguard children.* London: Department of Health

4 UKCC. 1996. Guidelines for Professional Practice. London: UKCC

5 D v. NSPCC [1977] 1 All ER 589

6 Department of Health. 1990. *An introductory guide to the Children Act for the NHS.* London: HMSO

7 List 99 is a list held by the Department for Education and Employment of those considered unsuitable to work with children. It has always been a statutory list.

8 Department of Health. Press Notice 2 October 2000

9 *The Times*, 29 October 1993

10 *The Times*, 6 November 1993

11 Gregoriadis L and Peek L. 2001. Baby starved to death on fruit diet. *The Times*, 14 July 2001

12 Re C (a minor)(medical treatment – refusal of parental consent) [1997] 8 Med LR 166 CA

13 For example Re E(a minor)(wardship: medical treatment) Family Division [1993] 1 FLR 386

14 Cramb A. Father who smacked his daughter goes free. *The Daily Telegraph*, 10 June 1999

15 Dimond B. 2002. Teenage pregnancy and the law. *British Journal of Midwifery*, 10(2), 1005-8

Chapter 33
THE CARE OF THE MENTALLY DISORDERED

Like any other practitioner, the midwife could find herself dealing with patients who suffer from mental disorder. This includes both those suffering from a mental illness and also those who have learning disabilities. Because of the dangers of postnatal depression and puerperal fever to the mother and child it is essential that the midwife has a good understanding of the help which is to hand, the legal powers which exist if intervention is necessary and what action she should take. It is not the intention here to provide the midwife with a comprehensive account of the law relating to mental disorder, but rather to raise her awareness of the issue and to enable her to know how to seek further information.

At present the law relating to compulsory admission of mentally disordered patients is laid down in the Mental Health Act 1983. There are however currently discussions on major changes and a White Paper has been published. Draft legislation is at present awaited.

The philosophy behind the Mental Health Act 1983 is that where possible patients suffering from mental disorder should be treated without admission to psychiatric hospitals. If admission is required then it should be on the basis of informal admission. Only where there is no alternative to detention should the powers of compulsory admission in the Act be used.

Most patients would therefore be cared for in the community with assistance from the community psychiatric nurse with overall responsibility taken by the General Practitioner assisted by out-patient referrals to a Consultant psychiatrist. Mothers may require specialist help and advice if they are taking anti-psychotic or anti-depressant medication when they become pregnant. The midwife should ensure that she is aware of any possible contraindications for medication at all times during and after the pregnancy. If admission to hospital becomes necessary, most patients would agree to informal (i.e. voluntary) admission. The midwife should discuss with the patient and the hospital staff the antenatal care required by the mother and the arrangements to be made when labour commences trying to ensure that the mother's wishes are obtained and respected.

Unfortunately, one of the characteristics of some forms of mental disorder is an absence of insight and therefore it is necessary in certain exceptional circumstances to arrange for the admission of a person compulsorily to hospital for in-patient treatment. This may be necessary following confinement if it is suspected that the mother is suffering from puerperal disorder or severe postnatal depression. Most districts now have a mother and baby unit and the midwife should ensure that she is aware of the location of these, since it may be that, with assurance, the mother might be prepared to accept informal admission to such a unit if she knows that she can take the baby with her. If the midwife is aware that no such provision has been made, she could take up the issue with her supervisor and the Health Authority. It may be possible for admission to such a unit to be provided on the basis of an out of the catchment area referral.

DEFINITION OF MENTAL DISORDER

No person can be compulsorily detained under the Mental Health Act 1983 unless she is suffering from mental disorder as defined in the Act. The definition is set out in Box 33.1.

Box 33.1 Definition of mental disorder

Mental illness, arrested or incomplete development of mind, psychopathic disorder and any other disorder or disability of mind.

All the terms except 'mental illness' are further defined in the Act.

The Act makes if clear that a person cannot be dealt with under the Act as suffering from mental disorder 'by reason only of promiscuity or other immoral conduct, sexual deviancy or dependence on alcohol or drugs.' This means that if a woman is pregnant and abusing drugs she cannot be detained under the Mental Health Act 1983 unless she is shown to be suffering from mental disorder apart from the drug abuse.

COMPULSORY ADMISSION

There are three main sections for the compulsory admission of the mentally disordered person (other than through the courts). These are shown in Box 33.2.

Box 33.2 Compulsory admission for mental disorder

Section 4 emergency admission for assessment for up to 72 hours

Section 2 admission for assessment for up to 28 days

Section 3 admission for treatment for up to 6 months.

Section 4

This is an emergency admission section and enables a person to be detained for up to 72 hours on the basis of one medical recommendation. It must be established that it is of urgent necessity for the admission for assessment and that compliance with the provisions for two medical recommendations would involve undesirable delay. The patient can be detained under Section 4 for up to 72 hours. The requirements for Sections 2 and 4 are shown in Box 33.3.

Box 33.3 Medical requirements for Sections 2 and 4

a. The patient is suffering from mental disorder of a nature or degree which warrants the detention of the patient in a hospital for assessment (or for assessment followed by medical treatment) for at least a limited period; and

b. he ought to be so detained in the interests of his own health or safety or with a view to the protection of other persons.

The applicant is usually an approved social worker though, as with the other two Sections, it could be the 'nearest relative'. The approved social worker is 'approved' because she/he has undergone a special training in mental health. In applying for a Section 4 admission the approved social worker has to explain why a second medical recommendation for admission could not be obtained. The application is made to the managers of the appropriate hospital and the application gives authority to ambulance men or police to transfer the patient to the hospital.

Section 2

This is an application for assessment and under this the person can be detained for up to 28 days. There must be two medical recommendations, one of them from a doctor who is recognised as having the required expertise in psychiatric medicine, i.e. he is approved under Section 12 of the Act and is colloquially called a 'Section 12 doctor'. One of the two doctors should have had previous acquaintance with the patient and if this is not possible the approved social worker must explain the reasons why on the application form. The medical requirements shown in Box 33.3 must be present.

Section 3

This is an admission for treatment and can last up to six months. Two medical recommendations are required but unlike Section 2 a specific form of mental disorder must be specified (see Box 33.4). The other requirements shown in Box 33.4 must be present. Again one of the medical recommendations must be by a section 12 approved doctor and preferably at least one of the doctors should have had previous acquaintance with the patient. The nearest relative should be consulted over the application by the approved social worker and has the right to object to the application being made.

Box 33.4 Medical requirements for Section 3 admission

a. He is suffering from mental illness, severe mental impairment, psychopathic disorder or mental impairment and his mental disorder is of a nature of degree which makes it appropriate for him to receive medical treatment in a hospital; and

b. In the case of psychopathic disorder or mental impairment, such treatment is likely to alleviate or prevent a deterioration of his condition; and

c. It is necessary for the health or safety of the patient or for the protection of other persons that he should receive such treatment and it cannot be provided unless he is detained under this section.

Definition of nearest relative

The relative who is 'nearest' is defined by statute (Section 26 of the Mental Health Act 1983). Where the patient is married it would be the spouse. A cohabitee would count as the nearest relative where the couple had been living together for a period of not less than six months. A person other than a relative could be classified as a relative if he/she had been ordinarily living with the patient for at least five years.

TREATMENT FOR MENTAL DISORDER

Compulsory treatment for mental disorder can be given under the Act to the patient detained under either Section 2 or Section 3, but not to the patient who is detained under Section 4. This is so even though Section 2 is described as admission for assessment.

Box 33.5 shows the treatments which can be given and the conditions required.

Box 33.5 Treatment for mental disorder

Section 57 Surgery destroying brain tissue, hormonal implants to control sexual urge. The patient must consent and the understanding of the patient to consent should be certified by three persons appointed by the Mental Health Act Commission, one of whom must be a registered medical practitioner. The latter must certify that the treatment should be given.

Section 58 Medication after three months and electroconvulsive therapy. The patient must either consent or a second opinion must be obtained from an

▶

independent doctor appointed by the Mental Health Act Commission.

Section 63 Any treatment not covered by Section 57 and 58 which is given for mental disorder under the direction of the responsible medical officer.

Section 62 Enables the provisions of the above Sections to be dispensed with in an emergency situation.

It should be noted that if medication is required after 3 months and the mother is either unable or unwilling to give consent, a second opinion doctor must be called in to decide if the treatment should be given. He has a duty to examine the patient, determine whether the patient is incapable of giving consent or is refusing consent, talk to the responsible medical officer about the proposed treatment, and decide whether the treatment should be given against the patient's will. Before he decides he must consult with two persons: one a nurse who is professionally concerned with the treatment of the patient, the other who is neither doctor nor nurse who is also professionally concerned with the patient. This latter person could be a midwife if she is sufficiently involved with the patient. The second opinion advisory doctor (SOAD) merely has to record on the statutory form (Form 39) the names of the nurse and the other professional whom he has consulted. He does not have to record what their advice was. If the midwife were to be the second professional to be consulted it would be advisable for her to ensure that she records in her patient records the content of her advice to the SOAD.

The midwife must of course take particular precautions to ensure that any treatment being given for mental disorder will not be harmful to the pregnancy or breastfeeding.

In one case[1] (which is discussed in Chapter 7) the judge decided that the woman, who was suffering from paranoid schizophrenia, was detained in a psychiatric hospital under Section 3 and was refusing to have a Caesarean operation, could be given a Caesarean operation under Section 63 of the Mental Health Act 1983 as being treatment for mental disorder. This decision is highly disputed and since the decision in Re MB[2] and in the case of St George's Hospital[3] is unlikely to be followed.

COMMON LAW POWERS

If life-saving treatment is required for the patient who is admitted under Section 4 then it could be given under the powers which exist at common law under the Re F ruling. (For further discussion on this see Chapter 7.)

Again, any treatment must take into account the pregnancy or if the mother is feeding the baby.

THE INFORMAL IN-PATIENT

If the mother is already in hospital as an informal patient and wishes to take her own discharge and it would be dangerous to her health or safety or to other people for her to do so, she could be detained. See Boxes 33.6 and 33.7.

Box 33.6 Holding power of the nurse (Section 5(4))

This enables a nurse qualified in mental disorder to prevent an informal patient who is being treated for mental disorder from leaving the hospital. The detention can exist for up to 6 hours but it will end as soon as the patient's own doctor (or his nominee) arrives to see the patient. He may then, following an examination of the patient, decide to detain the patient further.

Box 33.7 Power of doctor to detain an in-patient (Section 5(2))

This enables the patient's doctor or his nominee to detain the patient for up to 72 hours to enable an application to be considered for admission under the Mental Health Act 1983. It may be that after the doctor has examined the patient it is decided that compulsorily admission is not necessary and the section will then end and the patient will become informal. Alternatively, following examination by the patient's own doctor and by another doctor and the approved social worker an application is made under Section 2 or Section 3.

RENEWAL

Section 4, Section 2, Section 5(4) and Section 5(2) are not renewable. A patient on Section 2 who needs to be detained for longer can be further detained on Section 3. Section 3 can be renewed for a further six months and then for one year at a time. The procedure for the renewal is that the responsible medical officer in charge of the patient's care examines the patient, within the period of two months ending with the date the Section is due to end and, if it appears to him that the specific condition of mental disorder is present and the other conditions required by Section 20 are present, he must furnish to the managers a report to that effect and the patient's detention is then renewed. The managers in their review can decide that the patient should be discharged.

APPEALS AGAINST DETENTION

The patient can appeal to a Mental Health Review Tribunal (MHRT) for discharge or to the managers of the hospital. There are set times for applying to the MHRT but not to the managers. The nearest relative also has the right to apply to an MHRT if his/her attempt to discharge the patient under Section 23 has been barred by the responsible medical officer under Section 25. Either patient or nearest relative can apply to the MHRT if the specific form of mental disorder is reclassified under Section 16.

Where a patient has not himself applied for a Mental Health Review Tribunal hearing during the first six months and after that at least once every three years, the managers of the hospital have a duty to refer the patient to the MHRT. (In the case of those under 16 years, the time limit is every year.)

It may be that, if the midwife has remained in close contact with the patient during a period of detention, a report and/or oral evidence might be required from the midwife at the hearing giving her views upon the discharge.

INFORMATION TO THE PATIENT

One of the duties on the managers introduced by the 1983 Act is to ensure that the patient receives both in writing and orally information relating to her Section, the right to apply to the managers and the Mental Health Review Tribunal, and the rules relating to consent to treatment. This duty is usually delegated by the managers to the nursing staff or the medical records staff. Leaflets are available giving the information for each of the different Sections and these are available in a wide variety of languages. A midwife who has a client detained in hospital should ask to see the leaflet so that she herself understands the implications of the Section the patient is under.

Information to the nearest relative

The information which is given to the patient must also be given in writing to the nearest relative. However the patient has a statutory right to object to this information being given to the nearest relative.

The managers

In respect of an NHS trust these are the non-executive board members and only they, with their co-opted members can carry out the function of hearing appeals to the managers by the patient against detention or renewing the patient's detention following a report from the responsible medical officer. Other functions in respect of the Mental Health Act can be delegated to officers.

THE MENTAL HEALTH ACT COMMISSION

In 1983 a watchdog for detained patients was established, known as the Mental Health Act Commission. It consists of about 90 different professionals and lay people whose jurisdiction is to visit the detained patients and to take up any complaints from them where they are not satisfied by the response from the managers, or any other complaint relating to the exercise of powers and duties under the Mental Health Act. It also has statutory duties in relation to the withholding of mail in the special hospitals (i.e. Broadmoor, Rampton and Ashworth). It also has a duty every other year to provide a report to the Secretary of State which he must place before each House of Parliament.

CODE OF PRACTICE

The Secretary of State has a duty to prepare a Code of Practice. A third edition has been published and midwives who are involved in the care of mothers with a mental disorder would find this a useful tool of reference.

Caesareans and mental disorder

There have been examples where pregnant women being treated for mental disorder under the Mental Health Act 1983 have been compelled to undergo a Caesarean section. These are considered in Chapter 7 where the guidance from the Court of Appeal is discussed.

Protection of vulnerable adults

Legislation establishing lists of those who are a potential danger to children and vulnerable adults, and statutory requirements to consult these lists, are considered in Chapter 32. Midwives caring for women with learning disabilities have a responsibility as part of their duty of care to take into account their level of capacity to make decisions and should ensure that their standards of information giving and communication with the women take into account the disabilities. In November 2001 an Oxford midwife who shouted at a mother and her partner, both of whom had a learning disability, told them that their newborn twins would be taken away from them by social services, was removed from the Register following a hearing before the UKCC Professional Conduct Committee.

FUTURE CHANGES

Major changes to our present mental health law are currently being proposed. An expert committee was set up by the government in 1998 under the chairmanship of Professor Richardson to review the Mental Health Act 1983. Its terms of reference included the degree to which the current legislation needs updating, and to ensure that there is a proper balance between safety (both of individuals and the wider community) and the rights of individual patients. It was required to advise the government on how mental health legislation should be shaped to reflect contemporary patterns of care and treatment and to support its policy as set out in Modernising Health Services.[4] The Expert Committee presented its preliminary proposals, which set out the principles on which any future legislation should be based, in April 1999, and its full report was published in November 1999.[5] The government presented its proposals for reform in 1999, with a final date for response by 31st March 2000.[6] The proposals include the reasons for proposed changes and cover the following topics:

- Guiding principles for a new mental health act
- Processes of applying compulsory powers
- Criteria for compulsory care and treatment
- The new tribunal's remit
- Discharge and aftercare
- Interface with the criminal justice system
- Treatment
- Safeguards.

At the time of writing, a bill is awaited for legislation to progress through Parliament.

NATIONAL SERVICE FRAMEWORKS

The government has published National Service Frameworks for different specialties to ensure that there is a minimum standard of provision across the country. The National Service Frameworks for Mental Health were published in 1999 and set standards in five areas:

- Standard one: Mental health promotion
- Standards two and three: Primary care and access to services
- Standards four and five: Effective services for people with severe mental illness
- Standards six: Caring about carers
- Standard seven: Preventing suicide

The implementation of these standards will be overseen by the Commission for Health Improvement on its inspection visits to hospitals.

CONCLUSION

Major changes are to take place in the care of the mentally disordered. It is essential that the rights of the mentally disordered pregnant woman are safeguarded and appropriate provision made for the care of the mother and baby. Midwives have an important role to play in ensuring that high standards are set and implemented and in order to secure this a good understanding of the mental health laws is essential. They also need to ensure that the rights of the mentally ill pregnant women are protected, particularly in relation to the law of consent and compulsory Caesareans (see Chapter 7).

QUESTIONS AND EXERCISES

1. You are concerned that a patient of yours who is extremely depressed and is 36 weeks pregnant might be in need of assistance. You have discussed this with her but she refuses to see her General Practitioner or seek other help. What action do you take?

2. You visit a mother who gave birth two days ago, and she seems very disturbed and irrational. You are worried about her mental health. She has made it clear that she would refuse to see her General Practitioner and would not be prepared to consider informal admission for treatment. What action do you take and what is your legal liability?

References

1 Tameside and Glossop Acute Services Trust v. CH [1996] 31 BMLR 93

2 Re MB (an adult: medical treatment) [1997] 2 FLR 426

3 St George's Healthcare NHS Trust v. S; R. v. Collins ex parte S [1998]; 44 BMLR 160 CA

4 Department of Health. 1998. *Modernising Mental Health Services*. London: HMSO

5 Department of Health. 1999. *Expert Committee Review of the Mental Health Act 1983*. London: HMSO

6 Department of Health. 1999. *Reform of the Mental Health Act 1983*. London: HMSO

Chapter 34
COMPLEMENTARY THERAPIES

The popularity of complementary and alternative therapies has increased dramatically over recent years both within and outside the NHS. Midwives are increasingly likely to be caring for women who are interested in using in place of or in addition to orthodox treatments a wide variety of complementary and alternative therapies. This chapter briefly sets out the law relating to complementary therapy practice in relation to midwifery practice and considers the following topics:

– Definition of complementary therapies

– Clients who are involved in a complementary therapy:

    disclosure to the midwife

    ignorance on the part of the midwife

– The midwife as complementary therapist

    agreement of employer

    consent of the woman

    defining standards

– Use of complementary therapies in midwifery

– National developments

More detailed analysis of the law for the practitioner in a complementary therapy and the legal implications of many different therapies are to be found in a book by this author.[1] The RCM has also issued a position paper on complementary therapies and the midwife.[2]

Midwives are affected by the increase in the popularity of complementary therapies in two ways:

- Some are undertaking training in a therapy regarded as complementary to conventional medicine.

- Others are aware that the mothers they care for are consulting practitioners in complementary medicine therapies and may be taking homeopathic or herbal remedies or other treatment at the same time as receiving orthodox treatments.

DEFINITION OF COMPLEMENTARY THERAPIES

'Complementary' is defined as: completing: together making up a whole... of medical treatment, therapies, etc... (Pamphlet of the British Complementary Medicine Association (BCMA)[3]) It is thus seen to work in parallel with orthodox medicine. The BCMA therefore states that therapy groups which are represented by the BCMA advise and encourage patients to see their doctor wherever appropriate. The House of Lords select committee on science and technology held an inquiry into complementary medicine. It reported[4] in November 2000 and recommended that there should be regulations of complementary and alternative medicines and there should be further research to evaluate their effectiveness. It divided such therapies into three groups:

a. Professionally organised therapies, where there is some scientific evidence of their success, though seldom of the highest quality, and there are recognised systems for treatment and training of practitioners. This group includes acupuncture, chiropractic, herbal medicine, homeopathy and osteopathy.

b. Complementary medicines where evidence that they work is generally lacking but which are used as an adjunct rather than a replacement for conventional therapies, so that lack of evidence may not matter so much. Included in this group are Alexander Technique, aromatherapy, nutritional medicine, hypnotherapy and Bach and other flower remedies.

c. Techniques that offer diagnosis as well as treatment, but for which scientific evidence is almost completely lacking. This group cannot be supported and includes naturopathy, crystal therapy, kinesiology, radionics, dowsing and iridology.

The Select Committee of the House of Lords considered that some remedies such as acupuncture and aromatherapy should be available on the NHS, and NHS patients should have wider access to osteopathy and chiropractics. The implementation of these recommendations will lead to fundamental changes in how complementary and alternative therapies are viewed in relation to orthodox medicine and within the NHS.

519

THE CLIENT IN COMPLEMENTARY THERAPY

DISCLOSURE TO THE MIDWIFE

When a woman is referred to a midwife in the NHS, then information relating to that person's care within the NHS would also be given. Thus the midwife should have basic information about the client in order to determine the care which is required by the woman. In addition, the midwife would usually have access to health records kept on the woman, to ensure that her care is compatible with other treatment that she is receiving.

In contrast, where the woman is receiving treatment from a complementary therapist, there is usually no official way in which this information can be made known to the midwife other than through the woman. The midwife therefore relies upon the openness of the woman in disclosing information which may be relevant to the care and treatment provided during the pregnancy.

Clearly the importance of this communication between woman and midwife will depend upon the relevance of the complementary therapy to the pregnancy. Some therapies may have little effect; others, such as acupuncture and homeopathy, may have a significant effect on the recommendations the midwife may make. If there is a conflict between the two treatments, then the midwife and therapists need to discuss this with the woman who should be given the choice over which course to pursue.

IGNORANCE ON THE PART OF THE MIDWIFE

Does it matter if the midwife has no knowledge of the complementary therapy which the patient is undergoing? The answer is that it may have an important effect, and had the midwife been aware of certain information about the therapy she may have advised the woman differently. Where harm has occurred, expert evidence on causation would be required to show whether anything the midwife had done could have caused that harm. It is hoped that in reviewing the practice of the midwife, it would be revealed that the woman had been receiving treatment from other persons. In the light of this, any liability on the part of each of these persons could be analysed. Reasonable practice would require that once a midwife ascertains that the woman is receiving alternative or complementary therapies, then the midwife should make all reasonable inquiries (eg. from the complementary therapist or from others who could be reasonably be expected to point out any contraindications) so that the woman and baby are reasonably safe.

THE MIDWIFE AS COMPLEMENTARY MEDICINE THERAPIST

AGREEMENT OF EMPLOYER

It is recognised that many midwives are considering the use of complementary therapies in the care of mothers and babies. If a midwife obtains a training in a complementary therapy, she should ensure that she obtains the agreement of the employer before she uses this skill as part of her practice as a midwife. If she fails to do this and causes harm to the patient whilst using her complementary therapy skills, then her employer could argue that she was not acting in course of employment when she caused the harm. It is therefore not vicariously liable for the harm, but the midwife must accept personal liability for the harm which has been caused. (In the light of a recent case such an argument by the employer may not succeed: see the discussion on vicarious liability in Chapter 13.)

If the NHS trust gives expressed or implied consent to complementary therapies being used by a midwife then her work in this field could be seen as being in the course of employment, in which case the NHS trust would be vicariously liable for the harm which has been caused. On the other hand, if the NHS trust were unaware of the complementary therapy work, then it may refuse to accept vicarious liability for any harm caused by her complementary therapy, arguing that the work was not performed in the course of her employment as a practitioner (see Chapter 13 on vicarious liability). In this case the midwife would be personally liable.

It is also essential for the midwife to obtain the consent of the employer if she intends to use her complementary therapy skills privately during working hours. In the case of Watling v. Gloucester County Council Employment[5] an occupational therapist was dismissed when he saw private patients for alternative therapy during working hours. His application for unfair dismissal failed. He had been warned by his employers not to conduct his private business during his working hours and lunch times were for a break, not for private work.

CONSENT OF THE WOMAN

It is also essential that the woman should explicitly give consent before the midwife is allowed to use any complementary therapies on her. The basic principles of obtaining consent apply (see Chapter 7) but since a woman would not normally expect a midwife to be providing complementary therapies, it is imperative that the midwife gives full details of all that is involved and makes it absolutely clear that the mother is fully entitled to receive the treatment usually provided by the midwife even though she refuses the complementary medicine treatment and care. It is preferable to obtain the consent in writing and to put in a leaflet the information which the woman should be told about the treatment.

DEFINING STANDARDS

One of the difficulties of some complementary therapies is that there may not be a clear definition of the expected standard of care. If harm were to occur to a woman and the woman wished to claim compensation, she would have to establish that the midwife, in using her complementary therapy skills, failed to use the reasonable standard of care which she was entitled to expect from her. This may not be easy to prove. Reference must be made to the various bodies providing accreditation for individual therapies on what would be regarded as the reasonable standards of their specific therapy in those particular circumstances.

The issue of the standards within Chinese medicine arose in a recent case.

Box 34.1 Standard of care of a complementary therapist[6]

S, who was suffering from a skin condition, consulted a practitioner of traditional Chinese herbal medicine. After taking nine doses of the herbal remedy, S became ill and later died of acute liver failure, which was attributable to a rare and unpredictable reaction to the remedy. His widow brought proceedings against the practitioner but failed. The High Court held that on the evidence before it the actions of the herbalist had been consistent with the standard of care appropriate to traditional Chinese herbal medicine in accordance with established requirements.

In May 2001[7] a woman was awarded £6,500 in her case against a hypnotist. She alleged that she had become a suicidal zombie as a result of being hypnotised on stage, which reawakened the trauma of childhood sex abuse. The judge held that a suggestion by the hypnotist that she should imagine going back to being a child was negligent. This could be seen as age regression, which is expressly forbidden in a Home Office Circular in 1989 which states that no stage performance should include age regression.

ADVICE OF THE UKCC

In Paragraph 37 of the Midwife's Code of Practice[8] the UKCC provides the advice shown in Box 34.2.

Box 34.2 Paragraph 37 of the Midwife's Code of Practice

Some practising midwives, having gained a qualification in a complementary or alternative therapy, may want to apply their additional knowledge and skill in their practice. This may involve the use of substances such as essential oils, or

> specific equipment. It is essential that practice in these respects, as in all others, is based upon sound principles and upon all available knowledge and skill. You must obtain consent from the mother to the use of such therapies. Your professional accountability applies in the use of such therapies as in any other area of practice.

The UKCC advice on the administration of homeopathic or herbal substances is discussed in Chapter 20.

USE OF COMPLEMENTARY THERAPIES IN MIDWIFERY

There are several general works describing the role which complementary therapies can play in nursing and midwifery.[9] Denise Tiran has also described the use of aromatherapy for pregnancy and childbirth.[10] Mandy Curry describes the introduction of complementary therapies into the Peterborough Maternity Unit,[11] and the importance of ensuring that standards and practices of staff within a maternity service are maintained at a high and safe level. The March 2002 issue of *The Practising Midwife* (Volume 5 Number 3) focuses on the use of complementary therapies and their use antenatally and during labour. Articles include the use of chiropractic, self-hypnosis, cranio-sacral therapy and massage in midwifery and the development of a database on the use of complementary therapies in midwifery by Maggie Evans.

ACUPUNCTURE IN PREGNANCY

One of the obvious therapies which complements orthodox practice is that of acupuncture. Michele Denny described the setting up of an acupuncture clinic within the NHS to provide acupuncture in pregnancy.[12] The clinic offered treatment for backache, sciatica, muscle and ligament pain, nausea and vomiting, carpal tunnel syndrome, constipation, headaches and heartburn. She concluded, following an audit of the service, that women were enthusiastic about the service and wanted the acupuncture service to be offered for labour and the puerperium. She suggested that if funding could be secured, a specialist clinical midwife could be employed to promote the benefits of complementary therapies to pregnant and childbearing women.

AROMATHERAPY IN CHILDBIRTH

Ethel Burns and others[13] undertook a study to assess a cohort of mothers who all used aromatherapy during childbirth. The authors concluded that aromatherapy oils had the potential to reduce anxiety, fear or pain and suggest that the integration of aromatherapy into mainstream practice is worth exploring as a means of enabling midwives to gain greater confidence in their holistic skills and improve the quality of midwifery care. However, the authors realised that further research including randomised controlled trials were required.

Spiritual midwifery care[14] is recommended by Jennifer Hall, not in the sense of organised religion, but as part of the holistic care of the woman required by the Midwives Rules. Rosemary Ann Garratt also explores holistic woman-centred care through the use of complementary therapies in the healing role of the midwife.[15] Pat Hung explores traditional Chinese customs and practices for the postnatal care of Chinese mothers.[16] Psychotherapy is considered by Diane Gosden and Ann Saul[17] to have a valuable part to play in midwifery, but they warn against the midwife becoming too interventionist and disempowering of the woman.

However, the findings of many of these studies are not supported by the rigorous research which is now required for orthodox medicine.

NATIONAL DEVELOPMENTS

There is no doubt about the interest which now exists in complementary or alternative therapies. It is estimated that a third of the population have tried its remedies or visited its practitioners.[18] The Health Education Authority has published an A to Z guide which covers 60 therapies.[19] Much research needs to be done on the efficacy of these therapies and the Health Authority Council has approved a research project to be undertaken by the National Association of Health Authorities and Trusts into the prevalence of complementary therapies and their services for patients, purchasers and providers. The Health Authority Council has appointed a steering and working group to co-ordinate the project which will be undertaken by Blueprint Consultancy.[20]

The Prince of Wales suggested the setting up of a group to consider the current positions of orthodox, complementary and alternative medicine in the UK and how far it would be appropriate and possible for them to work more closely together. Four working groups looking at

– research and development

– education and training

– regulation, and

– delivery mechanisms

were established under a steering group chaired by Dr Manon Williams, Assistant Private Secretary to HRH The Prince of Wales. It reported in 1997 and made extensive recommendations.[21] These include encouraging more research and the dissemination of its results; emphasising the common elements in the core curriculum of all healthcare workers, both orthodox and complementary and alternative medicine; establishing statutory self-regulatory bodies for those professions which could endanger patient safety; and identifying areas of conventional medicine and nursing which are not meeting patients' needs at present. It also recommended the establishment of an Independent Standards Commission for Complementary and Alternative Medicine. An information pack for primary care on complementary medicine has been sponsored by the Department of Health.[22] The pack was initiated after a survey found that 1 in 4 adults would use alternative therapies at some point in their lives. The Select Committee on Science and Technology of the House of Lords[23] (see above) considered that some remedies such as acupuncture and aromatherapy should be available on the NHS, and NHS patients should have wider access to osteopathy and chiropractics. The implementation of these recommendations will lead to fundamental changes in how complementary and alternative therapies are viewed in relation to orthodox medicine and within the NHS.

In September 2001 the Medicines Control Agency (MCA) called upon the UK traditional Chinese medicines sector to improve the quality and safety standards of its medicines.[24] The MCA has started consultations with the ethnic medicine sector with the intention of extending the list of potent or toxic ingredients which are not permitted in unlicensed herbal medicines in order that the public should be protected. The MCA has issued guidance on traditional ethnic medicines and its compliance with the law.[25]

CONCLUSIONS

There is every likelihood that the interest and demand for complementary therapy will continue to grow and women will demand that these therapies should be provided within the NHS. In the past some GP fund holders have used their purchasing power to buy such therapies for their patients. It remains to be seen what effect the abolition of GP fundholding and the establishment of primary care groups and primary care trusts (in Wales Local Health Boards) will have on the availability of complementary therapies within the NHS. The British Medical Association at its conference in 2000 recommended that acupuncture should be available on the NHS. Following the recommendations of the House of Lords Select Committee on Science and Technology there will be more requirements for research-based evidence of the clinical effectiveness of many complementary therapists so practitioners are likely to become involved in this area.

QUESTIONS AND EXERCISES

1. You have decided that you would like to undertake a training in aromatherapy and eventually use it as part of your practice as a midwife. What actions would you take to ensure that your plans are compatible with your professional role as a registered midwife?

2. Identify the ways in which the knowledge that a woman was receiving complementary therapy treatment could affect the tests, care or treatment which you give that person.

3. Do you consider that those complementary therapists who so wished, should be permitted to have registered status under the Health Professions Council? If not, what criteria would you lay down for a profession to receive registered status?

4. Which complementary therapies do you consider could be seen as most effective in supporting a woman during and after her pregnancy?

References

1 Dimond B. 1998. *The Legal Aspects of Complementary Therapy Practice*. Edinburgh: Churchill Livingstone

2 Royal College of Midwives. 1999. Complementary therapies and midwifery. London: RCM

3 Further information can be obtained from the BCMA at Exmoor Street, London W10 6DZ

4 House of Lords Select Committee on Science and Technology. *6th Report: Complementary and Alternative Medicine*. 21 November 2000 Session 1999-2000

5 Watling v. Gloucester County Council Employment Tribunal EAT/868/94 17 March 1995, 23 November 1994, Lexis transcript

6 Shakoor (Administratrix of the Estate of Shakoor (Deceased)) v. Situ (T/A Eternal Health Co). *The Independent*, May 25 2000

7 Horsnell M. Abused woman wins case against hypnotist. *The Times*, 26 May 2001

8 UKCC. 1998. *Midwives Rules and Code of Practice*. London: UKCC

9 Rankin-Box A. 1998. *Complementary Therapies: A guide for Nursing and the Caring Profession*. London: Croom-Helm; Tiran D, Mack S (eds). 1995. *Complementary Therapies for Pregnancy and Childbirth*. London: Balliere Tindall

10 Tiran D. 2000. *Clinical Aromatherapy for Pregnancy and Childbirth*. 2nd edition. Edinburgh: Churchill Livingstone

11 Curry M. 1998. Complementing Practice. *Practising Midwife*, 1(5), 32-4

12 Denny M. 1999. Acupuncture in Pregnancy. *Practising Midwife*, 2(4), 29-31

13 Burns E, Blamey C and Lloyd AJ. 2000. Aromatherapy in childbirth: an effective approach to care. British Journal of Midwifery, 8(10), 639-43

14 Hall J. 2000. Spiritual midwifery care: old practice for a new millenium. *British Journal of Midwifery*, 8(2), 82

15 Garratt RA. 2001. The midwife as healer. *Complementary Therapies in Nursing and Midwifery*, 7(4), 197-201

16 Hung P. 2001. Traditional Chinese customs and practices for the postnatal care of Chinese mothers. *Complementary Therapies in Nursing and Midwifery*, 7(4), 202-6

17 Gosden D and Saul A. 1999. Reflections on the use of psychotherapy in midwifery. *British Journal of Nursing*, 7(9), 543-6

18 Laurance J. 1996. Alternative Health: An honest alternative or just magic? *The Times*, 5 February 1996

19 Health Education Authority. 1995. *A-Z guide on complementary therapies*

20 For further details contact Yvonne Mouncer, Regional Development Manager, NAHAT

21 Foundation for Integrated Medicine. 1997. *Integrated Healthcare: A Way Forward for the Next Five Years*

22 Department of Health. *Complementary Medicine Information Pack for Primary Care*. www.doh.gov.uk

23 House of Lords Select Committee on Science and Technology. *6th Report: Complementary and Alternative Medicine*. 21 November 2000 Session 1999-2000

24 Department of Health. 2001. Press Release 2001/0448 Concern over quality and safety standards of traditional Chinese medicines

25 Medicines Control Agency. *Traditional ethnic medicines, public health and compliance with medicines law*; www.mca.gov.uk

HUMAN RIGHTS ACT 1998

SCHEDULE 1: THE ARTICLES

PART I

THE CONVENTION
RIGHTS AND FREEDOMS

ARTICLE 2

RIGHT TO LIFE

1. Everyone's right to life shall be protected by law. No one shall be deprived of his life intentionally save in the execution of a sentence of a court following his conviction of a crime for which this penalty is provided by law.

2. Deprivation of life shall not be regarded as inflicted in contravention of this Article when it results from the use of force which is no more than absolutely necessary:

(a) in defence of any person from unlawful violence;

(b) in order to effect a lawful arrest or to prevent the escape of a person lawfully detained;

(c) in action lawfully taken for the purpose of quelling a riot or insurrection.

ARTICLE 3

PROHIBITION OF TORTURE

No one shall be subjected to torture or to inhuman or degrading treatment or punishment.

ARTICLE 4

PROHIBITION OF SLAVERY AND FORCED LABOUR

1. No one shall be held in slavery or servitude.

2. No one shall be required to perform forced or compulsory labour.

3. For the purpose of this Article the term "forced or compulsory labour" shall not include:

(a) any work required to be done in the ordinary course of detention imposed according to the provisions of Article 5 of this Convention or during conditional release from such detention;

(b) any service of a military character or, in case of conscientious objectors in countries where they are recognised, service exacted instead of compulsory military service;

(c) any service exacted in case of an emergency or calamity threatening the life or well-being of the community;

(d) any work or service which forms part of normal civic obligations.

ARTICLE 5

RIGHT TO LIBERTY AND SECURITY

1. Everyone has the right to liberty and security of person. No one shall be deprived of his liberty save in the following cases and in accordance with a procedure prescribed by law:

(a) the lawful detention of a person after conviction by a competent court;

(b) the lawful arrest or detention of a person for non-compliance with the lawful order of a court or in order to secure the fulfilment of any obligation prescribed by law;

(c) the lawful arrest or detention of a person effected for the purpose of bringing him before the competent legal authority on reasonable suspicion of having committed an offence or when it is reasonably considered necessary to prevent his committing an offence or fleeing after having done so;

(d) the detention of a minor by lawful order for the purpose of educational supervision or his lawful detention for the purpose of bringing him before the competent legal authority;

(e) the lawful detention of persons for the prevention of the spreading of infectious diseases, of persons of unsound mind, alcoholics or drug addicts or vagrants;

(f) the lawful arrest or detention of a person to prevent his effecting an unauthorised entry into the country or of a person against whom action is being taken with a view to deportation or extradition.

2. Everyone who is arrested shall be informed promptly, in a language which he understands, of the reasons for his arrest and of any charge against him.

3. Everyone arrested or detained in accordance with the provisions of paragraph 1(c) of this Article shall be brought promptly before a judge or other officer authorised by law to exercise judicial power and shall be entitled to trial within a reasonable time or to release pending trial. Release may be conditioned by guarantees to appear for trial.

4. Everyone who is deprived of his liberty by arrest or detention shall be entitled to take proceedings by which the lawfulness of his detention shall be decided speedily by a court and his release ordered if the detention is not lawful.

5. Everyone who has been the victim of arrest or detention in contravention of the provisions of this Article shall have an enforceable right to compensation.

ARTICLE 6

RIGHT TO A FAIR TRIAL

1. In the determination of his civil rights and obligations or of any criminal charge against him, everyone is entitled to a fair and public hearing within a reasonable time by an independent and impartial tribunal established by law. Judgment shall be pronounced publicly but the press and public may be excluded from all or part of the trial in the interest of morals, public order or national security in a democratic society, where the interests of juveniles or the protection of the private life of the parties so require, or to the extent strictly necessary in the opinion of the court in special circumstances where publicity would prejudice the interests of justice.

2. Everyone charged with a criminal offence shall be presumed innocent until proved guilty according to law.

3. Everyone charged with a criminal offence has the following minimum rights:

(a) to be informed promptly, in a language which he understands and in detail, of the nature and cause of the accusation against him;

(b) to have adequate time and facilities for the preparation of his defence;

(c) to defend himself in person or through legal assistance of his own choosing or, if he has not sufficient means to pay for legal assistance, to be given it free when the interests of justice so require;

(d) to examine or have examined witnesses against him and to obtain the attendance and examination of witnesses on his behalf under the same conditions as witnesses against him;

(e) to have the free assistance of an interpreter if he cannot understand or speak the language used in court.

ARTICLE 7

NO PUNISHMENT WITHOUT LAW

1. No one shall be held guilty of any criminal offence on account of any act or omission which did not constitute a criminal offence under national or international law at the time when it was committed. Nor shall a heavier penalty be imposed than the one that was applicable at the time the criminal offence was committed.

2. This Article shall not prejudice the trial and punishment of any person for any act or omission which, at the time when it was committed, was criminal according to the general principles of law recognised by civilised nations.

ARTICLE 8

RIGHT TO RESPECT FOR PRIVATE AND FAMILY LIFE

1. Everyone has the right to respect for his private and family life, his home and his correspondence.

2. There shall be no interference by a public authority with the exercise of this right except such as is in accordance with the law and is necessary in a democratic society in the interests of national security, public safety or the economic well-being of the country, for the prevention of disorder or crime, for the protection of health or morals, or for the protection of the rights and freedoms of others.

ARTICLE 9

FREEDOM OF THOUGHT, CONSCIENCE AND RELIGION

1. Everyone has the right to freedom of thought, conscience and religion; this right includes freedom to change his religion or belief and freedom, either alone or in community with others and in public or private, to manifest his religion or belief, in worship, teaching, practice and observance.

2. Freedom to manifest one's religion or beliefs shall be subject only to such limitations as are prescribed by law and are necessary in a democratic society in the interests of public safety, for the protection of public order, health or morals, or for the protection of the rights and freedoms of others.

ARTICLE 10

FREEDOM OF EXPRESSION

1. Everyone has the right to freedom of expression. This right shall include freedom to hold opinions and to receive and impart information and ideas

without interference by public authority and regardless of frontiers. This Article shall not prevent States from requiring the licensing of broadcasting, television or cinema enterprises.

2. The exercise of these freedoms, since it carries with it duties and responsibilities, may be subject to such formalities, conditions, restrictions or penalties as are prescribed by law and are necessary in a democratic society, in the interests of national security, territorial integrity or public safety, for the prevention of disorder or crime, for the protection of health or morals, for the protection of the reputation or rights of others, for preventing the disclosure of information received in confidence, or for maintaining the authority and impartiality of the judiciary.

ARTICLE 11

FREEDOM OF ASSEMBLY AND ASSOCIATION

1. Everyone has the right to freedom of peaceful assembly and to freedom of association with others, including the right to form and to join trade unions for the protection of his interests.

2. No restrictions shall be placed on the exercise of these rights other than such as are prescribed by law and are necessary in a democratic society in the interests of national security or public safety, for the prevention of disorder or crime, for the protection of health or morals or for the protection of the rights and freedoms of others. This Article shall not prevent the imposition of lawful restrictions on the exercise of these rights by members of the armed forces, of the police or of the administration of the State.

ARTICLE 12

RIGHT TO MARRY

Men and women of marriageable age have the right to marry and to found a family, according to the national laws governing the exercise of this right.

ARTICLE 14

PROHIBITION OF DISCRIMINATION

The enjoyment of the rights and freedoms set forth in this Convention shall be secured without discrimination on any ground such as sex, race, colour, language, religion, political or other opinion, national or social origin, association with a national minority, property, birth or other status.

ARTICLE 16

RESTRICTIONS ON POLITICAL ACTIVITY OF ALIENS

Nothing in Articles 10, 11 and 14 shall be regarded as preventing the High Contracting Parties from imposing restrictions on the political activity of aliens.

ARTICLE 17

PROHIBITION OF ABUSE OF RIGHTS

Nothing in this Convention may be interpreted as implying for any State, group or person any right to engage in any activity or perform any act aimed at the destruction of any of the rights and freedoms set forth herein or at their limitation to a greater extent than is provided for in the Convention.

ARTICLE 18

LIMITATION ON USE OF RESTRICTIONS ON RIGHTS

The restrictions permitted under this Convention to the said rights and freedoms shall not be applied for any purpose other than those for which they have been prescribed.

PART II

THE FIRST PROTOCOL

ARTICLE 1

PROTECTION OF PROPERTY

Every natural or legal person is entitled to the peaceful enjoyment of his possessions. No one shall be deprived of his possessions except in the public interest and subject to the conditions provided for by law and by the general principles of international law. The preceding provisions shall not, however, in any way impair the right of a State to enforce such laws as it deems necessary to control the use of property in accordance with the general interest or to secure the payment of taxes or other contributions or penalties.

ARTICLE 2

RIGHT TO EDUCATION

No person shall be denied the right to education. In the exercise of any functions which it assumes in relation to education and to teaching, the State shall respect the right of parents to ensure such education and teaching in conformity with their own religious and philosophical convictions.

ARTICLE 3

RIGHT TO FREE ELECTIONS

The High Contracting Parties undertake to hold free elections at reasonable intervals by secret ballot, under conditions which will ensure the free expression of the opinion of the people in the choice of the legislature.

PART III

THE SIXTH PROTOCOL

ARTICLE 1

ABOLITION OF THE DEATH PENALTY

The death penalty shall be abolished. No one shall be condemned to such penalty or executed.

ARTICLE 2

DEATH PENALTY IN TIME OF WAR

A State may make provision in its law for the death penalty in respect of acts committed in time of war or of imminent threat of war; such penalty shall be applied only in the instances laid down in the law and in accordance with its provisions. The State shall communicate to the Secretary General of the Council of Europe the relevant provisions of that law.

CONGENITAL DISABILITIES (CIVIL LIABILITY) ACT 1976

(1976 c.28; 46 Halsbury's Statutes (3rd Edn.) 1837)
Amended by 1977 Unfair Contract Terms Act

1. CIVIL LIABILITY TO A CHILD BORN DISABLED

(1) If a child is born disabled as the result of such an occurrence before its birth as is mentioned in subsection (2) below, and a person (other than the child's own mother) is under this section answerable to the child in respect of the occurrence, the child's disabilities are to be regarded as damage resulting from the wrongful act of that person and actionable accordingly at the suit of the child.

(2) An occurrence to which this section applies is one which -
(a) affected either parent of the child in his or her ability to have a normal, healthy child; or
(b) affected the mother during her pregnancy, or affected her or the child in the course of its birth, so that the child is born with disabilities which would not otherwise have been present.

(3) Subject to the following subsections, a person (here referred to as 'the defendant') is answerable to the child if he was liable in tort to the parent or would, if sued in due time, have been so; and it is no answer that there could not have been such liability because the parent suffered no actionable injury, if there was a breach of legal duty which, accompanied by injury, would have given rise to the liability.

(4) In the case of an occurrence preceding the time of conception, the defendant is not answerable to the child if at that time either or both of the parents knew the risk of their child being born disabled (that is to say, the particular risk created by the occurrence); but should it be the child's father who is the defendant, this subsection does not apply if he knew of the risk and the mother did not.

(5) The defendant is not answerable to the child, for anything he did or omitted to do when responsible in a professional capacity for treating or advising the parent, if he took reasonable care having due regard to then received professional opinion applicable to the particular class of case; but this does not mean that he is answerable only because he departed from received opinion.

(6) Liability to the child under this section may be treated as having been excluded or limited by contract made with the parent affected, to the same extent and subject to the same restrictions as liability in the parent's own case; and a contract term which could have been set up by the defendant in an operation by the parent, so as to exclude or limit his liability to him or her, operates in the defendant's favour to the same, but no greater, extent in an action under this section by the child.

(7) If in the child's action under this section it is shown that the parent affected shared the responsibility for the child being born disabled, the damages are to be reduced to such extent as the court thinks just and equitable having regard to the extent of the parent's responsibility.

2. LIABILITY OF A WOMAN DRIVING WHEN PREGNANT

A woman driving a motor vehicle when she knows (or ought reasonably to know) herself to be pregnant is to be regarded as being under the same duty to take care for the safety of her unborn child as the law imposes on her with respect to the safety of other people; and if in consequence of her breach of that duty her child is born with disabilities which would not otherwise have been present, those disabilities are to be regarded as damage resulting from her wrongful act and actionable accordingly at the suit of the child.

3. DISABLED BIRTH DUE TO RADIATION

(1) Section 1 of this Act does not affect the operation of the Nuclear Installations Act 1965 as to liability for, and compensation in respect of, injury or damage caused by occurrences involving nuclear matter or the emission of ionising radiations.

(2) For the avoidance of doubt anything which -
(a) affects a man in his ability to have a normal, healthy child; or
(b) affects a woman in that ability, or so affects her when she is pregnant that her child is born with disabilities which would not otherwise have been present, is an injury for the purposes of that Act.

(3) If a child is born disabled as the result of an injury to either of its parents caused in breach of a duty imposed by any of sections 7 to 11 of that Act (nuclear persons, etc.) the child's disabilities are to be regarded under the subsequent provisions of that Act (compensation and other matters) as injuries caused on the same occasion, and by the same breach of duty, as was the injury to the parent.

(4) As respects compensation to the child, section 13(6) of that Act (contributory fault of person injured by radiation) is to be applied as if the reference there to fault were to the fault of the parent.

(5) Compensation is not payable in the child's case if the injury to the parent preceded the time of the child's conception and at that time either or both of the parents knew the risk of their child being born disabled (that is to say, the particular risk created by the injury).

4. INTERPRETATION AND OTHER SUPPLEMENTARY PROVISIONS

(1) References in this Act to a child being born disabled or with disabilities are to its being born with any deformity, disease or abnormality, including predisposition (whether or not susceptible of immediate prognosis) to physical or mental defect in the future.

(2) In this Act -
(a) 'born' means born alive (the moment of a child's birth being when it first has a life separate from its mother), and 'birth' has a corresponding meaning; and
(b) 'motor vehicle' means a mechanically propelled vehicle intended or adapted for use on roads.

(3) Liability to a child under section 1 or 2 of this Act is to be regarded -
(a) as respects all its incidents and any matters arising or to arise out of it; and
(b) subject to any contrary context or intention, for the purpose of construing references in enactments and documents to personal or bodily injuries and cognate matters, as liability for personal injuries sustained by the child immediately after its birth.

(4) No damages shall be recoverable under either of those sections in respect of any loss of expectation of life, nor shall any such loss be taken into account in the compensation payable in respect of a child under the Nuclear Installations Act 1965 as extended by section 3, unless (in either case) the child lives for at least 48 hours.

(5) This Act applies in respect of births after (but not before) its passing, and in respect of any such birth it replaces any law in force before its passing, whereby a person could be liable to a child in respect of disabilities with which it might be born; but in section 1 (3) of this Act the expression 'liable in tort' does not include any reference to liability by virtue of this Act, or to liability by virtue of any such law.

(6) References to the Nuclear Installations Act 1965 are to that Act as amended; and for the purposes of section 28 of that Act (power by Order in Council to extend the Act to territories outside the United Kingdom) section 3 of this Act is to be treated as if it were a provision of that Act.

5. CROWN APPLICATION

This Act binds the Crown. (N.B. The Act was passed on 22nd July, 1976.)

GLOSSARY

Midwifery terms taken from definitions contained in the Midwives Rules

Emergency
A situation in which a sudden, unexpected event occurs relating to the health of the mother or baby which requires immediate attention

Health authority
In England and Wales: Meaning as in The Health Authorities Act 1995
In Scotland: A Health Board
In Northern Ireland: A Health and Social Services Board

Local Supervising Authority
A body prescribed by Section 15(1) of the 1997 Act as being a Local Supervising Authority for midwives

Midwives Directive
Council Directive No 80/155/EEC concerning the co-ordination of provisions laid down by law and the regulation of administrative action relating to the taking up and pursuit of activities of midwives as amended by European Union Directive No 89/594/EEC

Mother and baby
Means a woman and her baby whether before or after birth and a reference to 'mother and baby' shall be a reference to the woman and her unborn baby during the antenatal and intranatal periods and to the mother and her baby during the period from the birth of the baby to the end of the postnatal period, and 'mother' and 'baby' shall be construed accordingly

Postnatal period
A period of not less than ten and not more than twenty-eight days after the end of labour, during which the continued attendance of a midwife on the mother and baby is requisite

Practising midwife
A midwife who attends professionally upon a woman during the antenatal, intranatal and/or postnatal period or who holds a post for which a midwifery qualification is essential and who notifies her intention to practise to the Local Supervising Authority

Supervisor of Midwives
The person appointed by the Local Supervising Authority in accordance with Section 15(3) of the 1997 Act

Other terms used

Accusatorial - System of court proceedings where the two sides contest the issues (contrast with inquisitorial)

Actionable per se - A court action where the plaintiff does not have to show loss, damage or harm to obtain compensation eg. an action for trespass to the person

Actus reus - The physical elements which make up the definition of a crime

Adversarial - The approach adopted in an accusatorial system

Advocate - A person who pleads for another: it could be paid and professional, such as a barrister or solicitor, or it could be a lay advocate either paid or unpaid

Affidavit - A statement given under oath

Appellate court - A court which hears appeals from lower courts eg. Court of Appeal and House of Lords

Arrestable offence - An offence defined in Section 24 of the Police and Criminal Evidence Act 1984 which gives to the citizen the power of arrest in certain circumstances without a warrant

Assault - A threat of unlawful contact (trespass to the person)

Bailee - A person who undertakes to care for the property of another

Bailment - The transfer of property from a bailor to a bailee

Bailor - One who leaves property in the care of another

Barrister - A lawyer qualified to take a case in court

Battery - An unlawful touching (see trespass to the person)

Bench - The magistrates, Justice of the Peace

Bolam Test - The test laid down by Judge McNair in the case of Bolam v. Friern HMC on the standard of care expected of a professional in cases of alleged negligence

Bona fide - In good faith

Breach - Breaking, usually of a legal duty

Burden of proof - The duty of a party to litigation to establish the facts, or in criminal proceedings the duty of the prosecution to establish both the actus reus and the mens rea

Case citation - The reference to an earlier reported case made possible because of the reference system, eg. 1981 1 All ER 267 means the first volume of the All England Reports for 1981 at page 267 which is the reference for the case of Whitehouse v. Jordan, where Whitehouse is the plaintiff, Jordan the defendant and 'v' stands for versus, i.e. against. Other law reports include:

AC   Appeals Court
QB   Queens Bench Division
WLR   Weekly Law Reports

Cause of action - The facts that entitle a person to sue

Certiorari - An action taken to challenge an administrative or judicial decision (literally: to make more certain)

Civil action - Proceedings brought in the civil courts; civil refers to matters which are non-criminal, i.e. they pertain to the civil courts.

Civil wrong - An act or omission which can be pursued in the civil courts by the person who has suffered the wrong (see torts)

Claimant - A person who brings an action in the civil courts (term now used instead of plaintiff)

Committal proceedings - The hearing which takes place in the Magistrates Court to determine if the case should go to the Crown Court for trial by jury

Common law - Law derived from the decisions of judges, case law, judge-made law

Conditional fee system - A system whereby client and lawyer can agree that payment of fees is dependent upon the outcome of the court action

Conditions - Terms of a contract (see warranties)

Constructive knowledge - Knowledge which can be obtained from the circumstances

Continuous service - The length of service which an employee must have served in order to be entitled to receive certain statutory or contractual rights

Contract - An agreement enforceable in law

Contract for services - An agreement enforceable in law whereby one party provides services, not being employment, in return for payment or other consideration from the other

Contract of service - A contract for employment

Coroner - A person appointed to hold an inquiry (inquest) into a death in unexpected or unusual circumstances

Criminal - Refers to matters which pertain to the criminal courts

Criminal wrong - An act or omission which can be pursued in the criminal courts

Damage - Harm which has occurred

Damages - Compensation payable as the result of a tort or civil wrong

Declaration - A ruling by the court, setting out the legal situation

Dissenting judgement - A judge who disagrees with the decision of the majority of judges

Distinguished (of cases) - The rules of precedent require judges to follow decisions of judges in previous cases, where these are binding upon them. However in some circumstances it is possible to come to a different decision because the facts of the earlier case are not comparable to the case now being heard, and therefore the earlier decision can be 'distinguished'

Defamation - The publication of a statement which tends to lower a person in the estimation of right thinking members of society generally. If spoken it is known as slanderous; if in permanent form, a libel

Domiciliary - At the home

Ethics - the science of morals, moral principles and rules of conduct

Eugenics - the science of the production of fine offspring

Euthanasia - Bringing about gentle and easy death, mercy killing

Ex gratia - without admitting liability (usually refers to a payment by a prospective defendant)

Ex parte - On one side only, where the other side is not a party to the action

Expert witness - Evidence given by a person whose general opinion, based on training or experience, is relevant to some of the issues in dispute

Gynaecology - The branch of medicine which devotes itself to the care and prevention of genital tract disorders in women and which for the most part is not concerned with pregnancy*

Re F ruling - A professional who acts in the best interests of an incompetent person who is incapable of giving consent, does not act unlawfully if he follows the accepted standard of care according to the Bolam Test

Guardian ad litem - A person with a social work and childcare background who is appointed to ensure that the court is fully informed of the relevant facts which relate to a child and that the wishes and feelings of the child are clearly established. The appointment is made from a panel set up by the local authority

HSC - Health Service Circular issued by Department of Health

Hearsay - Evidence which has been learnt from another person

Hierarchy - The recognised status of courts which results in lower courts following the decisions of higher courts (see precedent). Thus decisions of the House of Lords must be followed by all lower courts unless they can be distinguished (see above)

Honourary - Without payment

In camera - Court proceedings heard in private

Indemnity - Security against loss or damage, compensation for loss occurred

Indictable - Can be tried on an indictment (i.e. before the crown court - some crimes are triable either way, i.e. before the crown court and summarily before magistrates)

Indictment - A written accusation against a person, charging him with a serious crime, triable by jury

Injunction - An order of the court restraining a person

Inquisitorial - A system of justice whereby the truth is revealed by an inquiry into the facts conducted by the judge, eg. coroner's court

Invitation to treat - The early stages in negotiating a contract, eg. an advertisement, or letter expressing interest. An invitation to treat will often precede an offer which when accepted leads to the formation of an agreement which, if there is consideration and an intention to create legal relations, will be binding

Judiciary - Judges

Judicial review - An application to the High Court for a judicial or administrative decision to be reviewed and an appropriate order made, eg. declaration

Justice of the peace - A lay magistrate, i.e. not legally qualified, who hears summary (minor) offences and sometimes indictable (serious) offences in the magistrates court in a group of three (bench)

Litigation - Law suits, legal actions

Live birth - The birth of a child born alive (Section 41 of 1953 Act)

Magistrate - A person (see JP and stipendiary) who hears summary (minor) offences or indictable offences which can be heard in the magistrates court

Mens rea - The mental element required in most crimes. Crimes which do not require this mental element are known as crimes of strict liability

Misconduct - conduct unworthy of a registered nurse, midwife or health visitor, as the case may be, and includes obtaining registration by fraud (Rule 1(2)(k) Professional Conduct Rules SI 1993 No 893)

Negligence(1) - A breach by the defendant of a legal duty to take care not to injure the plaintiff or cause him loss

Negligence(2) - The attitude of mind of a person committing a civil wrong as opposed to intentionally

Next friend - A person who brings a court action on behalf of a minor

Non-executive - A person who does not hold office, used in relation to NHS board members who are directors but who do not hold office within the authority

Notifiable - A disease which must be notified to the authorities by law

Nuisance - A wrong which interferes with the use and enjoyment of a person's land

Obstetrics - The field of medicine dealing with the care of women during pregnancy, labour and delivery and the postpartum period*

Offer - A proposal made by a party which if accepted can lead to a contract. It often follows an invitation to treat

542

Ombudsman - A Commissioner (eg. health, local government) appointed by the government to hear complaints

Plaintiff - The person bringing an action in the civil courts (term now replaced by claimant)

Plea in mitigation - A formal statement to the court aimed at reducing the sentence to be pronounced by the judge

Postpartum - Occurring after childbirth or pertaining to the period following delivery or childbirth*

Practice - Direction guidance issued by the head of the court to which they relate on the procedure to be followed

Precedent - An earlier case which may be binding upon the judge

Prima facie - At first sight, or sufficient evidence brought by one party to require the other party to provide a defence

Privilege - In relation to evidence, being able to refuse to disclose it to the court

Privity - The relationship which exists between parties as the result of a legal agreement

Professional misconduct - Conduct unworthy of a nurse, midwife or health visitor

Proof - Evidence which secures the establishment of a plaintiff's or prosecution's or defendant's case

Prosecution - The pursuing of criminal offences in court

Proxy decision making - Making a decision on behalf of another

Quantum - How much? i.e. the amount of compensation claimed, agreed or awarded

Ratio - The reasoning behind the decision in a court case

Reasonable doubt - To secure a conviction in criminal proceedings the prosecution must establish beyond reasonable doubt the guilt of the accused

Res ipsa loquitur - The thing speaks for itself

Sanctions - Penalties, remedies following civil or criminal wrong

Solicitor - A lawyer who is qualified on the register held by the Law Society

Stillborn child - A child which has issued forth from its mother after the twenty-fourth week of pregnancy and which did not at any time after being completely expelled from its mother breathe or show any other signs of life, and the expression 'stillbirth' shall be construed accordingly (Section 41 Births and Deaths Registration Act 1953)

Standard of proof - The level that the party who has the burden of proof must satisfy, eg. on a balance of probabilities (civil courts); beyond all reasonable doubt (criminal courts)

Stipendiary magistrate - A legally qualified magistrate who is paid (i.e. has a stipend)

Strict liability - Liability for a criminal act where the mental element does not have to be proved; in civil proceedings liability without establishing negligence

Subpoena - An order of the court requiring a person to appear as a witness (subpoena ad testificandum) or to bring records/documents (subpoena duces tecum)

Summary offence - a lesser offence which can only be heard by magistrates

Statute - An Act of Parliament cited by the year and chapter number eg. Nurses, Midwives and Health Visitors Act 1997 chapter x

Statutory instrument - Orders and regulations having binding force. They must usually be laid before Parliament and will usually become law if they are confirmed by a simple resolution of both Houses. (affirmative resolution). Some become law after they have been laid for a prescribed period unless they are annulled by resolution of either House (negative resolution)

Summary - Relating to proceedings before the Magistrates

Summary judgement - A procedure whereby the plaintiff can obtain judgement without the defendant being permitted to defend the action

Surrogacy - An arrangement whereby a person carries a child for another mother or couple

Tort - A civil wrong, excluding breach of contract. It includes: negligence, trespass (to the person, goods or land), nuisance, breach of statutory duty and defamation

Trespass to the person - A wrongful direct interference with another person. Harm does not have to be proved

Trustee - One who holds property in trust for another (eg. has duties to care for it)

Ultra vires - Outside the powers given by law (eg. of a statutory body or company)

Vicarious liability - The liability of an employer for the negligence of his employee whilst acting in the course of employment

Void - Invalid or not legally binding

Voidable - Can be made void

Volenti non fit injuria - To the willing there is no wrong (i.e. where there is consent there is no injury)

Ward of court - A minor placed under the protection of the High Court, which assumes responsibility for him or her and all decisions relating to his or her care must be made in accordance with the directions of the court

Warranties - terms of a contract which are considered to be less important than the terms described as conditions: breach of a condition entitles the innocent party to see the contract as ended, i.e. repudiated by the other party, breach of warranties entitles the innocent party to claim damages

Wednesbury principle - The court will intervene to prevent or remedy abuses of power by public authorities if there is evidence of unreasonableness or perversity. Principle laid down by the Court of Appeal in the case of Associated Provincial Picture House Ltd v. Wednesbury Corporation 1948 1 KB 233

Without prejudice - Without detracting from or without disadvantage to. The use of the phrase prevents the other party using the information to the prejudice of the one providing it

Writ - A document which is issued by the court and served on the defendant to commence a civil action (now known as a claim form)

* Definitions taken from Churchill's Medical Directory, Churchill Livingstone 1989

RECOMMENDED FURTHER READING

Beddard R. 1992. *Human Rights and Europe*. 3rd edition. Cambridge: Grotius Publications Ltd

Brazier M. 1992. *Medicine, Patients and the Law*. Harmondsworth: Penguin

Brazier M (ed). 1998. *Street on Torts*. 8th edition. London: Butterworths

British Medical Association. 2001. *Consent, Rights and Choices in Health Care for Children and Young People*. London: BMJ Books

Clarkson CMV and Keating HM. 1990. *Criminal Law Text and Materials*. 2nd edition. London: Sweet and Maxwell

Dale GE and Appelbe J. 1993. *Pharmacy, Law and Ethics*. 5th edition. London: The Pharmaceutical Press

Dimond BC. 1996. *Legal Aspects of Child Health Care*. London: Mosby

Dimond BC. 1997. *Legal Aspects of Occupational Therapy*. Oxford: Blackwell Scientific Publications

Dimond BC. 1997. *Legal Aspects of Care in the Community*. London: Macmillan Press

Dimond BC. 1998. *Legal Aspects of Complementary Therapy Practice*. Edinburgh: Churchill Livingstone

Dimond BC. 1999. *Legal Aspects of Physiotherapy*. Oxford: Blackwell Science

Dimond BC. 1999. *Patients Rights, Responsibilities and the Nurse: Central Health Studies*. 2nd edition. Lancaster: Quay Publishing

Dimond BC. 2001. *Legal Aspects of Nursing*. 3rd edition. Hemel Hempstead: Prentice Hall

Ellis N. 1994. *Employing Staff*. 5th edition. London: BMJ Books

English National Board. 1992. *Preparation for Supervisors of Midwives Open Learning Programme*. London: ENB

Finch J. 1994. *Speller's Law Relating to Hospitals*. 7th edition. London: Chapman and Hall Medical

Gann R. 1993. *The NHS A to Z*. 2nd edition. Winchester: The Help for Health Trust

Ham C. 1991. *The New National Health Service*. Birmingham: NAHAT

Henderson C (ed). 2001. *Mayes' Midwifery*. 13th edition. London: Balliere Tindall

Hendrick J. 2000. *Law and Ethics in Nursing and Healthcare*. London: Stanley Thomas (Publishers) Ltd

Heywood JI (ed). 1999. *The UKCC Code of Conduct: a critical guide*. London: Nursing Times Books

Hoggett B. 1994. *Mental Health Law*. London: Sweet and Maxwell

Howarth DR and O'Sullivan JA. 2000. *Hepple, Howarth and Matthews Tort: Cases and Materials*. 5th edition. London: Butterworths

Hunt G and Wainwright P (eds). 1994. *Expanding the Role of the Nurse*. Oxford: Blackwell Scientific Publications

Hurwitz B. 1998. *Clinical Guidelines and the Law*. Abingdon: Radcliffe Medical Press

James PS. 1992. *Introduction to English Law*. London: Butterworths

Jones R. 1994. *Mental Health Act Manual*. 4th edition. London: Sweet and Maxwell

Kennedy I and Grubb A. 2000. *Medical Law and Ethics*. 3rd edition. London: Butterworths

Kidner R. 1993. *Blackstone's Statutes on Employment Law*. 3rd edition. London: Blackstones

Kloss D. 2000. *Occupational Health Law*. 3rd edition. Oxford: Blackwell Scientific Publications

Korgaonhar G and Tribe D. 1995. *Law for Nurses*. London: Cavendish Publishing Ltd

Maclean A. 2001. *Briefcase of Medical Law*. London: Cavendish Publishing Ltd

Mandelstam M. 1998. *An A-Z of Community Care Law*. London: Jessica Kingsley Publishers

Markesinis BS and Deakin SF. 1999. *Tort Law*. 4th edition. Oxford: Clarendon Press

Mason D and Edwards P. 1993. *Litigation: A risk management guide for midwives*. London: Royal College of Midwives

Mason JK and McCall-Smith A. 1994. *Law and Medical Ethics*. London: Butterworths

McHale J and Fox M with Murphy J. 1997. *Health Care Law*. London: Sweet and Maxwell

McHale J and Tingle J. 2001. *Law and Nursing*. 2nd edition. Oxford: Butterworth-Heinemann

Miers D and Page A. 1990. *Legislation*. 2nd edition. London: Sweet and Maxwell

Montgomery J. 1997. *Health Care Law*. Oxford: Oxford University Press

Morgan D and Lee RG. 1991. *Human Fertilisation and Embryology Act 1990*. London: Blackstone Press Limited

Pyne RH. 1991. *Professional Discipline in Nursing, Midwifery and Health Visiting*. 2nd edition. Oxford: Blackwell Scientific Publications

Rowson R. 1990. *An Introduction to Ethics for Nurses*. Harrow: Scutari Press

Royal College of Midwives. 1993. *Examples of effective midwifery management.* London: RCM

Royal College of Midwives. 1993. *The Midwife: Her legal status and accountability.* London: RCM

Rumbold G. 1993. *Ethics in Nursing Practice.* 2nd edition. London: Balliere Tindall

Selwyn N. 1993. *Selwyn's Law of Employment.* 8th edition. London: Butterworths

Silverton L. 1998. *The Art and Science of Midwifery.* London: Pearson Education

Smith JC and Keenan R. 1992. *English Law.* 10th edition. London: Pitman

Springhouse Corporation. 1992. *Nurse's Handbook of Law and Ethics.* Illinois: Springhouse Corporation

Stauch M and Wheat K with Tingle J. 1998. *Sourcebook on Medical Law.* London: Cavendish Publishing Ltd

Steiner J. 1992. *Textbook on EC Law.* 3rd edition. London: Blackstone Press

Stone J and Matthews J. 1996. *Complementary Medicine and the Law.* Oxford: Oxford University Press

Symon A. 2001. *Obstetric Litigation from A to Z.* Wiltshire: Mark Allen Publishing

Thompson R and Thompson B. 1993. *Dismissal: A basic introduction to your legal rights.* London: Robin Thompson and Partners and Brian Thompson and Partners.

Thompson R and Thompson B. 1993. *Equal Pay.* London: Robin Thompson and Partners and Brian Thompson and Partners.

Thompson R and Thompson B. 1993. *Health and Safety at Work.* London: Robin Thompson and Partners and Brian Thompson and Partners.

Thompson R and Thompson B. 1993. *Injuries at Work and Work Related Illnesses.* London: Robin Thompson and Partners and Brian Thompson and Partners.

Thompson R and Thompson B. 1993. *Women at Work.* London: Robin Thompson and Partners and Brian Thompson and Partners.

Tingle J and Cribb A (eds). 1995. *Nursing Law and Ethics.* Oxford: Blackwell Science

Tschudin V and Marks Maran D. 1993. *Ethics: A Primer for Nurses.* London: Balliere Tindall

Vincent C (ed). 1995. *Clinical Risk Management.* London: BMJ Books

Wyndham-Kay J (Chairman). 1991. *Report of Royal College of Midwives' Commission on Legislation relating to Midwives.* London: RCM

Young AP. 1989. *Legal Problems in Nursing Practice.* 2nd edition. London: Harper and Rowe

Young AP. 1994. *Law and Professional Conduct in Nursing.* 2nd edition. Harrow: Scutari Press

White R, Carr P and Lowe N. 1991. *A Guide to the Children Act 1989*. Oxford: Butterworths

Reference should also be made to the many articles on different legal aspects of midwifery practice which can be found in *The Practising Midwife*, *The British Journal of Midwifery*, the *Midwives Chronicle*, *Midwifery Matters*, *Midwife* and similar journals for registered practitioners in general.

The Midwives Information and Resource Service (MIDIRS) provides an extremely useful guide to articles relevant to midwifery published in other journals.

A bibliography of general and specialist books on midwifery, nursing and medical books is available from Meditec, Nursing Book Service York House, 26 Bourne Road, Coldersworth, Lincolnshire NG33 5JE.

INDEX